Long-Term Neurodevelopmental Outcomes of the NICU Graduate

Editors

IRA ADAMS-CHAPMAN
SARA B. DEMAURO

CLINICS IN PERINATOLOGY

www.perinatology.theclinics.com

Consulting Editor
LUCKY JAIN

September 2018 • Volume 45 • Number 3

ELSEVIER

1600 John F. Kennedy Boulevard • Suite 1800 • Philadelphia, Pennsylvania, 19103-2899

http://www.theclinics.com

CLINICS IN PERINATOLOGY Volume 45, Number 3
September 2018 ISSN 0095-5108, ISBN-13: 978-0-323-64145-6

Editor: Kerry Holland
Developmental Editor: Casey Potter

Clinics in Perinatology (ISSN 0095-5108) is published quarterly by Elsevier Inc., 360 Park Avenue South, New York, NY 10010-1710. Months of issue are March, June, September, and December. Business and Editorial Offices: 1600 John F. Kennedy Blvd., Ste. 1800, Philadelphia, PA 19103-2899. Customer Service Office: 3251 Riverport Lane, Maryland Heights, MO 63043. Periodicals postage paid at New York, NY and additional mailing offices. Subscription prices are $299.00 per year (US individuals), $548.00 per year (US institutions), $351.00 per year (Canadian individuals), $670.00 per year (Canadian institutions), $433.00 per year (international individuals), $670.00 per year (international institutions), $100.00 per year (US students), and $195.00 per year (Canadian and international students). International air speed delivery is included in all Clinics subscription prices. All prices are subject to change without notice. **POSTMASTER:** Send address changes to *Clinics in Perinatology*, Elsevier Health Sciences Division, Subscription Customer Service, 3251 Riverport Lane, Maryland Heights, MO 63043. **Customer Service: Telephone: 1-800-654-2452** (U.S. and Canada); **1-314-447-8871** (outside U.S. and Canada). **Fax: 1-314-447-8029. E-mail: journalscustomerservice-usa@elsevier.com** (for print support); **journalsonlinesupport-usa@elsevier.com** (for online support).

Reprints. For copies of 100 or more, of articles in this publication, please contact the Commercial Reprints Department, Elsevier Inc., 360 Park Avenue South, New York, NY 10010-1710. Tel. 212-633-3874; Fax: 212-633-3820; E-mail: reprints@elsevier.com.

Clinics in Perinatology is also published in Spanish by McGraw-Hill Interamericana Editores S.A., P.O. Box 5-237, 06500 Mexico D.F., Mexico.

Clinics in Perinatology is covered in *MEDLINE/PubMed (Index Medicus) Current Contents, Excepta Medica, BIOSIS and ISI/BIOMED.*

Contributors

CONSULTING EDITOR

LUCKY JAIN, MD, MBA

George W. Brumley Jr Professor and Chair, Emory University School of Medicine, Department of Pediatrics, Chief Academic Officer, Children's Healthcare of Atlanta, Executive Director, Emory and Childrens Pediatric Institute, Atlanta, Georgia, USA

EDITORS

IRA ADAMS-CHAPMAN, MD, MPH

Associate Professor, Department of Pediatrics, Division of Neonatology, Medical Director, Developmental Progress Clinic, Watkins Jennings Scholar in Neuroscience, Emory University School of Medicine, Children's Healthcare of Atlanta, Atlanta, Georgia, USA

SARA B. DeMAURO, MD, MSCE

Assistant Professor, Department of Pediatrics, Division of Neonatology, University of Pennsylvania Perelman School of Medicine, Program Director, Neonatal Follow-up, The Children's Hospital of Philadelphia, Philadelphia, Pennsylvania, USA

AUTHORS

IRA ADAMS-CHAPMAN, MD, MPH

Associate Professor, Department of Pediatrics, Division of Neonatology, Medical Director, Developmental Progress Clinic, Watkins Jennings Scholar in Neuroscience, Emory University School of Medicine, Children's Healthcare of Atlanta, Atlanta, Georgia, USA

NICKIE N. ANDESCAVAGE, MD

Assistant Professor, Department of Pediatrics, The George Washington University, Children's National Medical Center, Washington, DC, USA

GLEN P. AYLWARD, PhD, ABPP

Emeritus Professor of Pediatrics and Psychiatry, Divisions of Developmental and Behavioral Pediatrics and Psychology, SIU School of Medicine, Springfield, Illinois, USA

WANDA D. BARFIELD, MD, MPH, RADM

U.S. Public Health Service, Division of Reproductive Health, National Center for Chronic Disease Prevention and Health Promotion, Centers for Disease Control and Prevention, Atlanta, Georgia, USA

ALICE C. BURNETT, PhD

Premature Infant Follow-Up Program, The Royal Women's Hospital, Victorian Infant Brain Studies, Murdoch Children's Research Institute, Department of Pediatrics, University of Melbourne, Department of Neonatal Medicine, The Royal Children's Hospital, Parkville, Victoria, Australia

ANDREA C. CARCELEN, MPH
PhD Candidate, International Health Department, Johns Hopkins Bloomberg School of Public Health, Baltimore, Maryland, USA

BRIAN CARTER, MD
Professor, Division of Neonatology, Department of Pediatrics, Children's Mercy-Kansas City, University of Missouri-Kansas City School of Medicine, Kansas City, Missouri, USA

FRANCES A. CARTER, BA
Research Assistant, Department of Psychology, Center for Early Childhood Research, The University of Chicago, Chicago, Illinois, USA

JEANIE L.Y. CHEONG, MD
Professor, Premature Infant Follow-Up Program, Neonatal Services, The Royal Women's Hospital, Department of Obstetrics and Gynaecology, University of Melbourne, Parkville, Victoria, Australia; Victorian Infant Brain Studies, Murdoch Children's Research Institute, Newborn Research, The Royal Women's Hospital, Melbourne, Victoria, Australia

SARA B. DeMAURO, MD, MSCE
Assistant Professor, Department of Pediatrics, Division of Neonatology, University of Pennsylvania Perelman School of Medicine, Program Director, Neonatal Follow-up, The Children's Hospital of Philadelphia, Philadelphia, Pennsylvania, USA

LEX W. DOYLE, MD
Professor, Premature Infant Follow-Up Program, The Royal Women's Hospital, Departments of Pediatrics and Obstetrics and Gynaecology, University of Melbourne, Parkville, Victoria, Australia; Victorian Infant Brain Studies, Murdoch Children's Research Institute, Newborn Research, The Royal Women's Hospital, Melbourne, Victoria, Australia

ANDREA F. DUNCAN, MD, MSClinRes
Associate Professor, Department of Pediatrics, Division of Neonatal-Perinatal Medicine, University of Texas Health Science Center at Houston, Houston, Texas, USA

BALAJI GOVINDASWAMI, MBBS, MPH
Chief, Division of Neonatology, Pediatrics, Santa Clara Valley Medical Center: Hospital & Clinics, Director, Neonatal Intensive Care Unit, San Jose, California, USA; Clinical Professor (Affiliated) of Pediatrics, Stanford University School of Medicine, Palo Alto, California, USA

MATTHEW HICKS, MD, PhD
Neonatologist, Developmental Pediatrician, Assistant Professor, Department of Pediatrics, Neonatal Intensive Care Unit, University of Alberta, Diagnosis and Treatment Centre, Royal Alexandra Hospital, Edmonton, Alberta, Canada

PRIYA JEGATHEESAN, MD
Division of Neonatology, Pediatrics, Santa Clara Valley Medical Center: Hospital & Clinics, Neonatal Intensive Care Unit, San Jose, California, USA; Assistant Clinical Professor (Affiliated) of Pediatrics, Stanford University School of Medicine, Palo Alto, California, USA

HOWARD W. KILBRIDE, MD
Professor, Division of Neonatology, Department of Pediatrics, Children's Mercy-Kansas City, University of Missouri-Kansas City School of Medicine, Kansas City, Missouri, USA

ANGELA LEON HERNANDEZ, MD
Assistant Professor of Pediatrics, Neonatology Division, Emory University School of Medicine, Atlanta, Georgia, USA

MELISSA A. MATTHEWS, MD
Assistant Professor, Department of Pediatrics, Division of Neonatal-Perinatal Medicine, University of Texas Health Science Center at Houston, Houston, Texas, USA

CATHERINE MORGAN, PhD
Cerebral Palsy Alliance, Child and Adolescent Health, The University of Sydney, Sydney, New South Wales, Australia

MICHAEL E. MSALL, MD
Professor of Pediatrics, Section of Developmental and Behavioral Pediatrics, Kennedy Research Center on Intellectual and Neurodevelopmental Disabilities, The University of Chicago Comer Children's Hospital, Woodlawn Social Services Center, Chicago, Illinois, USA

SUDHA RANI NARASIMHAN, MD, IBCLC
Division of Neonatology, Pediatrics, Santa Clara Valley Medical Center: Hospital & Clinics, Neonatal Intensive Care Unit, San Jose, California, USA; Assistant Clinical Professor (Affiliated) of Pediatrics, Stanford University School of Medicine, Palo Alto, California, USA

IONA NOVAK, PhD
Cerebral Palsy Alliance, Child and Adolescent Health, The University of Sydney, Sydney, New South Wales, Australia

MATTHEW NUDELMAN, MD
Division of Neonatology, Pediatrics, Santa Clara Valley Medical Center: Hospital & Clinics, Neonatal Intensive Care Unit, San Jose, California, USA

JOY E. OLSEN, PhD
Victorian Infant Brain Studies, Murdoch Children's Research Institute, Neonatal Services, The Royal Women's Hospitals, Parkville, Australia

MYRIAM PERALTA-CARCELEN, MD, MPH
Interim Division Director, Division of Developmental and Behavioral Pediatrics, Professor, Department of Pediatrics, The University of Alabama at Birmingham, Birmingham, Alabama, USA

JUSTIN SCHWARTZ, MD
Division of Developmental and Behavioral Pediatrics, Assistant Professor, Department of Pediatrics, The University of Alabama at Birmingham, Birmingham, Alabama, USA

ELIZABETH K. SEWELL, MD, MPH
Assistant Professor, Department of Pediatrics, Emory University School of Medicine, Children's Healthcare of Atlanta, Atlanta, Georgia, USA

ALICIA J. SPITTLE, PhD
Associate Professor, Physiotherapy, University of Melbourne, Victorian Infant Brain Studies, Murdoch Children's Research Institute, Neonatal Services, The Royal Women's Hospitals, Parkville, Australia

ANNE SYNNES, MDCM, MHSc
Neonatologist, Director, Neonatal Follow-Up Program, British Columbia's Women's Hospital, Clinical Professor, University of British Columbia, Vancouver, British Columbia, Canada

JOHN A.F. ZUPANCIC, MD, ScD
Department of Neonatology, Beth Israel Deaconess Medical Center, Associate Professor of Pediatrics, Division of Newborn Medicine, Harvard Medical School, Boston, Massachusetts, USA

Contents

Technological advances in neonatal-perinatal medicine have led to a steady increase in the survival of preterm infants. Although the increase in survival is a remarkable success, children born preterm remain at high risk for brain injury and long-term neurodevelopmental deficits. Children born preterm may have abnormal muscle tone or movements, cognitive deficits, language impairments, and behavioral problems. This article reviews neurodevelopmental outcomes and factors that influence outcomes in preterm children during early childhood.

Despite improved survival of preterm infants, there has not been an equivalent improvement in long-term neurodevelopmental outcomes. Adverse neurodevelopmental outcome rates and severity are inversely related to the degree of prematurity, but only 1.6% are born very preterm and the motor, cognitive, behavioral, and psychiatric disabilities in the large moderate and late preterm population have a greater impact. The disability-free preterm adult has a lower educational achievement and income but similar health-related quality of life to term controls. Reducing the long-term neurodevelopmental impact of prematurity is the next frontier of neonatal care.

Infants born preterm are at increased risk of cerebral palsy (CP), with the risk increasing with decreasing gestational age. Although preterm children are at increased risk of CP compared with their term-born peers, most preterm children do not have CP, and thus, it is important to have a standardized process for detecting those children at high risk of CP early. A combination of clinical history, neuroimaging, and physical examination is recommended to ensure early, accurate diagnosis. Early detection of CP is essential for timely early intervention to optimize outcomes for children and their families.

Although very preterm birth and very low birthweight are recognized risk factors for longer-term developmental difficulties, there is a wide spectrum of outcomes for children and adolescents born preterm. Biological and social variables have the potential to explain this variability. Although current understanding of these influences and how they interact is incomplete, perinatal factors are related to permanent neurosensory impairments, such as cerebral palsy, blindness, and deafness. Cognitive and academic outcomes are variably associated with biological and social variables across development, and the most robust correlates of behavior and mental health difficulties include early behavioral problems and family influences.

To understand the trajectories of risk and resilience in the vulnerable preterm and neonatal brain, clinicians must go beyond survival and critically examine on a population basis the functional outcomes of children, adolescents, and adults across their life course. Evaluations must go well beyond Bayley assessments and counts of neonatal morbidities, such as bronchopulmonary dysplasia, retinopathy of prematurity, sonographic brain injury, sepsis, and necrotizing enterocolitis. Proactively providing support to families and developmental and educational supports to children can optimize academic functioning and participation in adult learning, physical and behavioral health activities, community living, relationships, and employment.

Prematurity is a significant risk factor for impaired neurodevelopmental outcomes. These include motor, cognitive, language, behavioral, and socioemotional competence. Long-term overall function depends on healthy socioemotional functioning. The vulnerability of the preterm brain during critical periods of development contributes to behavioral and socioemotional problems in preterm children. Attention deficit/hyperactivity disorder (ADHD) and autism spectrum disorder (ASD) clinical features are more frequent in preterm children compared with their full-term counterparts; however, true rates of ASD and ADHD vary across studies. Early detection of behavioral and socioemotional problems in preterm children would enable timely early intervention to improve long-term functional outcomes.

Behavioral and emotional problems are one of the most frequent chronic conditions diagnosed among children born prematurely. The high prevalence of these pathologies is a matter of concern not only because of their

PROGRAM OBJECTIVE

The goal of *Clinics in Perinatology* is to keep practicing perinatologists, neonatologists, obstetricians, practicing physicians and residents up to date with current clinical practice in perinatology by providing timely articles reviewing the state of the art in patient care.

TARGET AUDIENCE

Perinatologists, neonatologists, obstetricians, practicing physicians, residents and healthcare professionals who provide patient care utilizing findings from *Clinics in Perinatology.*

LEARNING OBJECTIVES

Upon completion of this activity, participants will be able to:
1. Review neurodevelopmental outcomes in early childhood and of preterm children at and beyond school age.
2. Discuss the public health Implications of very preterm birth and the impact of prematurity on behavioural, social, and emotional development.
3. Recognize advances in prevention of prematurity.

ACCREDITATION

The Elsevier Office of Continuing Medical Education (EOCME) is accredited by the Accreditation Council for Continuing Medical Education (ACCME) to provide continuing medical education for physicians.

The EOCME designates this enduring material for a maximum of 15 *AMA PRA Category 1 Credit*(s)™. Physicians should claim only the credit commensurate with the extent of their participation in the activity.

All other health care professionals requesting continuing education credit for this enduring material will be issued a certificate of participation.

DISCLOSURE OF CONFLICTS OF INTEREST

The EOCME assesses conflict of interest with its instructors, faculty, planners, and other individuals who are in a position to control the content of CME activities. All relevant conflicts of interest that are identified are thoroughly vetted by EOCME for fair balance, scientific objectivity, and patient care recommendations. EOCME is committed to providing its learners with CME activities that promote improvements or quality in healthcare and not a specific proprietary business or a commercial interest.

The planning committee, staff, authors and editors listed below have identified no financial relationships or relationships to products or devices they or their spouse/life partner have with commercial interest related to the content of this CME activity:

Ira Adams-Chapman, MD, MPH; Nickie N. Andescavage, MD; Glen P. Aylward, PhD, ABPP; Wanda D. Barfield, MD, MPH; Alice C. Burnett, PhD; Andrea C. Carcelen, MPH; Brian Carter, MD; Frances A. Carter, BA; Jeanie L.Y. Cheong, MD; Sara B. DeMauro, MD, MSCE; Lex W. Doyle, MD; Andrea F. Duncan, MD, MSClinRes; Balaji Govindaswami, MBBS, MPH; Matthew Hicks, MD, PhD; Kerry Holland; Lucky Jain, MD, MBA; Priya Jegatheesan, MD; Alison Kemp; Howard W. Kilbride, MD; Angela Leon Hernandez, MD; Melissa A. Matthews, MD; Catherine Morgan, MD; Michael E. Msall, MD; Sudha Rani Narasimhan, MD; Iona Novak, MD; Matthew Nudelman, MD; Joy E. Olsen, MD; Myriam Peralta-Carcelen, MD, MPH; Casey Potter; Justin Schwartz, MD; Elizabeth K. Sewell, MD, MPH; Alicia J. Spittle, MD; Anne Synnes, MDCM, MHSc; Subhalakshmi Vaidyanathan; John A.F. Zupancic, MD, ScD.

UNAPPROVED/OFF-LABEL USE DISCLOSURE

The EOCME requires CME faculty to disclose to the participants:
1. When products or procedures being discussed are off-label, unlabelled, experimental, and/or investigational (not US Food and Drug Administration [FDA] approved); and
2. Any limitations on the information presented, such as data that are preliminary or that represent ongoing research, interim analyses, and/or unsupported opinions. Faculty may discuss information about pharmaceutical agents that is outside of FDA-approved labelling. This information is intended solely for CME and is not intended to promote off-label use of these medications. If you have any questions, contact the medical affairs department of the manufacturer for the most recent prescribing information.

TO ENROLL

To enroll in the *Clinics in Perinatology* Continuing Medical Education program, call customer service at 1-800-654-2452 or sign up online at http://www.theclinics.com/home/cme. The CME program is available to subscribers for an additional annual fee of 244.40 USD.

METHOD OF PARTICIPATION

In order to claim credit, participants must complete the following:

1. Complete enrolment as indicated above.
2. Read the activity.
3. Complete the CME Test and Evaluation. Participants must achieve a score of 70% on the test. All CME Tests and Evaluations must be completed online.

CME INQUIRIES/SPECIAL NEEDS

For all CME inquiries or special needs, please contact elsevierCME@elsevier.com.

CLINICS IN PERINATOLOGY

THE CLINICS ARE AVAILABLE ONLINE!
Access your subscription at:
www.theclinics.com

Foreword

The Business of Predicting Long-Term Neonatal Outcomes

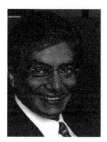

Lucky Jain, MD, MBA
Consulting Editor

No other area of medicine faces a prognostic challenge of this magnitude: predicting what the future holds for a newborn two or three decades later, and linking it definitively to information available around birth. Indeed, real-life outcomes can be very different from predictions based on neurodevelopmental studies done early on in infancy or even in preschool years. In a 2011 study evaluating the relationship of gestational age at birth and mortality in young adulthood, Crump and colleagues[1] provided strong evidence that for neonates born early, higher risk of death in adulthood resurfaces after being largely undetectable in intervening years. Preterm birth was associated with increased mortality in young adults even among individuals born late preterm. Crump and colleagues[1] had the advantage of longitudinal data from a large Swedish cohort with nearly 674,820 individuals. Most newborn follow-up studies don't have this luxury and suffer from small sample size and/or inadequate data.

The Neonatal Research Network supported by the Eunice Kennedy Shriver National Institute of Child Health and Human Development has done a great job of reporting outcomes from a large cohort of extremely preterm infants, and a recent study by Adams-Chapman and colleagues[2] exemplifies this. However, such networks are expensive to maintain, and outcomes data are limited to the data registries maintained.

One alternate approach then is to focus on school outcomes using existing educational data. In the United States, a large cache of testing data became available after Criterion-Referenced Competency Tests (CRCT) were adopted across the country. In states where results of the standardized school testing results and health data (vital statistics and hospital discharge data) can be deterministically linked, one can begin studying the long-term impact of perinatal events on a child's ability to acquire education. There is no limit to this approach since standardized testing is now commonplace in high schools and beyond (Scholastic Assessment Test, SAT; Graduate Record Examinations, GRE; and similar). Several years ago, we used this approach to report on perinatal origins of first grade academic failure and the role of prematurity (**Fig. 1**).[3] We

Clin Perinatol 45 (2018) xv–xvi
https://doi.org/10.1016/j.clp.2018.06.002
0095-5108/18/© 2018 Published by Elsevier Inc.

perinatology.theclinics.com

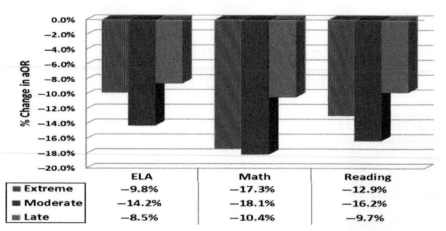

	ELA	Math	Reading
▓ Extreme	−9.8%	−17.3%	−12.9%
▓ Moderate	−14.2%	−18.1%	−16.2%
▓ Late	−8.5%	−10.4%	−9.7%

Fig. 1. Change in adjusted odds ratio (aOR) of failure of CRCT components according to gestational age category. ELA, English, language, arts. (*From* Williams B, Dunlop A, Kramer M, et al. Perinatal origins of first grade academic failure: role of prematurity and maternal factors. Pediatrics 2013;131:699; with permission.)

found that being born preterm versus term increased a child's chances of failing in each of the three components of CRCT when controlling for maternal age at birth, maternal education, maternal race/ethnicity, child's gender, and year of birth. Likelihood of failure was inversely related to gestational age with a significant dose-response pattern.

This issue of the *Clinics in Perinatology* addresses many of the challenges and opportunities for clinician-scientists engaged in this field. Drs Adams-Chapman and De-Mauro are to be congratulated for a superb issue of the *Clinics in Perinatology* compiling articles from top experts in the field. As always, I am grateful to the authors for their valuable contributions and to my publishing partners at Elsevier (Kerry Holland and Casey Jackson) for their help in bringing this valuable resource to you.

Lucky Jain, MD, MBA
Emory and Childrens Pediatric Institute
Emory University School of Medicine, and
Children's Healthcare of Atlanta
1760 Haygood Drive, W409
Atlanta, GA 30322, USA

E-mail address:
ljain@emory.edu

REFERENCES

1. Crump C, Sundquist K, Winkleby MA. Gestational age at birth and mortality in young adulthood. JAMA 2011;306:1233–40.
2. Adams-Chapman I, Heyne RJ, DeMauro SB, et al, Neurodevelopmental Impairment Among Extremely Preterm Infants in the Neonatal Research Network. Follow-up Study of the Eunice Kennedy Schriver National Institute of Child Health and Human Development Neonatal Research Network. Pediatrics 2018.
3. Williams B, Dunlop A, Kramer M, et al. Perinatal origins of first grade academic failure: role of prematurity and maternal factors. Pediatrics 2013;131:693–700.

Preface

Neurodevelopmental Outcomes of the Preterm Infant

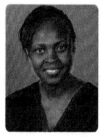 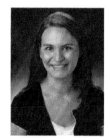

Ira Adams-Chapman, MD, MPH   Sara B. DeMauro, MD, MSCE
Editors

Neonatology has witnessed monumental declines in neonatal mortality and neonatal morbidities over the past several decades. Advances in neonatal care have directly translated into decreases in many of the morbidities known to be associated with adverse neurodevelopmental outcomes, such as neonatal infection and intraventricular hemorrhage. Researchers have helped us better understand the relationship between the inflammatory response associated with many neonatal morbidities and the risk for brain injury in these vulnerable neonates. Concomitant with these critical improvements in short-term outcomes, the longer-term neurodevelopmental outcomes of prematurely born children have also started to improve.

Historically, neurodevelopmental outcome studies have focused on evaluating the presence or absence of moderate/severe impairment at 2 years corrected age. Severe disability is commonly defined as moderate/severe cerebral palsy, severe cognitive delay, and/or bilateral blindness, though precise definitions of these components and means of assessing them vary widely. Although these data have been incredibly valuable for helping neonatologists understand the outcomes of their patients and impact of novel interventions, we are learning that many other important outcomes cannot be appropriately evaluated until school age. These include intellectual performance, motor coordination, and behavior/attention problems. Furthermore, it is important to recognize the full spectrum of neurodevelopmental outcomes, including milder degrees of impairment, which can have a significant influence on everyday functioning and quality of life. Last, illness in the preterm child can have a profound and long-lasting impact on the family, which we are only just beginning to understand.

In this review, the associations between major neonatal morbidities and risk of adverse neurodevelopmental outcomes in preterm infants are reviewed. In addition, we profile current outcome data in early childhood and at school age. Many

Clin Perinatol 45 (2018) xvii–xviii
https://doi.org/10.1016/j.clp.2018.06.001
0095-5108/18/© 2018 Published by Elsevier Inc.

prematurely born children are at risk for behavioral problems that impact short-term and long-term outcomes. The impact on the family is also examined as it relates to the individual patient and as a public health problem. In addition, we address how prematurity affects functioning and participation in activities of daily living throughout the life spectrum. Ultimately, efforts to continually decrease neonatal morbidities and prevent premature birth will be the most effective strategies for improving the neurodevelopmental outcomes of this vulnerable population.

Ira Adams-Chapman, MD, MPH
Department of Pediatrics/
Division of Neonatology
Developmental Progress Clinic
Emory University School of Medicine
Children's Healthcare of Atlanta
2015 Uppergate Drive
Atlanta, GA 30303, USA

Sara B. DeMauro, MD, MSCE
Department of Pediatrics/
Division of Neonatology
University of Pennsylvania
Perelman School of Medicine
Neonatal Follow-up
Children's Hospital of Philadelphia
3401 Civic Center Boulevard
Room 2NW15
Philadelphia, PA 19104, USA

E-mail addresses:
iadamsc@emory.edu (I. Adams-Chapman)
demauro@email.chop.edu (S.B. DeMauro)

Neurodevelopmental Outcomes in Early Childhood

Andrea F. Duncan, MD, MSClinRes*, Melissa A. Matthews, MD

KEYWORDS

• Preterm • Neurodevelopment • Early childhood • Developmental outcomes

KEY POINTS

- Survival of preterm infants is improving, but high risk for neurodevelopmental deficits remains.
- Guidelines exist for earlier assessment and diagnosis of cerebral palsy before 6 months of age.
- High-prevalence/low severity dysfunctions are increasing.
- A longer duration of follow-up is needed.

INTRODUCTION

Technological advances in neonatal-perinatal medicine have led to a steady increase in the survival of preterm infants (**Table 1**). Indeed, survival of children at the very lowest gestations (22–24 weeks) has increased from 30% in 2000 to 2003% to 36% in 2008 to 2011.[1] Although the increase in survival is a remarkable success, children born preterm remain at high risk for brain injury and long-term neurodevelopmental deficits. As survival rates have improved over the past decades, there is an increased focus on long-term morbidity associated with preterm birth. Recently, the fact that rates of extremely preterm (<28 weeks of gestation) infant survival without neurodevelopmental impairment (NDI) have increased from 16% to 20% between the years 2000 and 2011 has been celebrated.[2] Despite this, the rate of moderate to severe NDI at 2 years of age remains exceptionally high among children at the lowest gestational ages (GAs). Of infants born at 22 weeks GA, 85% to 90% have severe NDI, with a similar outcome reported at 23 weeks GA.[3] In infants born less than 25 weeks GA, there has not been a significant improvement in neurodevelopmental outcomes in recent studies.[3,4] However, longer follow-up of these infants is needed to understand the full impact of preterm birth at the limits of viability. Additionally, even though more

Disclosure Statement: There are no commercial or financial disclosures, conflicts of interest, or funding sources to report.
Department of Pediatrics, Division of Neonatal-Perinatal Medicine, University of Texas Health Science Center at Houston, 6431 Fannin Street, MSB 3.242, Houston, TX 77030, USA
* Corresponding author.
E-mail address: Andrea.F.Duncan@uth.tmc.edu

Clin Perinatol 45 (2018) 377–392
https://doi.org/10.1016/j.clp.2018.05.001
0095-5108/18/© 2018 Elsevier Inc. All rights reserved.
perinatology.theclinics.com

Table 1
Survival of children born extremely preterm

Year	Survival Rate, %
1943–1945	0
1980–1985	10
2006–2011	65

Data from Gong A, Johnson YR, Livingston J, et al. Newborn intensive care survivors: a review and a plan for collaboration in Texas. Matern Health Neonatol Perinatol 2015;1:24.

infants at extremely low GAs are surviving, most preterm births occur in the moderate preterm (32–33 weeks' gestation) to the late preterm (34–36 weeks' gestation) range.[5,6] Although the survival rate in this cohort is greater than 99%, there is an increased risk for NDI in this group.[5,7–9]

Because of the high risk of neurodevelopmental deficits, survival without NDI at 2 years of age has become a common benchmark for success. The Eunice Kennedy Shriver National Institute of Child Health and Development Neonatal Research Network defines NDI as having one or more of the following at 2 years: moderate to severe cerebral palsy (CP), profound hearing loss requiring amplification in both ears, profound visual impairment with visual acuity less than 20/200 in both eyes, moderate to profound cognitive delay on the Bayley Scales of Infant Development 3rd edition (Bayley-III) assessment (Cognitive Composite score of <54–84), and/or a Gross Motor Function Classification System (GMFCS) level of greater than 2 on a 5-point scale.[1] A GMFCS score of 2 or greater translates functionally to a child who cannot walk or pull to stand and may or may not have head control or the ability to sit unsupported. Infant-related factors associated with survival without NDI in early childhood include female sex, higher birth weight or gestation, larger head size, and absence of neonatal morbidities and interventions.[10] Although these early benchmarks, such as NDI, are extremely important, particularly for research purposes, it must be remembered that most neurodevelopmental deficits suffered by preterm children are mild to moderate. These deficits result in a significant functional burden. In addition, preterm children are more likely to have language deficits, and far more likely to have behavioral deficits than their term-born counterparts, which may adversely impact motor, cognition, language development, and testing.[11,12] Such deficits may not be considered in research outcomes using common definitions of NDI, although they must be considered clinically. Furthermore, many developmental deficits in cognition, emotional and behavioral development, and social adaptive functioning may emerge at older ages in the absence of NDI in toddlerhood.[12,13] These "high-prevalence/low severity dysfunctions" occur in 50% to 70% of very low birth weight infants (<1500 g) and are increasing-especially in children born most premature-and include attention-deficit/hyperactivity disorder, executive function deficits, visuomotor problems, learning disabilities, and behavior problems.[12]

This demonstrates a need for longer follow-up of all infants born preterm. This article reviews neurodevelopmental outcomes for children born preterm, with a focus on early childhood.

FACTORS IMPACTING NEURODEVELOPMENTAL OUTCOMES

The factors that influence neurodevelopment in infants born preterm are multifactorial, contributing to the complexity of follow-up research and variations in reported outcomes (**Box 1**). Certain perinatal and postnatal factors confer a higher risk for long-term neurodevelopmental deficits. These include severe intraventricular hemorrhage,

---

Box 1
Factors affecting neurodevelopmental outcomes in preterm children

Birth weight less than 750 g or less than 25 weeks' gestation

Periventricular hemorrhage (grades III and IV) or infarction

Periventricular leukomalacia

Persistent ventricular dilation

Neonatal seizures

Chronic lung disease

Neonatal meningitis

Subnormal head circumference at discharge

Parental drug abuse

Poverty and parental deprivation

Coexisting congenital malformation

Data from Wilson-Costello DE, Payne AH. Early childhood neurodevelopmental outcomes of high-risk neonates. In: Fanaroff and Martin's neonatal-perinatal medicine: diseases of the fetus and infant. Philadelphia: Elsevier/Saunders; 2015. p. 1018–31.

---

periventricular leukomalacia, persistent fetal circulation, infections including meningitis and pneumonia resulting in respiratory failure, seizures, severe respiratory distress syndrome, and extremes of birth weight or GA (see **Box 1**).[14]

Preterm infants are born at a time when their brains are particularly susceptible to injury. There is significant growth and organization that occurs during the second and third trimesters. Early insults during this time may adversely affect several processes involved in brain development including neuronal migration, synaptogenesis, myelination, cytologic maturation, and cell receptor development.[10] Additionally, preterm birth and iatrogenic factors inherent to neonatal intensive care unit (NICU) care lead to increased free radical generation in the presence of decreased antioxidant capacity in preterm infants, further compounding brain injury during this vulnerable period of brain development.[15]

Factors affecting developmental outcomes begin antenatally and continue after birth. Exposure to antenatal steroids has long been shown to reduce neonatal morbidity and mortality including respiratory distress syndrome and intraventricular hemorrhage.[16] However; it is unclear if antenatal steroids have a clear benefit for neurodevelopmental outcomes. Some studies suggest an associated reduction in NDI in exposed infants born 23 to 25 weeks GA.[4,16] A significant antecedent to adverse neurodevelopmental outcomes is the presence of a perinatal infection. Intrauterine infection has been associated with a nine-fold increase in the incidence of CP in full-term infants.[12] Increased odds of NDI are also described in extremely preterm infants exposed to chorioamnionitis.[17] However, data related to the importance of intrauterine infection are unclear, particularly given the difficulty in diagnosis of intrauterine infection and the limited predictability of outcomes in preterm infants.

Postnatally, the extent of NDI may be affected in part by GA and extent of brain maturity at birth, the magnitude of the initial injury, and recurrent insults during the recovery and reorganization phase.[12] For example, birth asphyxia can lead to significant brain injury, but recurrent hypoxia compounds the damage to vulnerable neurons during the recovery phase. Additional comorbid conditions, such as bronchopulmonary dysplasia, retinopathy of prematurity, and necrotizing enterocolitis, are associated with a several-fold increase in NDI for extremely low birth weight infants.[10,12]

The NICU environment might also impact neurodevelopmental outcomes. Although this concept remains controversial, there are studies to suggest that loud sounds and bright lights can have harmful effects on development. Conversely, decreased auditory input, particularly maternal sounds, is thought to negatively impact speech and language development.[10,18,19] It seems that auditory input is important to development, but the degree and origin of input still need to be determined.

Several other factors have been shown to play a role in adverse neurodevelopmental outcomes. Genetic factors, male gender, intrauterine growth restriction, location of birth, nutrition, high-frequency ventilation, surgery, and drug abuse are a few such factors.[10,12] Additional factors after discharge, such as maternal education, access to medical services, and socioeconomic status, also impact neurodevelopmental outcomes. These demographic factors highlight the importance of including detailed population information and a term equivalent control group in studies of early childhood outcomes in preterm children.

MOTOR OUTCOMES

Motor deficits in children born preterm are generally recognized earlier than other NDIs. Abnormal motor development, such as muscle asymmetries, hypotonia, and hypertonic extensor movements are identified before 40 weeks postmenstrual age in some infants.[8,12] In addition, preterm infants may display more extensor activity in infancy than those born term. This may be secondary to nursing postures and medical morbidities, such as chronic lung disease.[12] Children born preterm may also have transient neurologic deficits that resolve by 12 months, with rates ranging from 40% to 80%.[14] These deficits may include poor head control, generalized hypotonia or hypertonia, inability to sit at 8 months, or mild increases in extremity tone.

CP is the most common childhood physical disability, present in 0.21% of the general population in high-income countries.[20] CP is present in 9% to 20% of children born extremely preterm, and a greater proportion of preterm infants present with milder motor impairments.[10,21] The four types of CP are shown in **Table 2**. These types may develop and change during the first 2 years of life. It is of critical importance to remember that CP is often associated with significant and disabling comorbid conditions (**Table 3**).[20] Diplegia and hemiplegia are most common in preterm children, with spastic CP accounting for more than 90% of CP in preterm children.[14] Spastic CP is defined by increased tone with a velocity-dependent increase in resistance to passive

Table 2	
Types and distribution of cerebral palsy	
Type	**Percentage**
Spastic	85–91
Dyskinetic[a]	4–7
Ataxic	4–6
Hypotonic	2

[a] Includes dystonia and athetosis.

Data from Novak I, Morgan C, Adde L, et al. Early, accurate diagnosis and early intervention in cerebral palsy: advances in diagnosis and treatment. JAMA Pediatr 2017;171(9):897–907.

Table 3	
Comorbid conditions associated with cerebral palsy	
Condition	**Percentage**
Chronic pain	75
Intellectual disability	49
Epilepsy	35
Musculoskeletal problems (ie, hip displacement)	28
Behavioral disorders	26
Sleep disorders	23
Functional blindness	11
Hearing impairment	4

Data from Novak I, Morgan C, Adde L, et al. Early, accurate diagnosis and early intervention in cerebral palsy: advances in diagnosis and treatment. JAMA Pediatr 2017;171(9):897–907; and Novak I, Hines M, Goldsmith S, et al. Clinical prognostic messages from a systematic review on cerebral palsy. Pediatrics 2012;130(5):e1285–312.

movement. Assessment of passive tone using very slow stretch may therefore underestimate the degree of resistance. Hyperreflexia, protracted presence of primitive reflexes, abnormal Babinski response, abnormal posture, or abnormal movement may be present. These may be characterized in the lower extremities by equines foot position, a crouching gait, internal lower extremity rotation, and hip adduction. Upper limb findings may include arm flexion with fisting of hands, cortical thumbs, and poor coordination of finger movements.[14] Bilateral spastic CP may result in contractures.

Classically, the first 12 to 24 months of life was considered to be a "silent period" during which CP could not be accurately diagnosed. Experts now agree that the belief in a silent period is outdated, because a designation of CP or high-risk for CP may be accurately given before 6 months of corrected age.[20] Novak and colleagues[20] recently described the most predictive tools for detecting CP before and after 5 months of corrected age. Before 5 months, the most predictive tools are the Prechtl General Movements Assessment, the Hammersmith Infant Neurologic Examination (HINE), and MRI at term age with sensitivities of 98%, 90%, and 86%, respectively. However, the Prechtl Assessment has a low specificity and although the specificity of MRI is good, its sensitivity is comparatively lower.[10] After 5 months' corrected age, the most predictive tools for detecting CP are MRI and the HINE with 86% to 89% and 90% sensitivity, respectively. The HINE is used as a neurologic assessment from 2 months through 24 months.[22] The authors also note that the trajectory of HINE scores combined with abnormal MRI findings is more accurate than individual clinical assessments.[20,23] It is therefore recommended that a combination of medical history, standardized motor assessment, and neuroimaging is used when making a diagnosis of CP by 6 months corrected age.

If CP is suspected but cannot be definitively diagnosed, an interim diagnosis of high risk of CP should be given until the diagnosis may be confirmed.[20] Using the specific CP moniker is of import, because infants with CP have improved functional outcomes in response to different interventions than the interventions provided with concerns for developmental delay or autism. Early referral to CP-specific early intervention is critical to improve functional outcomes, as is continued, coordinated care including medical, neuromotor, and developmental monitoring to provide appropriate care in consideration of current diagnoses and comorbidities that may develop. A temporary diagnosis of high-risk CP requires that the child have motor dysfunction (essential criterion) and at least one of the other two additional criteria, which include abnormal MRI (with or without serial cranial ultrasound [CUS] examinations) neuroimaging and a clinical history conferring risk for development of CP (**Table 4**).[20] The MRI findings most predictive of CP and clinical findings conferring risk are detailed in **Table 3**. CUS is also frequently used in NICUs to detect intraventricular hemorrhage, intraparenchymal hemorrhage, and ventriculomegaly among other things. Although cystic periventricular leukomalacia on CUS is a strong predictor for CP, there are infants without abnormalities on CUS that later develop neurodevelopmental deficits.[12] Additionally, it is reported that preterm individuals with normal CUS have decreased cortical gray matter volume and increased ventricle size on MRI during adulthood compared with full-term control subjects.[12] Spasticity may develop after 1 year of age, and children who

Table 4	
Neuroimaging and clinical findings associated with cerebral palsy	
Abnormal Neuroimaging Associated with Cerebral Palsy	
White matter injury	Cystic periventricular leukomalacia
	Periventricular hemorrhagic infarctions
Cortical and deep gray matter lesions	Basal ganglia or thalamic lesions
	Parasagittal injury
	Multicystic encephalomalacia
	Stroke
Abnormal brain development	Lissencephaly
	Pachygyria
	Cortical dysplasia
	Polymicrogyria
	Schizencephaly
Preconception	History of stillbirths or miscarriages
	Low socioeconomic status
	Assisted reproduction
	Abnormal genetic
	Copy number variations
Pregnancy	Prematurity
	Abnormal genetic findings
	Birth defects
	Multiple birth
	Male sex
	Maternal thyroid disease
	Preeclampsia
	Infection
	Intrauterine growth restriction
	Substance abuse
Perinatal	Acute intrapartum hypoxia-ischemia
	Seizures
	Hypoglycemia
	Jaundice
	Infection
Postnatal	Stroke
	Infection
	Surgical complications
	Brain injury before 24 mo

Data from Novak I, Morgan C, Adde L, et al. Early, accurate diagnosis and early intervention in cerebral palsy: advances in diagnosis and treatment. JAMA Pediatr 2017;171(9):897–907.

later develop CP may demonstrate hypotonia in very early life.[14,20] Spasticity during the first 3 months of life is a poor prognostic sign.[14] Because spasticity may develop later, the absence of spasticity early does not preclude a diagnosis of spastic CP. In addition, infants may simultaneously have multiple motor disorders, with spasticity and dystonia often occurring together. An increase in voluntary movements may be associated with an improvement or worsening of symptoms.[20]

The severity of CP is difficult to accurately assess in infants younger than 2 years, because their motor skills are developing, the presence/absence of hypertonicity may change over time, and this is a period of extremely rapid brain growth and experience/use-dependent neuronal reorganization in response the environment, including interventions and therapy.[20]

Cautious prediction of CP severity should be made using standardized tools, such as the HINE, coupled with neuroimaging data and clinical history.[20,22] At 2 years of age and after, the severity of CP may be accurately classified using the five-level GMFCS, Extended & Revised.[24] The GMFCS is an age-based, five-level system that defines motor functioning based on a child's self-initiated movement, and emphasizes sitting, walking, and general mobility. The levels are determined by the presence or absence of functional limitations including the need for mobility devices and the quality of usual movements.

Appropriate counseling is important when giving a diagnosis of CP, because parental understanding of the disease may not take the entire spectrum of disease into account. Large population studies from high-income countries indicate that two in three individuals with CP will walk, that three in four will talk, and one in two will have normal intelligence.[20]

Isolated and minor motor disorders, such as minor neuromotor dysfunction and developmental coordination disorder, which is found in approximately one-third of all preterm children, are more common than CP.[14,25] Children with developmental coordination disorder do not have neurosensory or cognitive impairments. Instead, children with developmental coordination disorder demonstrate fine and gross motor delays that cause difficulties or clumsiness with tasks, such as using pencils or silverware or performing routine motor tasks of daily living.[26] Minor neuromotor dysfunction is more subtle than CP or other, more severe motor impairments. It covers a wide range, such as difficulties with coordination, learning, and fine motor function.[25] Generally, it does not occur in isolation, and subtle deficits may compound together to cause greater academic struggles. With a prevalence of 40% in some studies, there are currently no ideal predictors of minor neuromotor dysfunction.[8,25] So-called minor motor disorders have been associated with general decrease in function and cognitive and behavioral deficits at school age.[27]

VISUAL AND HEARING OUTCOMES

Although vision and hearing deficits are the least common of the neurodevelopmental deficits found in children born preterm, they are far more common in this group than among the population at large. Medical morbidities, such as retinopathy of prematurity and brain injury, may adversely affect visual acuity. A severe visual deficit is defined as functional bilateral blindness, including visual acuity of 20/200 or worse, an inability to perceive light, or the ability to perceive light only.[4,21,28–33] Rates of severe visual impairment in preterm children range from 0% to 5%[28,30,32]; milder impairment, such as strabismus and myopia, occur in 9% to 25% of these children.[34–36] More than one-third of children born extremely low birth weight needs glasses, a rate three times higher than that seen in children born term.[12]

In general, researchers have defined severe hearing deficits as bilateral loss of functional hearing that is not corrected with amplification.[28] Few studies have included audiologic cutpoints, defining profound loss as greater than 90 dBHL.[28] In most large studies of children born extremely preterm, rates of severe or profound hearing loss are less than 2.5%.[4,21,28–30,32]

Although hearing and vision deficits are rare in children born preterm, 25% of hearing impairment and 35% of all visual impairment in the United states is accounted for by preterm birth.[28,37] In addition, most children born extremely and very low birth weight express a deficit in visuomotor function, although these are commonly diagnosed at somewhat older ages, when such tasks as copying, pegboard completion, spatial processing, visuosequential memory, and spatial organization are affected.[12,38–42] These deficits often exist even in the presence of normal IQ.[12] Of import, these problems have been noted at school age in children who had normal development at 3 years of age.[12,42] Visual function is also interrelated with other neurodevelopmental functions, because commingled deficits in visuospatial processing, spatial working memory, and attention have been found at 3 to 4 years of age in children born preterm.[12,43] Early and consistent assessment of visual and hearing function in children born preterm is therefore essential.

COGNITIVE OUTCOMES

Cognitive impairment (defined as a score >2 standard deviations below the mean on a standardized assessment) is the most common impairment seen in children born preterm between 18 and 30 months of age.[34,44] Rates of cognitive impairment vary by region and are inversely proportional to GA. In large studies of children born extremely preterm, moderate cognitive impairment has been demonstrated in 15% to 35% of children, severe impairment in 10% to 35%, and profound impairment in 10%.[21] Although motor outcomes are linked with specific areas of brain injury, early cognitive deficits are not as strongly predicted by brain region.[28]

Most large studies of neurodevelopmental outcomes in children born premature use the Bayley-III for assessment of cognitive outcomes before 3 years of age. Unfortunately, the value of early assessments of cognition in predicting cognitive functioning at school age and older is questionable.[28] In addition, defining the severity of cognitive dysfunction in early life may be difficult in preterm children, because use of standard test cutpoints without the presence of a term control group may not accurately reflect outcomes, given the propensity for lower mean scores than the normed average in this population with higher aggregation of scores in the lower range and fewer scores in the higher range.[28] The Bayley-III is also used extensively in clinical care to diagnose developmental delays and to determine subsequent qualification for early intervention services. Cognitive function is assessed by examining the following cognitive constructs: (1) sensorimotor development, (2) exploration and manipulation, (3) object relatedness, (4) concept formation, (5) memory, (6) habituation, (7) visual acuity, (8) visual preference, and (9) object permanence. These constructs are measured through assessment of age-related skills including counting, visual and tactile exploration, object assembly, puzzle board completion, matching colors, comparing masses, and representational/pretend play.

Bayley-III Cognitive Composite Scale scores range from 55 to 145 with scores of 100 ± 15 representing the mean ± 1 standard deviation.[45] Moderate cognitive dysfunction has previously been defined as a Bayley-III score of 2 to 3 standard deviations below the mean (a score of 55–70), with a severe deficit defined as a score less than 55.[28] Following the introduction of the Bayley-III, researchers found that rates of developmental delay were greatly decreased compared with those found using the previous edition of the test.[46–48] Concerns regarding the increased scores and possible underestimation of cognitive impairment have resulted in the cutpoints for cognitive impairment being shifted when using the Bayley-III. The Eunice Kennedy Shriver National Institute for Child Health and Development Neonatal Research Network now uses Bayley-III Cognitive Composite scores between 70 and 84 to define moderate cognitive impairment, scores less than 70 to define severe impairment, and scores less than 54 to define profound impairment.[21,44] Bayley-III scores do not provide indication of particular strengths of a given child or definition of specific, subtle areas of development that may be adversely impacting performance.[28] Age at assessment is of import, with studies examining children at 18 to 22 months finding higher rates of cognitive impairment than those assessing children later.[44] In addition, in preschool years, assessment of cognition necessarily relies on language, motor, and visual function; thus, a pure cognitive assessment is difficult to obtain.[28]

LANGUAGE OUTCOMES

Language deficits are common in premature infants in early childhood and may include abnormalities in receptive language, expressive language, and articulation.[49–54] As with other NDIs in preterm children, language deficiencies are often interconnected with other deficits including CP, hearing loss, behavioral abnormalities, and cognitive deficits.[49,55] In addition, various biologic and environmental factors may adversely influence language outcomes in preterm children (**Box 2**).[49,56] Auditory exposure to language is also critical for language development.[57] Development of the auditory cortex and speech development require an infant to be regularly exposed to speech.[57] Early language function is essential to social interaction and later school achievement.

Language is categorized in different domains. In early language development, expressive language (production) and receptive language (comprehension) are generally considered separately, and receptive language development precedes language production.[50] Phonologic awareness (understanding of speech sounds) may also be considered.[50] Phonologic awareness is of particular import during early language

---

Box 2
Factors influencing early language development in preterm children

Gestational age

Illness severity

Increased number of neonatal morbidities

Duration of hospitalization

Hearing status

Gender

Age at assessment

Socioeconomic risk factors

Environment

Feeding difficulties

Data from Vohr B. Speech and language outcomes of very preterm infants. Semin Fetal Neonatal Med 2014;19(2):78–83.

development but, to our knowledge, has not been largely studied in preterm children in early childhood to date.[50]

Numerous studies have consistently demonstrated that children born preterm have significantly lower expressive language ability than their term-born peers, although effect sizes seen are often varied. The heterogenous ages at assessment likely contributed to these findings, along with the numerous assessment tools used.[50] Language differences found remain after adjustment for disability and socioeconomic status.[53,58] Receptive language studies in preterm children are rare and largely performed at school age, rather than early childhood.[50,59,60]

BEHAVIORAL OUTCOMES

Children born preterm are up to four times more likely to have behavioral problems than children born at term.[61] Normal behavioral development is crucial to socioemotional functioning and has strong influences on the development of motor function, cognition, and language.[55] Most studies of behavioral outcomes in preterm children report on children at school age or adolescence; however, lower rates of social responsiveness have been demonstrated in preterm infants in early infancy.[62] The few studies of behavioral outcomes in preterm children during infancy and preschool age have demonstrated poor social/interactive skills, externalizing and internalizing disorders, emotional dysregulation, aggression, reduced attention, and hyperactivity.[63,64] There is also evidence that behavioral deficits identified in toddler years remain stable from early childhood through school age; and lower social competence in the preschool years is associated with more externalizing and internalizing behavior problems at 10 to 14 years of age.[65,66] However; longitudinal studies of behavior in preterm children are rare. In the last decade, researchers have put forth a "preterm behavioral phenotype" consisting of inattention, anxiety, and social difficulties.[67]

Although the exact cause of the behavioral abnormalities noted in premature infants is unknown, medical complications, home environment and socioeconomic factors, and perinatal brain injury have been implicated.[68] In a large recent study of children born less than 27 weeks' gestation at 18 to 22 months, Peralta-Carcelen and colleagues[55] demonstrated that 35% of children had behavioral problems, and 26% had deficits in socioemotional competence measured using the Brief Infant and Toddler Social and Emotional Assessment (BITSEA). Male sex, public insurance, maternal education of less high school, and lower maternal age were associated with behavioral problems. Socioemotional competence deficits were associated with lower birth weight, public insurance, mothers with less than a high school education, and abnormal neuromotor examination. In addition, language and cognitive scores on the Bayley-III significantly mediated the relationships between risk factors and behavioral and competence scores.

CUS and MRI at term equivalent have been associated with cognitive, psychomotor, and neurosensory delays at 18 to 24 months of age; however, there is a paucity of data describing early behavioral correlates to imaging findings.[69,70] Four-year-old children born extremely premature are more likely to have severe executive function deficits if they had global moderate-to-severe white matter injury signal abnormalities on standard T1- and T2-weighted MRI performed at term GA.[71] Executive function refers largely to cognitive processes, but behavioral abilities, such as self-regulation and inhibition, are vital to executive functioning.[72]

Abnormalities in specific brain regions may also have a role in behavioral outcomes. Cerebellar injury has been associated with developmental outcomes in premature infants. Corpus callosum length has been independently associated with poorer inhibition and emotional control at 4 years, and corpus callosum thickness has been correlated with white matter volume.[73,74]

Behavioral function may be assessed in early childhood using such tools as the BITSEA and the Child Behavior Checklist.[75,76] The BITSEA is a parent-completed rating scale for children 12 months, 0 days to 35 months, 30 days. It includes 42 items and yields standardized scores for the Problem and Competence Scales based on age and gender. The Problem Scale assesses for externalizing problems (disruptive or aggressive behaviors), internalizing problems (ie, anxiety, withdrawal), dysregulation, and maladaptive and atypical behaviors. Higher Problem Scale scores indicate more difficulties in these areas. The Competence Scale assesses the social emotional competencies that emerge at this age, such as symbolic and imitative play and cooperation. Lower Competence Scale scores indicate lower social emotional competencies. Total standardized scores and Positive Screen scores were assessed for each of the scales. A Competence Scale score of less than or equal to 13 or less than or equal to 15 (for boys and girls, respectively) and a Problem Scale greater than or equal to 15 indicates positive screens for children aged 18 to 23 months.

Behavioral and socioemotional deficits may impede learning, thus early assessment of behavioral functioning is critical so that appropriate intervention may be provided. Trials of parenting interventions in early childhood have demonstrated improvement in behavioral problems and improved behavioral competence among typically developing infants and children and preterm children.[77,78]

THE MODERATE AND LATE PRETERM INFANT

The increased rates of prematurity recently seen have been largely secondary to increased rates of moderate preterm (32–33 weeks of gestation) and late preterm (34–36 weeks of gestation) birth, because these children account for 84% of all preterm births.[6,79,80] Although the literature is still emerging in this area, studies demonstrate that children born moderate and late preterm are at increased risk for neurodevelopmental deficits. In a study of 1130 infants born 32 to 36 weeks of gestation, Johnson and colleagues[80] demonstrated children born moderate to late preterm to be at double the risk for neurodevelopmental disability at 2 years of age, with most deficits observed in the cognitive domain of function. Male sex, low socioeconomic status, and maternal preeclampsia were independent predictors of low cognitive scores. Studies of late preterm infants have demonstrated rates of CP 10 times greater than that of the general population.[9,81] Deficits in language and visuospatial ability have also been demonstrated.[7,9] These findings highlight the need to follow children born moderate and late preterm for neurodevelopmental deficits.

SUMMARY

Preterm children remain at high risk for neurodevelopmental deficits in early childhood, with the prevalence of milder deficits increasing. In addition, new guidelines for early assessment and diagnosis of CP are of particular import to these children. Currently, no standardization exists for follow-up of children born preterm, and practices vary among centers.[82] Most research studies to date have focused on outcomes before age 3, with many follow-up sites following children to that age or before. Access to appropriate, long-term follow-up care and resources for preterm infants after discharge from the NICU plays a critical role in improving and maintaining function over time, because early assessment and intervention improves neurodevelopmental outcomes.[83,84] These findings point not only to a need for standardization of follow-up, but to the import of longer follow-up, because children may have normal assessments during infancy, with deficits emerging over time as the child is challenged with more complex tasks. A normal early assessment does not exclude the possibility of impairments becoming unmasked at a later age, thus emphasizing the need for longer term, comprehensive follow-up of preterm infants.

Best Practices

What is the current practice?

Children born preterm are at increased risk for developmental delay in early childhood in motor, cognitive, language, and behavioral domains.

Best practice/guideline/care path objectives

Comprehensive developmental assessments are recommended for children born preterm.

Summary statement

Preterm children remain at high risk for neurodevelopmental deficits in early childhood, with the prevalence of milder deficits increasing. There is a need for standardized, longer term follow-up, because deficits may emerge over time.

REFERENCES

1. Younge N, Goldstein RF, Bann CM, et al, Eunice Kennedy Shriver National Institute of Child Health and Human Development Neonatal Research Network. Survival and neurodevelopmental outcomes among periviable infants. N Engl J Med 2017;376(7):617–28.
2. Rysavy MA, Li L, Bell EF, et al, Eunice Kennedy Shriver National Institute of Child Health and Human Development Neonatal Research Network. Between-hospital variation in treatment and outcomes in extremely preterm infants. N Engl J Med 2015;372(19):1801–11.
3. Cummings J, Committee on Fetus and Newborn. Antenatal counseling regarding resuscitation and intensive care before 25 weeks of gestation. Pediatrics 2015; 136(3):588–95.
4. Hintz SR, Kendrick DE, Wilson-Costello DE, et al, NICHD Neonatal Research Network. Early-childhood neurodevelopmental outcomes are not improving for infants born at <25 weeks' gestational age. Pediatrics 2011; 127(1):62–70.
5. Woythaler M, McCormick MC, Mao WY, et al. Late preterm infants and neurodevelopmental outcomes at kindergarten. Pediatrics 2015;136(3):424–31.
6. Shapiro-Mendoza CK, Lackritz EM. Epidemiology of late and moderate preterm birth. Semin Fetal Neonatal Med 2012;17(3):120–5.
7. Stene-Larsen K, Brandlistuen RE, Lang AM, et al. Communication impairments in early term and late preterm children: a prospective cohort study following children to age 36 months. J Pediatr 2014;165(6):1123–8.
8. Allen MC, Cristofalo EA, Kim C. Outcomes of preterm infants: morbidity replaces mortality. Clin Perinatol 2011;38(3):441–54.
9. McGowan JE, Alderdice FA, Holmes VA, et al. Early childhood development of late- preterm infants: a systematic review. Pediatrics 2011;127(6):1111–24.
10. Jarjour IT. Neurodevelopmental outcome after extreme prematurity: a review of the literature. Pediatr Neurol 2015;52(2):143–52.
11. Anderson PJ, Doyle LW. Cognitive and educational deficits in children born extremely preterm. Semin Perinatol 2008;32(1):51–8.

12. Aylward GP. Neurodevelopmental outcomes of infants born prematurely. J Dev Behav Pediatr 2014;35(6):394–407.
13. Joo JW, Choi JY, Rha DW, et al. Neuropsychological outcomes of preterm birth in children with no major neurodevelopmental impairments in early life. Ann Rehabil Med 2015;39(5):676–85.
14. Wilson-Costello DE, Payne AH. Early childhood neurodevelopmental outcomes of high-risk neonates. In: Martin RJ, Fanaroff AA, Walsh MC, editors. Neonatal-perinatal medicine: diseases of the fetus and infant. Philadelphia: Elsevier/Saunders; 2015. p. 1018–31.
15. Perrone S, Negro S, Tataranno ML, et al. Oxidative stress and antioxidant strategies in newborns. J Matern Fetal Neonatal Med 2010;23(Suppl 3):63–5.
16. Roberts D, Brown J, Medley N, et al. Antenatal corticosteroids for accelerating fetal lung maturation for women at risk of preterm birth. Cochrane Database Syst Rev 2017;(3):CD004454.
17. Pappas A, Kendrick DE, Shankaran S, et al. Chorioamnionitis and early childhood outcomes among extremely low-gestational-age neonates. JAMA Pediatr 2014; 168(2):137–47.
18. Vohr B, McGowan E, McKinley L, et al. Differential effects of the single-family room neonatal intensive care unit on 18- to 24-month Bayley scores of preterm infants. J Pediatr 2017;185:42–8.
19. Pineda R, Durant P, Mathur A, et al. Auditory exposure in the neonatal intensive care unit: room type and other predictors. J Pediatr 2017;183:56–66.
20. Novak I, Morgan C, Adde L, et al. Early, accurate diagnosis and early intervention in cerebral palsy: advances in diagnosis and treatment. JAMA Pediatr 2017; 171(9):897–907.
21. Hintz SR, Newman JE, Vohr BR. Changing definitions of long-term follow-up: should "long term" be even longer? Semin Perinatol 2016;40(6):398–409.
22. Romeo DM, Ricci D, Brogna C, et al. Use of the Hammersmith Infant Neurological Examination in infants with cerebral palsy: a critical review of the literature. Dev Med Child Neurol 2016;58(3):240–5.
23. Bosanquet M, Copeland L, Ware R, et al. A systematic review of tests to predict cerebral palsy in young children. Dev Med Child Neurol 2013;55(5):418–26.
24. Palisano RJ, Hanna SE, Rosenbaum PL, et al. Validation of a model of gross motor function for children with cerebral palsy. Phys Ther 2000;80(10):974–85.
25. Arnaud C, Daubisse-Marliac L, White-Koning M, et al. Prevalence and associated factors of minor neuromotor dysfunctions at age 5 years in prematurely born children: the EPIPAGE Study. Arch Pediatr Adolesc Med 2007;161(11):1053–61.
26. Wilson PH, Ruddock S, Smits-Engelsman B, et al. Understanding performance deficits in developmental coordination disorder: a meta-analysis of recent research. Dev Med Child Neurol 2013;55(3):217–28.
27. Ferrari F, Gallo C, Pugliese M, et al. Preterm birth and developmental problems in the preschool age. Part I: minor motor problems. J Matern Fetal Neonatal Med 2012;25(11):2154–9.
28. Rogers EE, Hintz SR. Early neurodevelopmental outcomes of extremely preterm infants. Semin Perinatol 2016;40(8):497–509.
29. Doyle LW, Roberts G, Anderson PJ, Victorian Infant Collaborative Study Group. Outcomes at age 2 years of infants < 28 weeks' gestational age born in Victoria in 2005. J Pediatr 2010;156(1):49–53.
30. Serenius F, Källén K, Blennow M, et al, EXPRESS Group. Neurodevelopmental outcome in extremely preterm infants at 2.5 years after active perinatal care in Sweden. JAMA 2013;309(17):1810–20.

31. Costeloe KL, Hennessy EM, Haider S, et al. Short term outcomes after extreme preterm birth in England: comparison of two birth cohorts in 1995 and 2006 (the EPICure studies). BMJ 2012;345:e7976.

32. Ishii N, Kono Y, Yonemoto N, et al, Neonatal Research Network, Japan. Outcomes of infants born at 22 and 23 weeks' gestation. Pediatrics 2013;132(1):62–71.

33. Doyle LW. Evaluation of neonatal intensive care for extremely-low-birth-weight infants. Semin Fetal Neonatal Med 2006;11(2):139–45.

34. Stephens BE, Vohr BR. Neurodevelopmental outcome of the premature infant. Pediatr Clin North Am 2009;56(3):631–46.

35. Vohr BR, Wright LL, Dusick AM, et al. Neurodevelopmental and functional outcomes of extremely low birth weight infants in the National Institute of Child Health and Human Development Neonatal Research Network, 1993-1994. Pediatrics 2000;105(6):1216–26.

36. Vohr BR, Wright LL, Dusick AM, et al. Center differences and outcomes of extremely low birth weight infants. Pediatrics 2004;113(4):781–9.

37. Allen MC. Neurodevelopmental outcomes of preterm infants. Curr Opin Neurol 2008;21(2):123–8.

38. Anderson PJ, Doyle LW, Victorian Infant Collaborative Study Group. Executive functioning in school-aged children who were born very preterm or with extremely low birth weight in the 1990s. Pediatrics 2004;114(1):50–7.

39. Loe IM, Chatav M, Alduncin N. Complementary assessments of executive function in preterm and full-term preschoolers. Child Neuropsychol 2015;21(3):331–53.

40. Chan E, Quigley MA. School performance at age 7 years in late preterm and early term birth: a cohort study. Arch Dis Child Fetal Neonatal Ed 2014;99(6):F451–7.

41. Burnett A, Davey CG, Wood SJ, et al. Extremely preterm birth and adolescent mental health in a geographical cohort born in the 1990s. Psychol Med 2014; 44(7):1533–44.

42. Dewey DG, Crawford SG, Creighton DE, et al. Long-term neuropsychological outcomes in very low birth weight children free of sensorineural impairments. J Clin Exp Neuropsychol 1999;21(6):851–65.

43. Vicari S, Caravale B, Carlesimo GA, et al. Spatial working memory deficits in children at ages 3-4 who were low birth weight, preterm infants. Neuropsychology 2004;18(4):673–8.

44. Vohr BR. Neurodevelopmental outcomes of extremely preterm infants. Clin Perinatol 2014;41(1):241–55.

45. Bayley N. Bayley scales of infant development-3rd edition. San Antonio (TX): The Psychological Corporation; 2006.

46. Lowe JR, Erickson SJ, Schrader R, et al. Comparison of the Bayley II Mental Developmental Index and the Bayley III Cognitive Scale: are we measuring the same thing? Acta Paediatr 2012;101(2):e55–8.

47. Anderson PJ, De Luca CR, Hutchinson E, et al, Victorian Infant Collaborative Group. Underestimation of developmental delay by the new Bayley-III Scale. Arch Pediatr Adolesc Med 2010;164(4):352–6.

48. Vohr BR, Stephens BE, Higgins RD, et al. Are outcomes of extremely preterm infants improving? Impact of Bayley assessment on outcomes. J Pediatr 2012; 161(2):222–8.

49. Vohr B. Speech and language outcomes of very preterm infants. Semin Fetal Neonatal Med 2014;19(2):78–83.

50. Barre N, Morgan A, Doyle LW, et al. Language abilities in children who were very preterm and/or very low birth weight: a meta-analysis. J Pediatr 2011;158(5): 766–74.e1.

51. Foster-Cohen SH, Friesen MD, Champion PR, et al. High prevalence/low severity language delay in preschool children born very preterm. J Dev Behav Pediatr 2010;31(8):658–67.
52. Ortiz-Mantilla S, Choudhury N, Leevers H, et al. Understanding language and cognitive deficits in very low birth weight children. Dev Psychobiol 2008;50(2):107–26.
53. van Noort-van der Spek IL, Franken MC, Weisglas-Kuperus N. Language functions in preterm-born children: a systematic review and meta-analysis. Pediatrics 2012;129(4):745–54.
54. Marston L, Peacock JL, Calvert SA, et al. Factors affecting vocabulary acquisition at age 2 in children born between 23 and 28 weeks' gestation. Dev Med Child Neurol 2007;49(8):591–6.
55. Peralta-Carcelen M, Carlo WA, Pappas A, et al. Behavioral problems and socioemotional competence at 18 to 22 months of extremely premature children. Pediatrics 2017;139(6) [pii:e20161043].
56. Duncan AF, Watterberg KL, Nolen TL, et al. Effect of ethnicity and race on cognitive and language testing at age 18-22 months in extremely preterm infants. J Pediatr 2012;160(6):966–71.e2.
57. McMahon E, Wintermark P, Lahav A. Auditory brain development in premature infants: the importance of early experience. Ann N Y Acad Sci 2012;1252:17–24.
58. Vohr BR. Language and hearing outcomes of preterm infants. Semin Perinatol 2016;40(8):510–9.
59. Luu TM, Ment LR, Schneider KC, et al. Lasting effects of preterm birth and neonatal brain hemorrhage at 12 years of age. Pediatrics 2009;123(3):1037–44.
60. Pritchard VE, Clark CA, Liberty K, et al. Early school-based learning difficulties in children born very preterm. Early Hum Dev 2009;85(4):215–24.
61. Hack M, Taylor HG, Schluchter M, et al. Behavioral outcomes of extremely low birth weight children at age 8 years. J Dev Behav Pediatr 2009;30(2):122–30.
62. Landry SH, Chapieski ML, Richardson MA, et al. The social competence of children born prematurely: effects of medical complications and parent behaviors. Child Dev 1990;61(5):1605–16.
63. Spittle AJ, Treyvaud K, Doyle LW, et al. Early emergence of behavior and social-emotional problems in very preterm infants. J Am Acad Child Adolesc Psychiatry 2009;48(9):909–18.
64. Frazier JA, Wood ME, Ware J, et al. Antecedents of the child behavior checklist-dysregulation profile in children born extremely preterm. J Am Acad Child Adolesc Psychiatry 2015;54(10):816–23.
65. Gray RF, Indurkhya A, McCormick MC. Prevalence, stability, and predictors of clinically significant behavior problems in low birth weight children at 3, 5, and 8 years of age. Pediatrics 2004;114(3):736–43.
66. Bornstein MH, Hahn CS, Haynes OM. Social competence, externalizing, and internalizing behavioral adjustment from early childhood through early adolescence: developmental cascades. Dev Psychopathol 2010;22(4):717–35.
67. Johnson S, Marlow N. Preterm birth and childhood psychiatric disorders. Pediatr Res 2011;69(5 Pt 2):11R–8R.
68. Conrad AL, Richman L, Lindgren S, et al. Biological and environmental predictors of behavioral sequelae in children born preterm. Pediatrics 2010;125(1):e83–9.
69. Hintz SR, Barnes PD, Bulas D, et al. Neuroimaging and neurodevelopmental outcome in extremely preterm infants. Pediatrics 2015;135(1):e32–42.
70. Woodward LJ, Anderson PJ, Austin NC, et al. Neonatal MRI to predict neurodevelopmental outcomes in preterm infants. N Engl J Med 2006;355(7):685–94.

71. Woodward LJ, Clark CA, Pritchard VE, et al. Neonatal white matter abnormalities predict global executive function impairment in children born very preterm. Dev Neuropsychol 2011;36(1):22–41.
72. Sokol B, Muller U, Carpendale J, et al. Self- and social-regulation: the development of social interaction, social understanding, and executive functions. New York: Oxford University Press; 2010.
73. Ghassabian A, Herba CM, Roza SJ, et al. Infant brain structures, executive function, and attention deficit/hyperactivity problems at preschool age. A prospective study. J Child Psychol Psychiatry 2013;54(1):96–104.
74. Panigraphy A, Wisnowski JL, Furtado A, et al. Neuroimaging biomarkers of preterm brain injury: toward developing the preterm connectome. Pediatr Radiol 2012;42(Suppl 1):S33–61.
75. Briggs-Gowan MJ, Carter AS, Irwin JR, et al. The Brief Infant-Toddler Social and Emotional Assessment: screening for social-emotional problems and delays in competence. J Pediatr Psychol 2004;29(2):143–55.
76. Achenbach TM, Rescorla LA. Manual for the ASEBA preschool forms and profiles. Burlington (VT): University of Vermont Department of Psychiatry; 2000.
77. Gardner F, Shaw DS, Dishion TJ, et al. Randomized prevention trial for early conduct problems: effects on proactive parenting and links to toddler disruptive behavior. J Fam Psychol 2007;21(3):398–406.
78. Landry SH, Smith KE, Swank PR, et al. A responsive parenting intervention: the optimal timing across early childhood for impacting maternal behaviors and child outcomes. Dev Psychol 2008;44(5):1335–53.
79. Fuchs K, Gyamfi C. The influence of obstetric practices on late prematurity. Clin Perinatol 2008;35(2):343–60.
80. Johnson S, Evans TA, Draper ES, et al. Neurodevelopmental outcomes following late and moderate prematurity: a population-based cohort study. Arch Dis Child Fetal Neonatal Ed 2015;100(4):F301–8.
81. Marret S, Ancel PY, Marpeau L, et al. Neonatal and 5-year outcomes after birth at 30-34 weeks of gestation. Obstet Gynecol 2007;110(1):72–80.
82. Gong A, Johnson YR, Livingston J, et al. Newborn intensive care survivors: a review and a plan for collaboration in Texas. Matern Health Neonatol Perinatol 2015;1:24.
83. Spittle A, Orton J, Anderson PJ, et al. Early developmental intervention programmes provided post hospital discharge to prevent motor and cognitive impairment in preterm infants. Cochrane Database Syst Rev 2015;(11):CD005495.
84. Novak I, McIntyre S, Morgan C, et al. A systematic review of interventions for children with cerebral palsy: state of the evidence. Dev Med Child Neurol 2013; 55(10):885–910.

Neurodevelopmental Outcomes of Preterm Children at School Age and Beyond

Anne Synnes, MDCM, MHSc[a],*, Matthew Hicks, MD, PhD[b]

KEYWORDS

- Preterm • Child development • Neuro development • Developmental disabilities
- Follow-up • Outcomes • Cognitive • Motor

KEY POINTS

- Prematurity is associated with motor, cognitive, behavioral, psychiatric, and other disabilities in adolescents and adults and the frequency and severity is inversely associated with gestational age at birth.
- Most teens and adults with prematurity-associated disabilities were born moderately or late preterm, but this group is less well studied compared with those born extremely preterm.
- Preterm adolescents and young adults have similar well-being and greater risk avoidance than controls.
- Disability-free preterm survivors attain a lower level of education and income than term-born peers but health-related quality of life is unaffected.

IMPORTANCE OF THE PROBLEM

Globally, approximately 15 million infants every year (11.1% of all births) are born preterm, at less than 37 completed weeks' gestation, with national rates varying from 5% to 18%.[1] As a result of the large number of preterm births and the increasing preterm birth survival rates, the long-term sequelae of prematurity will impact annually approximately 14 million children, their families, and societies. Unfortunately, the advances in survival have not been accompanied by an equal reduction in adverse outcomes.[2]

Disclosure Statement: Neither author has any conflicts of interest to disclose.
[a] Neonatal Follow-Up Program, British Columbia's Women's Hospital, University of British Columbia, Room 1R16, 4500 Oak Street, Vancouver, British Columbia V6H 3N1, Canada;
[b] Department of Pediatrics, Neonatal Intensive Care Unit, University of Alberta, 5027 Diagnosis and Treatment Centre, Royal Alexander Hospital, 10240 Kingsway Northwest, Edmonton, Alberta T5H 3V9, Canada
* Corresponding author.
E-mail address: asynnes@cw.bc.ca

Clin Perinatol 45 (2018) 393–408
https://doi.org/10.1016/j.clp.2018.05.002
0095-5108/18/© 2018 Elsevier Inc. All rights reserved.

perinatology.theclinics.com

Most children born preterm are doing very well with a very good quality of life. The goal of this review was to highlight the challenges that some preterm survivors face so that they will receive the necessary supports and that we can strive to continuously improve the antenatal, perinatal, postnatal, and childhood care of these children.

Although many trials and cohort studies of preterm populations evaluate outcomes at 18 to 24 months of age, they are limited in their ability to describe the full neurodevelopmental impact of prematurity. A review of prematurity-associated school-age and adult outcomes is therefore important. The focus in this review is on neurodevelopment because of its clinical significance and frequency. Other health outcomes have been reviewed by Luu and colleagues.[3]

Most preterm births are late preterm, defined as occurring between 34 0/7 weeks and 36 6/7 weeks' gestational age or moderate preterm, 32 0/7 to 33 6/7 weeks' gestational age. In the United States in 2015, only 1.59% were born very preterm at less than 32 weeks' gestation and 0.68% extremely preterm at less than 28 weeks' gestation.[4] The frequency and severity of adverse outcomes vary inversely with gestational age. The research methods to describe outcomes in the larger late preterm cohorts often differ from those used in the smaller very preterm cohorts. Very preterm and moderate–late preterm outcomes are therefore described separately.

RESEARCH CHALLENGES

Research on school-age neurodevelopmental outcomes in the preterm population is derived mostly from observational cohort studies. The reader must therefore consider the potential biases and limitations of the research methods. Population-based samples are preferred over multicenter or single-center cohorts to minimize referral biases. Small sample size may be a problem in single-center cohorts, especially when studying the lowest gestational ages. With variability in preterm care between sites and over time, the region and year(s) of birth of the cohort need to be considered. Attention must be paid to the denominator. Especially for the most premature babies with the highest mortality, the incidence of adverse outcome(s) varies significantly for the denominators live births compared with all births (live and stillbirths). Less obvious but equally significant is when the denominator includes only children who could complete a test or when children with a sensory, behavioral, or very severe impairment are excluded. Much of the data related to neurodevelopmental outcomes for adults born preterm come from national birth registries and large birth cohorts with linkage to intelligence testing at time of conscription at 18 or 19 years of age.[5] Adults with disabilities may be excluded from conscription and therefore observed associations likely underestimate the effect of prematurity on adult outcome. In addition, typically only male adults were registered in conscription databases and results therefore may not be relevant to female adults born preterm. When subjects of different gestational ages are lumped together, comparisons between studies with different gestational age cutoffs are difficult. Attrition bias is a major concern, as children lost to follow-up differ from those assessed.[6] Whereas greater than 90% follow-up is ideal, in longitudinal cohort studies this gets increasingly difficult as children get older. Finally, many studies that examine adult outcome do not use a healthy, nonadmitted term control group as a comparison for late preterm infants, which limits the conclusions that can be drawn from any analysis.[7]

WHY LOOK AT SCHOOL-AGE AND LONGER-TERM OUTCOMES?

Parents, families, health care providers, and society are interested in knowing what the long-term future holds for the infant born preterm, either to support the child and the child's family, provide counseling, assist with decision making, providing postdischarge services, or planning for health care service needs.[8] Compared with the limited repertoire of the infant and preschooler, at older ages the human brain is capable of a multitude of complex tasks that can be evaluated reliably and provide a good estimate of adult functioning. When studying the adult outcomes of children born preterm, the benefits of longer-term studies must be balanced against the clinical irrelevance of neonatal intensive care unit (NICU) practices from a generation ago, the increasing attrition biases as NICU graduates leave their parents' homes, and the cost and logistics of performing longitudinal studies that span over 20 years. Despite these challenges, there are a few remarkable cohort studies that have successfully maintained contact and engaged a high proportion of their subjects into adulthood.

By school age, the researcher has a larger range of assessment tools to choose from. Children's abilities or traits can be measured on a continuous or categorical scale for a variety of domains, such as cognitive, executive function, language, behavior, motor, hearing, and vision. Continuous outcomes can be described using a measure of central tendency (eg, means or median) and measure of spread (eg, standard deviation and interquartile range) for each domain or categorically/dichotomously (eg, "normal" and "abnormal"), which requires choosing cutoff points. Composite outcomes require defining multiple cutoff points and there is a lack of consensus on how to define these composite outcomes.[9] The World Health Organization's international classification of functioning, disability, and health shifts the focus from disease to health, and considers outcomes from the perspective of body structures and functions, individual activities, and participation, with a version for children and youth (ICF-CY).[10] The ICF-CY detailed classification system is conceptually promising but challenging to use.[10] Further development of core sets, such as those developed for cerebral palsy will be helpful.[11]

Predicting the pattern, frequency, and severity of adult outcomes improves with age as neurocognitive abilities mature. In early childhood, the Bayley Scales of Infant and Toddler Development, third edition and earlier versions, measure development rather than cognitive potential, which has a poor predictive ability for school-age cognitive abilities.[12] It is well accepted that correction for prematurity by calculating age from the expected date of delivery should be used rather than chronologic age based on birth date for the first 2 years of life. However, differences between corrected and chronologic age are still apparent at 5 years of age.[13] Cognitive impairment is overestimated by early measures, and impairment rates fall with increasing age at assessment. As shown by Marlow and colleagues,[14] using the EPICure very preterm cohort assessed at 30 months and 6 years of age, degree of disability is also not static, as 40% of those with a severe disability at 30 months changed category and 25% initially considered as disability-free were classified as having a moderate to severe disability. In the Caffeine for Apnea of Prematurity trial, mean intelligence quotient (IQ) scores were 20 points higher than the 18 months corrected age mental developmental index on the Bayley Scales of Infant Development, second edition.[15] Multiple studies with similar findings have therefore supported the conclusion that outcomes at school age or beyond are more valid.[16] Please see **Box 1** for a summary of the pros and cons of using school-age outcomes.

THE VERY PRETERM CHILD: OUTCOMES AT SCHOOL AGE AND BEYOND

Neurodevelopmental outcomes in the older child can be described either using a broad-stroke picture or by zooming in on specific skills. In early childhood, a global

---

Box 1
Pros and cons of using school-age outcomes

- Pros
  - Predictive of adult outcomes
  - Able to measure a variety of specific abilities
  - Able to measure patient-reported health-related quality of life
- Cons
  - Reflects neonatal care from an earlier era
  - Typically higher attrition rates
  - More difficult and often more costly to collect

---

description of neurodevelopmental outcome using a composite outcome including one or more of cerebral palsy, cognitive, language, or motor developmental delay or a visual or hearing impairment is common. This is less common at school age where the evaluations performed in a study reflect more a sample of skills rather than a comprehensive measure. The Victorian Infant Collaborative Study Group evaluated 8-year-old extremely preterm children and compared major neurosensory disabilities, defined as IQ less than − 2 SD, moderate or severe cerebral palsy, blindness or deafness, among 3 birth cohorts (1991–1992 vs 1997 vs 2005) and found rates unchanged at 18%, 15%, and 18% in these 3 time periods.[17] In a review of neurodevelopmental sequelae, recognizing that definitions varied, the 2 studies in which outcome was assessed at 5 years or beyond, 21% to 25% of subjects born extremely preterm at 26 weeks' gestation or less had sequelae.[18]

GLOBAL MEASURES OF OUTCOME

Other outcomes that have been used to give a global picture of neurodevelopment or health include the inability to work because of a medical disability, functional limitations, and quality of life. In a national registry of adults in Norway, Moster and colleagues,[19] described medical disability affecting working capacity as varying from 10.6% for adults born at 23 to 27 6/7 weeks' gestation to 2.4% for those born later preterm and 1.7% for term-born adults. A cohort of 241 very low birth weight (<1500 g birth weight) young adults from Cleveland, Ohio, reported similar health, wellness, and functioning compared with term-born controls but greater risk avoidance and less resilience.[20] Mental and emotional delays, restriction of activities of daily living, and self-care and chronic health disorders are more common in children born preterm than controls, which persists into adulthood.[20] Health-related quality of life when measured using parents as proxies, was lower in preschool and teenaged children born preterm.[21] Despite more functional limitations, extremely low birth weight teens and young adults rated their own quality of life as highly as controls.[21]

MOTOR OUTCOMES

Motor impairments are common in the preterm population. Cerebral palsy, the most severe form, is an umbrella term to describe a varied group of movement and posture disorders related to a static insult to the fetal or infant brain that may be accompanied by epilepsy and disorders of sensation, perception, cognition, communication, and behavior.[22] Prematurity is the most frequent cause of cerebral palsy, with an incidence of 9.1% in adults born at 23 to 27 weeks' gestation inclusive, 79 times higher than in term-born subjects.[23] However, developmental coordination disorder, a disorder of motor coordination not due to cerebral palsy, other medical conditions, or pervasive developmental disorder, that affects daily or academic functioning is also increased (odds ratio [OR] of 8.66 with a 95% confidence interval [CI] of 3.40–22.07) for very low birth weight infants compared with controls.[24] From a systematic review, in children born preterm, the incidence for mild-moderate motor impairment is 40.5% and for moderate impairment is 19.0%.[25] Compared with term-born children, motor skills are significantly lower in preterm children with a standardized mean difference (SMD) of −0.57 to −0.88 from infancy to 15 years of age.[24–26]

COGNITIVE OUTCOMES

Cognitive abilities, including intelligence, and academic performance are adversely affected by prematurity. In a Japanese cohort born at less than 28 weeks' gestation between 1992 and 2005, 31% had IQ scores <70 (< −2 SDs) at 6 years of age, although rates of 13% to 15% are more commonly reported in the extremely preterm population, with some reports of increasing impairment rates over time.[25,27–29] In a meta-analysis, prematurity had a significant impact on full-scale IQ (SMD −0.70) with a larger effect on performance (SMD −0.67) than verbal (SMD −0.53) IQ (**Table 1**).[30] Similar cognitive results were seen at all ages from preschool to adult.[30] The effect was greater for the more preterm population (see **Table 1**) and gestational age accounted for 39%, 38%, and 48% of the variance in full-scale IQ, verbal IQ, and performance IQ, respectively.[30] In children born preterm, cognitive scores are 11 to 12 points lower and in those free of disability, adjusting for sociodemographic variables, the mean IQ is 5 to 7 points lower (0.3–0.6 SD) than in controls.[30–33] Siblings of extremely low birth weight children have a higher IQ than their sibling in 84% of cases.[28] Cognitive function is complex, and aspects other than IQ need to be considered. Executive function encompasses the purposeful, goal-directed behaviors used to execute cognitive and other functions. Premature children with executive dysfunction have more difficulty with tasks such as initiating activities, organization, flexibility in generating ideas and problem solving, working memory, inhibition, and attention problems.[28,34] Weaknesses in working memory and visuo-motor integration have been documented as particular challenges in preterm survivors in multiple countries.[32] Working memory and processing speed are approximately 0.5 SD lower in preterm than term-born cohorts.[25] An advantaged home environment is associated with an improved cognitive trajectory from 20 months to 8 years of age.[31,33]

ACADEMIC OUTCOMES

Preterm children are 2.85 times more likely than their term-born peers to receive special education (see **Table 1**) and score significantly worse in arithmetic (SMD −0.6 to −0.78), reading (SMD −0.44 to −0.67), and spelling (SMD −0.52 to −0.76) (see **Table 1**).[30,35,36] Learning difficulties are reported in 50% to 70% of very low birth weight school-age children and inversely correlated with birth weight: 72% of children with a birth weight < 750 g, 53% with birth weight 750 to 1000 g and 13% of normal birth weight controls.[33,35] IQ is only one of several determinants of academic success. Academic achievement is often lower than anticipated by IQ in preterm children and may be explained by commonly identified weaknesses in attention, executive functioning, visual-motor skills, and verbal memory in preterm children.[33,34] Visual-motor integration (see **Table 1**), important for academic performance, which can be affected by the white matter pathways, is worse in the preterm population.[37]

Table 1
Domain-specific neurodevelopmental measures for extreme, very, and moderate to late preterm infants at school age and beyond

Domain	Extreme Preterm	Very Preterm	Moderate–Late Preterm	All Preterm
Global measures of outcome		[53]ASQ >2 SD below mean AOR 3.2 (1.9–5.4)[c]	[53]ASQ >2 SD below mean COR 2.1 (1.34–3.4)[c]	
Motor		[23]MABC < 5%ile OR 6.29 (4.37–9.05)[c] [23]MABC 5–15%ile OR 8.66 (3.40–22.07)[c] [26]MABC −0.65 (−0.70 to −0.60)[a] [26]BOTMP −0.57 (−0.68 to −0.46)[a]		[25]Motor −0.59 (−0.89 to −0.28)[a]
Cognitive	[25]Full-scale IQ −0.78 (−0.85 to −0.72)[c] [25]Performance IQ −0.89 (−1.05 to −0.72)[c] [25]Verbal IQ −0.67 (−0.83 to −0.51)[c]	[25]Full-scale IQ −0.73 (−0.78 to −0.67)[c] [25]Performance IQ −0.65 (−0.73 to −0.57)[c] [25]Verbal IQ −0.55 (−0.63 to −0.48)[c]	[25]Full-scale IQ −0.24 (−0.35 to −0.12) [25]Performance IQ −0.28 (−0.53 to −0.02)[c] [25]Verbal IQ −0.14 (−0.35 to 0.07)	[25]Full-scale IQ −0.70 (−0.73 to −0.66)[c] [25]Performance IQ −0.67 (−0.73 to −0.60)[c] [25]Verbal IQ −0.53 (−0.60 to −0.47)[c] [30]Preterm IQ difference −11.94 (10.47–13.42)[c] lower in preterms
Academic		[34]Math −0.60 (−0.74 to −0.46)[a] [34]Reading −0.48 (−0.60 to −0.34)[a] [34]Spelling −0.76 (−1.13 to −0.40)[a]		[25]Reading −0.51 (−0.67 to −0.35)[a] [25]Math −0.42 (−0.90 to 0.006) [25]Spelling −0.51 (−0.92 to −0.09) [35]Math −0.71[a] [35]Reading −0.44[a] [35]Spelling −0.52[a] [35]Special education RR 2.85 (2.12 to 3.84)[a]

Language		[39]Expressive −0.71 (−0.86 to −0.55)[a] Expressive Semantics −0.40 (−0.50 to −0.31)[a] [39]Receptive −0.83 (−0.97 to −0.69)[a] [39]Receptive semantics −0.59 (−0.79 to −0.40)[a] [39]Receptive grammar −0.44 (−0.72 to −0.17)[a]		[42]Simple language −0.45 (−0.59 to −0.30)[b] [42]Complex language −0.62 (−0.82 to −0.43)
Behavior	[25]ADHD OR 3.3 (2.0,5.6)[c]	[25]ADHD 3.7 (1.8 to 7.7)[c] [34]CBCL internalizing −0.20 (−0.48 to 0.08) [34]TRF internalizing −0.28 (−.45 to −0.12)[a] [34]CBCL attention −0.59 (−0.74 to −0.44)[a] [34]TRF attention −0.43 (−0.61 to −0.25)[a] [34]Executive Function verbal fluency −0.57 (−0.82 to −0.32)[a] [34]Executive Function working memory −0.36 (−0.47 to −0.20)[a] [34]Executive Function cognitive flexibility −0.49 (−0.66 to −0.33)[a]	[25]ADHD 1.3 (1.1 to 1.5)[c]	[25]ADHD 1.6 (1.3 to 1.8)[c] [25]Behavior −0.72 (−0.97 to −0.47)[c]
Sensory visual-motor integration (VMI)		[37]Beery VMI −0.69 (−0.80 to −0.58)[a]		

Outcomes expressed as standard deviation units (95% confidence interval). Simple language measured using the Peabody Picture Vocabulary test, Complex language measured using the Clinical Evaluation of language Fundamentals. Only analyses including populations with school age or beyond and when stratified by age, older school age reported.

Abbreviations: ADHD, attention deficit hyperactivity disorder; AOR, adjusted odds ratio; ASQ, Ages and Stages Questionnaire; BOTMP, Bruininks-Oseretsky Test of Motor Proficiency; CBCL, child behavior checklist; COR, crude odds ratio; MABC, Movement Assessment Battery for Children; OR, odds ratio; RR, relative risk; TRF, teacher report form.

[a] P<.01.
[b] P<.001.
[c] P value not provided.

SPEECH AND LANGUAGE

Language is important for communication, social, and academic success. In early childhood, language development is more delayed than motor or cognitive abilities.[38] At older ages, expressive language, receptive language processing, and articulation difficulties with deficits in phonologic short-term memory are seen.[2,39,40] In very preterm adolescents, receptive language improved with age, especially with greater maternal education, better sociodemographic situation, and intact neurosensory function, but complex language problems become more prevalent.[41,42]

BEHAVIOR

Behavior problems, peer relationships, psychopathology, and antisocial behavior are best assessed at school age or later, although differences in temperament and self-regulation can be assessed earlier. Differences between premature and term-born infants have been identified using the Brazelton Neonatal Behavioral Assessment Scale: at term corrected age, preterm infants have a pattern of behaviors that is more variable, and overall less competent than term-born controls.[43] Preterm infants show evidence of maturational delays on brainstem auditory evoked potentials, video-somnography, and autonomic function with some correlation with longer-term outcomes.[44,45] Approximately 40% of preterm infants have an overall atypical pattern of behavior with respect to processing sensory stimuli using the parent-completed Sensory Profile questionnaire and almost 90% have a probable or definite abnormality in one or more sensory processing domains (eg, oral, auditory, tactile, visual).[46] On the Infant Toddler Social and Emotional Assessment at 2 years of age, preterm infants have higher mean internalizing and dysregulation scores, a pattern also seen at older ages with higher rates of depression and anxiety.[47] In the EPICure study, internalizing emotional disorders were present in 9% of extremely preterm children compared with 2% in the term-born controls.[48] A typical preterm behavioral phenotype, described by Johnson and Wolke,[49] includes inattention, introversion, anxiety, rigidity, and risk aversion. Overall, children born very preterm score worse on behavioral assessment tools, which increases with age: primary school age SMD −0.34; 95% CI −0.45 to −0.23 and secondary school SMD −0.72; 95% CI −0.47 to −0.97.[25] Attention deficit hyperactivity disorder is diagnosed 2.6 to 6.0 times more commonly in extremely preterm infants, 1.6 times greater among all preterm children (see **Table 1**), and may be preceded by poor attention in the toddler and preschool years.[2,25,28] Ten times more children born preterm screen positive for autism spectrum disorder (ASD) and 4 times as many are diagnosed with ASD with a prevalence of 7.1% in an extremely preterm cohort.[2] Psychiatric disorders occur in approximately 25% of adolescents born preterm.[49]

SENSORY IMPAIRMENTS

Prematurity is an important risk factor for hearing and visual impairments and early screening and treatment of sensory impairments are important to optimize function. The incidence is much lower than the neurodevelopmental outcomes described previously. In a Canadian national cohort born at less than 29 weeks' gestation, 1.9% had a significant unilateral or bilateral severe visual impairment, 1.6% a bilateral visual impairment, and 2.6% had a hearing aid or cochlear implant with a similar incidence in other studies ranging from 0% to 4.6% for severe visual impairment and 0.9% to 5.2% for severe to profound hearing impairment.[2,38] Sensory impairments may co-occur with and hinder the assessment of cognition and neurodevelopment.

THE MODERATE TO LATE PRETERM CHILD: OUTCOMES AT SCHOOL AGE AND BEYOND

Children born at moderate, 32 0/7 to 33 6/7 weeks, and late, 34 0/7 weeks and 36 6/7 weeks, preterm gestation represent most surviving preterm infants, and they are an important contributor to overall disability associated with prematurity.[50] Indeed, most total disability associated with preterm birth is for the moderate and late preterm group, given the higher rates of delivery and survival at these gestations. In a large Swedish national birth cohort study that linked birth history with adult health and psychiatric outcomes, 74% of the risk of disability and 85% of the risk of a psychiatric disorder associated with prematurity was in the moderate and late preterm groups.[51,52] Please see **Table 1** for a summary of domain-specific neurodevelopmental measures for extreme, very, and moderate to late preterm infants at school age and beyond.

GLOBAL MEASURES OF OUTCOME

Developmental delay at school entry can be captured using screening tools, but these global measures may not be predictive of later measures of IQ and domain-specific function. In the large prospective cohort Lollypop study, the Ages and Stages Questionnaire was used at school entry to assess for developmental delay.[53] Children born moderately preterm had twice the prevalence of developmental delay as compared with full-term infants (8.3% vs 4.2%), and more frequently had problems with fine motor, communication, and personal-social functioning.[53] In that same cohort, moderate prematurity and low socioeconomic status had a multiplicative effect on risk of developmental delay.[54] Rates of resolution of motor and communication problems were similar for children born moderate preterm and full-term.[55] Moster and colleagues[19] used linkage of birth registries and national health databases in Norway to examine medical issues and disabilities of more than 900,000 adults. Adults born at 31 to 33 6/7 weeks' gestation or late preterm, respectively, had increased odds of cerebral palsy (OR 14.1 and 2.7), mental retardation (OR 2.1 and 1.6), and conditions that interfere with an ability to work (OR 2.2 and 1.4). In a similar, large birth cohort study in Sweden, preterm birth was associated with lower chance of completing university education and a lower net salary.[51] In both studies, risk of adverse outcome as an adult increased with decreasing gestational age in a "dose-dependent" or linear fashion. Please see **Box 2** for a highlight of adult outcomes for individuals born preterm.

MOTOR OUTCOMES

At school age, approximately one-third of children born moderately preterm have difficulty in the school environment, particularly with fine motor skills.[7,53,56] In a large

---

Box 2
Highlights of outcomes for adults born preterm

- Prematurity continues to be associated with motor, cognitive, behavioral, and other disabilities in adults
- Disability-free preterm survivors attain a lower level of education and income than term-born peers
- Outcomes are inversely associated with gestational age
- Very low birth weight young adults have well-being and greater risk avoidance than controls
- Health-related quality of life is not affected by prematurity

cohort of 7-year-old children born moderately preterm, 31% struggled with fine motor skills and 12% were identified as struggling in physical education classes.[56] Male sex was a significant risk factor for poor motor skill outcome in this group.[56] Similar to Moster and colleagues,[19] a large cohort study that linked outpatient and hospitalization data from the Northern California Kaiser Permanente Medical Care Program of more than 140,000 children born at or more than 30 weeks, decreasing gestational age was related to increased rates of cerebral palsy for both moderate and late prematurity.[57] Children born late preterm were at least 3 times more likely than those born at term to be diagnosed with cerebral palsy (hazard ratio, 3.39; 95% CI 2.54–4.52).[57]

COGNITIVE OUTCOMES

Standardized cognitive assessments are often performed during the school years and in several countries at time of registration for conscription at 18 or 19 years of age. Several researchers have linked birth data to these educational and administrative registries to study the effect of prematurity on cognitive outcome. In a large case-control study, the IQ scores in first grade of children born late preterm were compared with a random sample of children born at term.[58] Late preterm birth was associated with increased risk of lower full-scale IQ, adjusted OR 2.35 (95% CI 1.20–4.61) and performance IQ, adjusted OR 2.04 (95% CI 1.09–3.82) but no difference was seen with verbal IQ.[58] In the Avon longitudinal study, moderate and late preterm birth was associated with lower verbal IQ, performance IQ, and full-scale IQ scores at 11 years of age in univariate but not multivariate analysis.[59] However, children born moderate and late preterm had a 56% increased risk of receiving special education services, and this could not be explained by differences in IQ.[59] In a large cohort study in Norway that linked birth registry data to Conscript Service Intelligence scores, late preterm birth was associated with lower adult intelligence scores when controlling for social confounders and adult body size.[5] Intelligence test scores increased in a linear fashion with gestational age at birth, birth weight, and birth length up until 41 weeks.[5] In a similar study from Sweden that used birth registry data and IQ testing at time of conscription, there was a small "dose-response" between lower gestational age at delivery and lower IQ.[60] As with many other studies, socioeconomic status was an important modifier of the relationship between prematurity and IQ.[60] Using a comprehensive assessment at 31 years of age, Dalziel and colleagues[61] compared 126 adults who had been born moderately preterm with 66 adults born at term and found that there were no differences in cognitive, academic, psychological, or functional measures.

ACADEMIC OUTCOMES

The Kindergarten Cohort of the Early Childhood Longitudinal Study used US national standardized testing data to compare 970 preterm infants and 13,761 control subjects in elementary school.[62] Children born moderate preterm had scores that were lower than those born at term for reading and for math in several grades up to grade 5. In multivariate analysis, there was twice the risk of individualized education plans and special education enrollment for the moderate but not the late preterm group. Challenges persisted at fifth grade and, as noted in other studies, there was a linear association between gestational age and test scores.[56,62] In the United Kingdom Millennium Cohort study, educational and health data of more than 6000 children were linked to examine the effect of late preterm birth on school performance at 7 years of age.[63] Preterm birth was a risk for poor performance in the areas of reading, writing and mathematics, with children born at moderate prematurity at greater risk than those born late preterm, relative risk (RR) 1.71 (95%CI 1.15–2.54) versus RR 1.36 (95% CI 1.09–1.68).[63] In a study of more than 200,000 children in New York City that linked birth data and standardized educational testing at third grade, children born moderate and late preterm were found to have increased adjusted odds of special education placement in comparison with term children, adjusted odds ratio (AOR) 1.53 (95% CI 1.30–1.69) and AOR 1.34 (95% CI 1.29–1.40), respectively.[64] Children born preterm also had lower English and math standardized scores and there was a "dose-response" for each week of prematurity.[64] Similarly, in a population-based retrospective study of almost 18,000 children linking birth and school census data, MacKay et al, found an adjusted OR of 1.53 (95% CI 1.43–1.63) for having a special education placement for children born moderately preterm.[65] Children born moderate and late preterm accounted for most preterm children in special educational classes and, as with many other studies, male sex was also an important risk factor for special education placement.[65] In a follow-up study of children born moderately preterm who were not admitted to the NICU compared with children born at term, there was a higher need for special education placement, 7.7% versus 2.8%. In addition, children born at moderate and late preterm gestations were more likely to not advance a grade when compared with children born at term, 19% versus 8%.[66] This risk of failure to advance grades is consistent with adult registry studies that found that there is an increasing risk of not completing basic school with decreasing gestational age.[67]

BEHAVIORAL OUTCOMES

In follow-up studies that capture behavioral outcomes, parent or teacher questionnaires are often used at school age, and functional or psychological outcomes used for adults. In several studies, children born late preterm had increased risk of borderline clinical internalizing, clinical attention problems in first or second grade, and had higher scores in domains of inattention, hyperactivity, and total problems as determined by standardized parent and teacher report.[56,58,68] In large cohort studies that link birth data with medical and psychiatric adult data, adults born moderate and late preterm were at increased risk of having been diagnosed with a psychiatric, autism spectrum, or addictive disorder.[19,52] In all of the examined adverse outcomes, there was an inverse relationship between decreasing gestational age and increasing risk.[19,52] Risk of unemployment and criminal activity were not associated with preterm birth.[19,52]

SPEECH AND LANGUAGE OUTCOMES AND SENSORY IMPAIRMENTS

There are limited data systematically examining moderate and late preterm birth and speech and language and sensory outcomes at school age and beyond.

FACTORS AFFECTING OUTCOMES

Prematurity per se is not inevitably associated with adverse neurodevelopmental outcome.[69] The actively maturing preterm brain is, however, vulnerable to a variety of injuries and additional factors affecting brain maturation. An understanding of these factors is essential to reducing the neurodevelopmental sequelae of prematurity. Optimizing outcomes starts with good obstetric care to promote fetal growth and well-being. Intrauterine growth restriction or small for gestational age are associated with poorer outcomes in preterm infants.[53,70] When preterm delivery is necessary or unavoidable, use of antenatal corticosteroids, magnesium sulfate for fetal neuroprotection, and antibiotics among other evidence-based practices is beneficial.[71–73] Delivery in a hospital with the appropriate level of expertise in neonatal resuscitation and neonatal intensive care is beneficial.[74] Quality improvement interventions have reduced preterm complications associated with adverse neurodevelopmental outcomes.[75] Golden hour care management has reduced intraventricular hemorrhage.[76] Avoiding complications of prematurity and attention to everyday management supports healthy brain maturation. Bronchopulmonary dysplasia, infection, necrotizing enterocolitis, and severe retinopathy of prematurity are predictors of neurodevelopmental disability.[77] Interventions, such as postnatal steroids, painful procedures, and general anesthetics, are associated with adverse outcomes.[2] Caffeine for apnea of prematurity has shown benefit at 18 months of age and improved motor outcomes at 5 years of age.[78,79] The child's family and sociodemographic characteristics become increasingly important in the older child, especially for cognitive and language outcomes. A strong home environment is associated with resilience, and postnatal events, primarily parent-child interactions, may moderate prenatal effects through epigenetic changes.[80,81]

FUTURE DIRECTIONS

Efforts to reduce the incidence of preterm deliveries have not been successful to date and, therefore, reducing the long-term neurodevelopmental impacts of prematurity is the next frontier. This will require a multipronged approach with identification and reduction of risk factors, promotion of healthy brain maturation, consideration of the risks and benefits of neonatal interventions, and support for parents, caregivers, and the home environment. Exciting new preventive strategies include erythropoiesis-stimulating agents and extreme preterm care units.[2] Developmental care, minimizing procedural pain and repetitive noxious stimuli, and postdischarge early intervention strategies to support parents and families show promise.[2]

REFERENCES

1. Blencowe H, Cousens S, Chou D, et al. Born too soon: the global epidemiology of 15 million preterm births. Reprod Health 2013;10(Suppl 1):S2.
2. Rogers EE, Hintz SR. Early neurodevelopmental outcomes of extremely preterm infants. Semin Perinatol 2016;40:497–509.
3. Luu TM, Rehman Mian MO, Nuyt AM. Long-term impact of preterm birth: neurodevelopmental and physical health outcomes. Clin Perinatol 2017;44:305–14.
4. Martin JA, Hamilton BE, Osterman MJK, et al. National vital statistics reports births: final data for 2015. Natl Vital Stat Rep 2017;66:1–70.
5. Eide MG, Øyen N, Skj/Erven R, et al. Associations of birth size, gestational age, and adult size with intellectual performance: evidence from a cohort of Norwegian men. Pediatr Res 2007;62:636–42.
6. Tin W, Fritz S, Wariyar U, et al. Outcome of very preterm birth: children reviewed with ease at 2 years differ from those followed up with difficulty. Arch Dis Child Fetal Neonatal Ed 1998;79:83–7.
7. McGowan JE, Alderdice FA, Holmes VA, et al. Early childhood development of late-preterm infants: a systematic review. Pediatrics 2011;127:1111–24.
8. Kilbride HW, Aylward GP, Doyle LW, et al. Prognostic neurodevelopmental testing of preterm infants: do we need to change the paradigm? J Perinatol 2017;37:1–5.
9. Haslam MD, Lisonkova S, Creighton D, et al. Canadian Neonatal Network and the Canadian Neonatal Follow-Up Network. Severe neurodevelopmental impairment

in neonates born preterm: impact of varying definitions in a Canadian Cohort. J Pediatr 2018;197:75–81.

10. World Health Organization. International classification of functioning, disability and health: children and youth version. Geneva (Switzerland): WHO Press; 2007.

11. Schiariti V, Selb M, Cieza A, et al. International classification of functioning, disability and health core sets for children and youth with cerebral palsy: a consensus meeting. Dev Med Child Neurol 2015;57:149–58.

12. Hack M. Poor predictive validity of the Bayley scales of infant development for cognitive function of extremely low birth weight children at school age. Pediatrics 2005;116:333–41.

13. Van Veen S, Aarnoudse-Moens CSH, Van Kaam AH, et al. Consequences of correcting intelligence quotient for prematurity at age 5 years. J Pediatr 2016;173:90–5.

14. Marlow N, Wolke D, Bracewell M, et al. Neurologic and developmental disability at six years of age after extremely preterm birth. N Engl J Med 2005;352:9–19.

15. Schmidt B. Survival without disability to age 5 years after neonatal caffeine therapy for apnea of prematurity. JAMA 2012;307:275.

16. Hintz SR, Newman JE, Vohr BR. Changing definitions of long-term follow-up: should "long term" be even longer? Semin Perinatol 2016;40:398–409.

17. Cheong JLY, Anderson PJ, Burnett AC, et al. Changing neurodevelopment at 8 years in children born extremely preterm since the 1990s. Pediatrics 2017;139: e20164086.

18. Saigal S, Doyle LW. An overview of mortality and sequelae of preterm birth from infancy to adulthood. Lancet 2008;371:261–9.

19. Moster D, Lie RT, Markestad T. Long-term medical and social consequences of preterm birth. N Engl J Med 2008;359:262–73.

20. Hack M, Cartar L, Schluchter M, et al. Self-perceived health, functioning, and well-being of very low birth weight infants at age 20 years. J Pediatr 2007;15: 635–41.e2.

21. Zwicker JG, Harris SR. Quality of life of formerly preterm and very low birth weight infants from preschool age to adulthood: a systematic review. Pediatrics 2008; 121:e366–76.

22. Rosenbaum P, Paneth N, Leviton A. A report: the definition and classification of cerebral palsy April 2006. Dev Med Child Neurol Suppl 2007;109:8–14.

23. Edwards J, Berube M, Erlandson K, et al. Developmental coordination disorder in school-aged children born very preterm and/or at very low birth weight: a systematic review. J Dev Behav Pediatr 2011;32:678–87.

24. Williams J, Lee KJ, Anderson PJ. Prevalence of motor-skill impairment in preterm children who do not develop cerebral palsy: a systematic review. Dev Med Child Neurol 2010;52:232–7.

25. Allotey J, Zamora J, Cheong-See F, et al. Cognitive, motor, behavioural and academic performances of children born preterm: a meta-analysis and systematic review involving 64 061 children. BJOG 2018;125:16–25.

26. de Kieviet JF, Piek JP, Aarnoudse-Moens CS, et al. Motor development in very preterm and very low birth-weight children from birth to adolescence. JAMA 2009;302:2235.

27. Asami M, Kamei A, Nakakarumai M, et al. Intellectual outcomes of extremely preterm infants at school age. Pediatr Int 2017;59:570–7.

28. Aylward GP. Neurodevelopmental outcomes of infants born prematurely. J Dev Behav Pediatr 2014;35:394–407.

29. Synnes AR, Anson S, Arkesteijn A, et al. School entry age outcomes for infants with birth weight ≤800 grams. J Pediatr 2010;157:989–94.e1.

30. Kerr-Wilson CO, MacKay DF, Smith GCS, et al. Meta-analysis of the association between preterm delivery and intelligence. J Public Health (Oxf) 2012;34:209–16.
31. Vohr B. Follow-up care of high-risk infants. Pediatrics 2004;114(Supplement 5): 1377–97.
32. Saigal S, den Ouden L, Wolke D, et al. School-age outcomes in children who were extremely low birth weight from four international population-based cohorts. Pediatrics 2003;112:943–50.
33. Vohr BR. Neurodevelopmental outcomes of extremely preterm infants. Clin Perinatol 2014;41:241–55.
34. Aarnoudse-Moens CSH, Weisglas-Kuperus N, van Goudoever JB, et al. Meta-analysis of neurobehavioral outcomes in very preterm and/or very low birth weight children. Pediatrics 2009;124:717–28.
35. Twilhaar ES, de Kieviet JF, Aarnoudse-Moens CS, et al. Academic performance of children born preterm: a meta-analysis and meta-regression. JAMA Pediatr 2018; 172:361–7.
36. Saigal S, Hoult LA, Streiner DL, et al. School difficulties at adolescence in a regional cohort of children who were extremely low birth weight. Pediatrics 2000;105:325–31.
37. Geldof CJA, van Wassenaer AG, de Kieviet JF, et al. Visual perception and visual-motor integration in very preterm and/or very low birth weight children: a meta-analysis. Res Dev Disabil 2012;33:726–36.
38. Synnes A, Luu TM, Moddemann D, et al. Determinants of developmental outcomes in a very preterm Canadian cohort. Arch Dis Child Fetal Neonatal Ed 2017;102. F235.
39. Barre N, Morgan A, Doyle LW, et al. Language abilities in children who were very preterm and/or very low birth weight: a meta-analysis. J Pediatr 2011;158: 766–74.e1.
40. Ortiz-Mantilla S, Choudhury N, Leevers H, et al. Understanding language and cognitive deficits in very low birth weight children. Dev Psychobiol 2008;50:107–26.
41. Luu TM, Vohr BR, Allan W, et al. Evidence for catch-up in cognition and receptive vocabulary among adolescents born very preterm. Pediatrics 2011;128:313–22.
42. van Noort-van der Spek IL, Franken M-CJP, Weisglas-Kuperus N. Language functions in preterm-born children: a systematic review and meta-analysis. Pediatrics 2012;129:745–54.
43. Ferrari F, Grosoli M, Fontana G. Neurobehavioural comparison of low-risk preterm and full term infants at term conceptional age. Dev Med Child Neurol 1983;25: 450–8.
44. Kaga K, Hashira S, Marsh RR. Auditory brainstem responses and behavioural responses in pre-term infants. Br J Audiol 1986;20:121–7.
45. Cohen SE, Parmelee AH, Beckwith L, et al. Cognitive development in preterm infants: birth to 8 years. J Dev Behav Pediatr 1986;7:102–10.
46. Wickremasinghe AC, Rogers EE, Johnson BC, et al. Children born prematurely have atypical Sensory Profiles. J Perinatol 2013;33:631–5.
47. Spittle AJ, Treyvaud K, Doyle LW, et al. Early emergence of behavior and social-emotional problems in very preterm infants. J Am Acad Child Adolesc Psychiatry 2009;48:909–18.
48. Johnson S, Hollis C, Kochhar P, et al. Psychiatric disorders in extremely preterm children: longitudinal finding at age 11 years in the EPICure study. J Am Acad Child Adolesc Psychiatry 2010;49:453–63.e1.
49. Johnson S, Wolke D. Behavioural outcomes and psychopathology during adolescence. Early Hum Dev 2013;89:199–207.

50. Vohr B. Long-term outcomes of moderately preterm, late preterm, and early term infants. Clin Perinatol 2013;40(4):739–51.
51. Lindstrom K, Winbladh B, Haglund B, et al. Preterm infants as young adults: a Swedish national cohort study. Pediatrics 2007;120:70–7.
52. Lindstrom K, Lindblad F, Hjern A. Psychiatric morbidity in adolescents and young adults born preterm: a Swedish national cohort study. Pediatrics 2009;123: e47–53.
53. Kerstjens JM, De Winter AF, Bocca-Tjeertes IF, et al. Developmental delay in moderately preterm-born children at school entry. J Pediatr 2011;159:92–8.
54. Potijk MR, Kerstjens JM, Bos AF, et al. Developmental delay in moderately preterm-born children with low socioeconomic status: risks multiply. J Pediatr 2013;163:1289–95.
55. Hornman J, de Winter AF, Kerstjens JM, et al. Stability of developmental problems after school entry of moderately-late preterm and early preterm-born children. J Pediatr 2017;187:73–9.
56. Huddy CLJ. Educational and behavioural problems in babies of 32-35 weeks gestation. Arch Dis Child Fetal Neonatal Ed 2001;85:23–8.
57. Petrini JR, Dias T, McCormick MC, et al. Increased risk of adverse neurological development for late preterm infants. J Pediatr 2009;154:169–76.
58. Talge NM, Holzman C, Wang J, et al. Late-preterm birth and its association with cognitive and socioemotional outcomes at 6 years of age. Pediatrics 2010;126: 1124–31.
59. Odd DE, Emond A, Whitelaw A. Long-term cognitive outcomes of infants born moderately and late preterm. Dev Med Child Neurol 2012;54:704–9.
60. Ekeus C, Lindstrom K, Lindblad F, et al. Preterm birth, social disadvantage, and cognitive competence in Swedish 18- to 19-year-old men. Pediatrics 2010;125: e67–73.
61. Dalziel SR, Lambert A, McCarthy D, et al. Psychological functioning and health-related quality of life in adulthood after preterm birth. Dev Med Child Neurol 2007; 49:597–602.
62. Chyi LJ, Lee HC, Hintz SR, et al. School outcomes of late preterm infants: special needs and challenges for infants born at 32 to 36 weeks gestation. J Pediatr 2008;153:25–31.
63. Chan E, Quigley MA. School performance at age 7 years in late preterm and early term birth: a cohort study. Arch Dis Child Fetal Neonatal Ed 2014;99:F451–7.
64. Lipkind HS, Slopen ME, Pfeiffer MR, et al. School-age outcomes of late preterm infants in New York City. Am J Obstet Gynecol 2012;206:222.e1-6.
65. Mackay DF, Smith GCS, Dobbie R, et al. Gestational age at delivery and special educational need: retrospective cohort study of 407,503 schoolchildren. PLoS Med 2010;7:1–10.
66. van Baar AL, Vermaas J, Knots E, et al. Functioning at school age of moderately preterm children born at 32 to 36 weeks' gestational age. Pediatrics 2009;124: 251–7.
67. Mathiasen R, Hansen BM, Andersen A-MNN, et al. Gestational age and basic school achievements: a national follow-up study in Denmark. Pediatrics 2010; 126:e1553–61.
68. Talge NM, Holzman C, Van Egeren LA, et al. Late-preterm birth by delivery circumstance and its association with parent-reported attention problems in childhood. J Dev Behav Pediatr 2012;33:405–15.
69. Bonifacio S, Glass H, Chau V. Extreme premature birth is not associated with impaired development of brain microstructure. J Pediatr 2010;157:726–32.

70. Tanis JC, Van Braeckel KN, Kerstjens JM, et al. Functional outcomes at age 7 years of moderate preterm and full term children born small for gestational age. J Pediatr 2015;166:552–8.e1.
71. American Academy of Pediatrics. Antenatal corticosteroid therapy for fetal maturation. Pediatrics 2017;140:2016–8.
72. Magee L, Sawchuck D, Synnes A, et al. Magnesium sulphate for fetal neuroprotection. J Obstet Gynaecol Can 2011;33:516–29.
73. Puopolo KM, Beigi R, Silverman NS, et al. ACOG committee opinion: intrapartum management of intraamniotic infection. Obstet Gynecol 2017;130:95–101.
74. Chien LY, Whyte R, Aziz K, et al. Improved outcome of preterm infants when delivered in tertiary care centers. Obstet Gynecol 2001;98:247–52.
75. Lee SK, Shah PS, Singhal N, et al. Association of a quality improvement program with neonatal outcomes in extremely preterm infants: a prospective cohort study. CMAJ 2014;186:E485–94.
76. Reuter S, Messier S, Steven D. The neonatal golden hour - intervention to improve quality of care of the extremely low birth weight infant. S D Med 2014;67:397–403.
77. Patel R. Short- and long-term outcomes for extremely preterm infants. Am J Perinatol 2016;33(3):318–28.
78. Doyle LW, Schmidt B, Anderson PJ, et al. Reduction in developmental coordination disorder with neonatal caffeine therapy. J Pediatr 2014;165:356–9.e2.
79. Schmidt B, Roberts S, Davis P. Long-term effects of caffeine therapy for apnea of prematurity. N Engl J Med 2007;357:1893–902.
80. Monk C, Spicer J, Champagne F. Linking prenatal maternal adversity to developmental outcomes in infants: the role of epigenetic pathways. Dev Psychopathol 2012;24:1361–76.
81. Manley BJ, Roberts RS, Doyle LW, et al. Social variables predict gains in cognitive scores across the preschool years in children with birth weights 500 to 1250 grams. J Pediatr 2015;166:870–6.

Early Diagnosis and Treatment of Cerebral Palsy in Children with a History of Preterm Birth

Alicia J. Spittle, PhD[a,b,c,]*, Catherine Morgan, PhD[d],
Joy E. Olsen, PhD[b,c], Iona Novak, PhD[d], Jeanie L.Y. Cheong, MD[a,b,c]

KEYWORDS

• Cerebral palsy • Preterm • Neuroimaging • Early intervention

KEY POINTS

- Preterm children are at increased risk of cerebral palsy compared with term-born infants.
- Early diagnosis of cerebral palsy is possible within the first 6 months of life using a combination of clinical history, neuroimaging, and physical examination.
- Infants with cerebral palsy should be referred for cerebral palsy–specific early intervention, which includes task-specific training, environmental enrichment, and parental support.
- Infants with cerebral palsy should be screened for comorbidities including pain, epilepsy, sleep disorders, visual impairment, and hearing impairments to maximize outcomes.

INTRODUCTION

Cerebral palsy (CP) is a heterogeneous motor impairment seen in infants born across all gestational ages (GAs) but is more common in infants born preterm.[1,2] By definition CP is an umbrella term to describe "a group of permanent disorders of the development of movement and posture, causing activity limitation, that are attributed to non-progressive disturbances that occurred in the developing fetal or infant brain."[3] The

This work was supported by the National Health Medical Research Council (NHMRC) Center of Research Excellence in Newborn Medicine ID 1060733 (A.J. Spittle and J.Y. Cheong) and NHMRC Center of Research Excellence in Cerebral Palsy ID 1057997 (I. Novak, C. Morgan), NHMRC Career Development Fellowship ID 1053767 (A.J. Spittle), NHMRC Career Development Fellowship ID 1141354 (J.Y. Cheong), and the Victorian Government's Operational Infrastructure Support Program.
[a] Physiotherapy, University of Melbourne, 161 Barry Street, Parkville 3052, Australia; [b] Victorian Infant Brain Studies, Murdoch Children's Research Institute, 50 Flemington Road, Parkville 3052, Australia; [c] Neonatal Services, The Royal Women's Hospitals, Cnr Flemington Road and Grattan Street, Parkville 3052, Australia; [d] Cerebral Palsy Alliance, Child and Adolescent Health, The University of Sydney, Sydney NSW 2006, Australia
* Corresponding author. University of Melbourne, 7th Floor, Alan Gilbert Building, 161 Barry Street, Parkville 3052, Australia.
E-mail address: aspittle@unimelb.edu.au

Clin Perinatol 45 (2018) 409–420
https://doi.org/10.1016/j.clp.2018.05.011
0095-5108/18/© 2018 Elsevier Inc. All rights reserved.

incidence of CP in the general population varies throughout the world at a rate of 0.1% to 0.2% of live births in developed countries and is slightly higher in developing countries, with the risk of CP increasing with decreasing GA.[4,5] The prevalence of CP in a meta-analysis of 19 studies, with CP expressed by GA, is reported to be 14.6% (95% confidence interval [CI], 12.5–17.0) in extremely preterm children (born 22–27 weeks' gestation), 6.2% (95% CI, 4.9%–7.8%) in very preterm children (born 28–31 weeks' gestation), and 0.7% in the moderate to late preterm (32–36 weeks' gestation) compared with 0.11% (95% CI, 0.09–0.14) in term-born children.[6] Prematurity is a major risk factor for CP; in Australia between 1993 and 2009, a total of 43% of children with CP were born preterm.[7] Although it is clear that children born preterm are at an increased risk of CP, the biologic basis for the associations is unclear and likely to be multifactorial.[8] The preterm brain is particularly vulnerable because it is exposed to the extra-uterine environment during critical periods of brain development, and thus at risk of alterations in the "normal" trajectory of brain development.[1,9] However, there are other pathologic processes related to preterm birth and CP, and in many cases it is likely that there are several causal pathways involved, including genetics, early delivery, and pregnancy complications.[1,8] This article discusses evidence related to the risk factors for CP in children born preterm, making a diagnosis of CP and, importantly, early treatment and intervention to optimize outcomes for the preterm child with CP and their family.

DIAGNOSIS OF CEREBRAL PALSY

Recent clinical practice guidelines recommend that the diagnosis of CP or high risk of CP can be made within the first 6 months postterm age.[10] Traditionally diagnosis has been made much later, between the ages of 12 and 42 months, with many clinicians adopting a "wait and see" approach.[2] However, late diagnosis results in delayed referral to early intervention (EI) and can lead to increase in parent anxiety and grief.[10] The diagnosis of CP is based on clinical presentation rather than a single diagnostic tool. It is recommended that a combination of clinical history, neuroimaging, and standardized motor/neurologic assessments is used to make an early, accurate diagnosis of CP.[10]

CLINICAL HISTORY IN CHILDREN BORN PRETERM WITH CEREBRAL PALSY

Although the exact causal pathways for an individual with CP are often unknown, there are many factors associated with an increased risk of CP (**Table 1**).[11] The risk factors for CP differ for children born preterm compared with full-term children and include brain injury,[11] lower GA, small for GA,[12] infection, chorioamnionitis,[13] multiple births, male sex,[11] postnatal corticosteroids,[14] and early surgery.[15] There are several perinatal interventions that aim to prevent CP in children born preterm.[16] These neuroprotective interventions had been introduced into obstetric and neonatal care over the past decade and have had already had an impact on reducing the rates of CP.[17] Magnesium sulfate given to women at risk of preterm birth for neuroprotection of their fetus reduces the rate of CP,[18] and methylxanthine (caffeine) therapy used to prevent apnea of prematurity and thus reduce hypoxemia and bradycardia has also been shown to reduce rates of CP in infants born very preterm.[19] There is an urgent need for further randomized controlled trials of interventions addressing risk factors for CP in the antenatal and postnatal period.[16]

NEUROIMAGING AND CEREBRAL PALSY IN PRETERM CHILDREN

Given that brain injury is the best prognostic factor for CP in preterm children,[11] neuroimaging and visualization of the preterm infant's brain play a pivotal role in early

Table 1
Summary of protective factors and risk for cerebral palsy in children born preterm from systematic reviews

Protective Factors	Population	Benefit
Magnesium sulfate	GA <37 wk	Review of 5 RCTs (n = 6145 infants) showed a reduction in relative risk of CP (RR, 0.68; 95% CI, 0.54–0.87)[18]
Caffeine therapy	GA 500–1250 g	Review of 1 multicenter RCT (n = 937) showed a reduction in rates of CP (adjusted OR, 0.58; 95% CI, 0.39–0.87)[66]

Risk Factors	Population	Risk
Brain injury	GA <32 wk	Review of 12 cohort, case control, and RCTs reported a reduction in rates of CP (OR range, 2.4–43)[11]
Lower gestational age	GA <37 wk	Review of 8 studies reported rates of CP to be • 8.3% (95% CI, 5.5–12.6) in GA <28 wk • 4.3% (95% CI, 3.3–5.7) at 28–31 wk • 0.7% (95% CI, 0.5–1.0) at 32–36 wk[5]
Low birth weight	BW <2500 g	Review of 9 studies reported rates of CP to be • 5.6 (95% CI, 4.3–7.4) in BW <1000 g • 5.9 (95% CI, 5.3–6.6) at BW 1000–1499 g • 0.10 (95% CI, 0.9–1.1) at 1500–2499 g[5]
Small for gestational age	GA 32–36 wk	Review of 7 case control and cohort studies (n = 135,650) showed an increased risk (OR, 2.34; 95% CI, 1.43–3.82)[12]
Chorioamnionitis	GA <37 wk	Review of 19 case control and cohort studies of clinical chorioamnionitis showed an increased risk of CP (RR, 1.9; 95% CI, 1.4–2.5)[13]
Postnatal corticosteroid use	GA <32 wk	Review of 12 RCT trials (n = 1452) showed early use (<8 d) increased risk of CP (RR, 1.45; 95% CI, 1.06–1.98)[14]

Abbreviations: BW, birthweight; OR, odds ratio; RCT, randomized controlled trial; RR, risk ratio.

diagnosis of CP.[20] Neuroimaging modalities, such as cranial ultrasound (cUS) and brain MRI, are used to detect the patterns of brain injury in preterm children that correlate with patterns of impairment including CP. In fact, neuroimaging especially brain MRI has been recommended as one of the three tools with the best predictive validity for detecting CP before 5 months of age.[10] A systematic review of tests to predict CP reported that MRI performed at term-corrected age (in preterm infants) seemed to be a strong predictor of CP, with sensitivity ranging in individual studies from 86% to 100% and specificity ranging from 89% to 97%, and sensitivity of cUS 74% (95% CI, 63%–83%) and 92% (95% CI, 81%–96%), respectively.[21]

Cranial Ultrasound

cUS has been standard of care in many neonatal units since the 1970s. It has the advantage of being a bedside tool, and thus, the ability to have repeated examinations performed in sick preterm babies. Through several acoustic windows (the anterior, posterior, and mastoid fontanelles), cUS can detect major brain injury affecting the preterm infant, including intraventricular hemorrhage (IVH), hemorrhagic parenchymal infarction (HPI), posthemorrhagic ventricular dilatation, cerebellar hemorrhage, and cystic periventricular leukomalacia (PVL). Low-grade IVH (Papile grade 1 and 2) is associated with a low risk of CP, in the order of 6.8% to 8.1%.[2] However, the risk is higher with high-grade IVH. The risk for CP with grade 3 IVH (refers to bleeds that occupy >50% of the lateral ventricle with acute dilatation) varies in the literature, but the risk is highest if there is associated posthemorrhagic ventricular dilatation.[22,23] When there is an associated HPI (also known as Papile grade 4), the risk of CP increases to a mean positive predictive value of 47% (95% CI, 31%–64%).[23] The wide CI of predictive ability is related to the variability of size and site of lesion. It is possible to refine the prediction of the pattern of CP from the knowledge of the site of the HPI. Unilateral HPI is associated with spastic hemiplegia involving the contralateral side to the lesion, whereas bilateral lesions are associated with spastic quadriplegia. The risk of CP is highest where parenchymal infarcts or cysts are located in the occipital periventricular region, and involve more than one periventricular region.[24]

cUS is sensitive for detection of cystic PVL, but not so diffuse PVL, which is better visualized on MRI. The presence of cysts is predictive of CP (mean positive predictive value, 77%; 95% CI, 59%–89%).[23] The severity of CP is associated with the extent of the cysts. With localized cystic changes, there is an 85% chance of achieving independent walking. However, this is greatly reduced to less than 10% in the presence of extensive cysts.[25]

With increasing use of the mastoid window, cerebellar hemorrhages are more easily identified. Studies have shown that cerebellar hemorrhages detected on cUS tend to be larger than that seen on MRI. There are more limited data about its association with neurodevelopmental outcomes. Up to 58% of children with CP have cerebellar injury after IVH, and the risk of CP was higher with involvement of the medial part of the cerebellum.[26,27]

MRI

MRI has revolutionized the way the newborn brain is visualized. In the newborn, up to about 3 months of age, brain MRI is performed in natural sleep or with a dose of sedation using custom designed devices, such as beanbags and swaddling the infant. Past this age, children require a general anesthetic to assist in a successful MRI that is free from motion artifact.

Unlike cUS, MRI of the newborn brain is often done once the preterm baby is clinically stable. This is usually around term-equivalent age, although there are centers that are imaging preterm infants at a younger age. Although the lesions seen on cUS can also be identified on MRI, MRI is the best imaging modality to detect diffuse white matter injury. White matter injury is characterized by the presence of abnormal signal in the white matter, ventriculomegaly, smaller brain size, presence of cysts, decreased myelination, and corpus callosum thinning.[28] In a large cohort of infants born less than 30 weeks, the presence of moderate to severe white matter injury was associated with an increased odds ratio for CP (mean, 9.55; 95% CI, 3.22–28.3).[28] The presence of punctate white matter lesions on an earlier MRI, done at 31 to 33 weeks' postmenstrual age, was equally as predictive of motor outcome including CP.[29]

In addition to structural images, advanced MRI techniques have also been shown to predict later motor outcome in preterm infants. Preterm children with CP have abnormal microstructure (eg, lower fractional anisotropy) in key regions, such as the posterior limb of the internal capsule and centrum semiovale, compared with children without CP.[30]

STANDARDIZED MOTOR/NEUROLOGIC EXAMINATION

Given the definition of CP includes that a child has an impairment in the development of movement and posture that causes activity limitation, a physical examination is an essential part of the diagnosis picture. There have been several systematic reviews examining the best predictive assessment tools for motor impairment and CP, with the Prechtl General Movement Assessment (GMA) and Hammersmith Infant Neurologic Examination (HINE) demonstrating the best combination of sensitivity and specificity.[10,21,31]

General Movements

The quality of an infant's spontaneous movements reflects their central nervous system integrity,[32] and infants with CP demonstrate early movement abnormalities, often before term-equivalent age.[33,34] The GMA[35] evaluates infants' spontaneous whole-body movements (general movements [GMs]) according to age-specific characteristics, and is an ideal assessment for very preterm infants. This assessment is used from birth during the early neonatal period and is observational, so that medically fragile infants who may not tolerate the handling required from other neurodevelopmental instruments are assessed.

Abnormal GMs that are classified as cramped synchronized are an early marker for CP in very preterm infants.[33] Cramped synchronized GMs are rigid stop/start movements involving cocontraction of the limbs and trunk, with minimal rotation. For very preterm infants with cramped synchronized GMs before or at term-equivalent age, additional GMA are indicated to determine the risk of CP because transient cramped synchronized GMs may not necessarily precede CP. Studies of preterm infants with cramped synchronized GMA at more than one time point have reported specificity of 92% to 100% and sensitivity of 46% to 97% for CP diagnosis,[33,36] with higher risk when cramped synchronized GMs are evident close to term-equivalent age.[33] Therefore, the early prediction of CP is best when considered in context of a GMA trajectory. Ideally a GMA is conducted before term, at term-equivalent, and at 3 to 4 months' corrected age.[35] Infants with consistently abnormal GMA at these serial assessment time points are at the highest risk of CP. Conversely, for preterm infants who initially have an abnormal GMA followed by normal assessments (or consistently normal GMA), then CP is less likely, particularly given the high sensitivity of the GMA.[33]

The highest predictive validity of a single GMA is between 9 and 20 weeks' postterm age when fidgety GMs are present,[21] although the best time to observe these is between 12 and 16 weeks postterm before GMs are superseded by the infant's goal-directed movements.[37] Fidgety GMs are small amplitude, segmental movements throughout the whole body that occur in multiple directions.[35] In high-risk infants, absent fidgety GMA predicts CP with sensitivity of 98% and specificity of 94%.[38] In a meta-analysis of tests to predict CP, pooled sensitivity of the GMA was 98% (95% CI, 74–100) and specificity 91% (95% CI, 83–93).[21] For infants born very preterm, a fidgety age GMA is recommended for early detection of CP in conjunction with neuroimaging and (HINE) neurodevelopmental assessment.[10]

Because of the time-sensitive window for fidgety GMA, consideration of when very preterm infant follow-up occurs is important. An on-site clinic visit for GMA at 3 to 4 months is not always feasible because of geographic or other service/resource constraints and therefore technology, such as smartphone applications, can be used. Parents can upload a video of their infant's GMs using a smartphone application, such as Baby Moves,[39] for remote GMA before a clinic visit. If GMA is scored as absent fidgety, then other assessments are organized, such as brain MRI and additional neurodevelopmental assessment. Furthermore, if the GMA is considered borderline or ambiguous, another video is arranged for a more definitive assessment. Regardless, in cases where absent fidgety is scored, then a second fidgety age GMA should be obtained where possible to ascertain whether fidgety GMs have not yet appeared and assist with accurate CP diagnosis.[40]

Hammersmith Infant Neurologic Examination

The HINE is a standardized 26-item neurologic examination that is simple to perform in the clinical setting for infants 2 to 24 months.[41] A global score between 0 and 78 is obtained from scoring all items across five domains. Cranial nerve function, posture, movement quality, tone, and reflexes and reactions are assessed and a score between 0 and 3 is assigned for each item in each domain. This assessment was originally standardized on a sample of low-risk term infants between 12 and 18 months and an optimality score was defined based on scores obtained by 90% of the normal population. Subsequent studies validated use of the tool in high-risk infants including those with perinatal asphyxia,[42] and preterm populations.[43,44] In a group of preterm infants (<31 weeks GA) HINE scores greater than 64 between 9 and 18 months predicted walking ability at 2 years (sensitivity, 98%; specificity, 85%).[45] Neither GA nor age of assessment was associated with HINE scores. In a cohort of 103 very preterm infants who were assessed longitudinally with the HINE, ambulation at 2 years was predicted accurately as young as 3 months of age.[43] Cutoff scores of 50 at 3 months and 52 at 6 months predicted walking with 93% sensitivity and 100% specificity. Receiver operator curve analysis demonstrated that the most predictive items at all time points across the first year of life were movement quality and quantity and lateral tilting. In a large cohort of high-risk infants (n = 1541), term and preterm, HINE scores of less than 40 always predicted CP, whereas scores greater than 73 were never associated with a CP diagnosis at 2 years.[46] At 3 months HINE score less than 56 was highly predictive of a diagnosis of CP at 2 years (96% sensitivity; 85% specificity). The combined use of the HINE and GMA at 3 months improves early prediction of neurodevelopmental outcomes and can specifically discriminate between those infants most likely to have bilateral versus unilateral CP.[46]

TREATMENT

Essential to treatment commencing early is early detection of CP to ensure management of factors that mediate long-term outcomes, assist health professional and families in selecting appropriate treatment pathways, and to developing and testing new interventions.[10,11] The focus of treatment differs depending on whether an infant is diagnosed early (ie, within first 6 months postterm) versus late (ie, 24 months postterm). Early diagnosis allows for intervention to commence in a timely manner during the first year of life when there is rapid maturation and development of the musculoskeletal and central nervous systems. Limitations in EI for CP to date have been the result of late diagnosis; rather than intervention being preventive and proactive, it has focused on treatment of impairments once a problem has occurred. For an infant whether they have CP or are typically developing, learning to move involves practice and trial and error, shaped by the environment and experience of the task.[47] Essential to improving outcomes of children with CP is starting early to harness brain plasticity; however, if intervention is delayed and abnormal neural pathways developed, muscles may become weak and shorter and the child frustrated and/or disengaged. Treatment needs to focus on evidenced-based EI, parental support, management of comorbidities, and prevention of secondary complications.

Early Intervention

EI is generally defined as "multidisciplinary services provided to children from birth to 5 years of age to promote child health and well-being, enhance emerging competencies, minimize developmental delays, remediate existing or emerging disabilities, prevent functional deterioration and promote adaptive parenting and overall family function."[48] As soon as a preterm infant is diagnosed with CP, or high risk of CP if a firm diagnosis cannot be made, they should be referred to CP-specific EI. Although the evidence base is limited at this time,[49] interventions should be multidisciplinary, involve caregivers, support families, and be functionally based.

Cochrane Reviews consistently demonstrate that EI programs benefit preterm infants, particularly their cognitive development.[50] The effects on motor development are less clear with only small gains reported.[50] Most clinical trials of EI in preterm populations exclude infants with brain injuries, thus extrapolating the effects of EI for infants with CP is difficult. Traditionally, therapy interventions have focused on positioning and handling interventions that emphasize normalization of movement and tone reduction, such as neurodevelopmental therapy.[51] A landmark randomized controlled trial in 1988 compared matched doses of neurodevelopmental therapy with a curriculum-based EI program, Learningames, in a group of infants with spastic diplegia, 70% of whom were born preterm. Infants in the EI group had superior motor and cognitive Bayley scores after 6 months and walked earlier than the group receiving neurodevelopmental therapy.[52] Since then, developments in CP intervention research have favored an activity and functional approach to rehabilitation.

The aim of EI for infants with CP is to harness the neuroplasticity mechanisms at work in the developing brain, particularly activity-dependent plasticity. Recent systematic reviews have summarized the published evidence for EI for infants with CP and recommend several key principles based on clinical trials and developments in neuroscience.[49,53] Broadly speaking, it is recommended that approaches based on active parent engagement, environmental enrichment, and principles of motor learning (including task-specific training) ought to form the basis of motor interventions for infants with CP.[49] Rather than a generic "one size fits all" approach, therapy programs should be targeted to the individual child based on the type and topography of CP and family goals. For example, infants with an asymmetrical presentation who are likely to be diagnosed with hemiplegia benefit from early constraint-induced movement therapy.[54] Studies of treatment intensity tend to favor higher doses of activity-based therapy; however, more research is required in this area.[53]

Involving Caregivers and Family Support

Parents of preterm infants may experience trauma and ongoing depression related to the events surrounding the birth and medical history of their infant. Systematic review evidence indicates that interventions for parents that incorporate cognitive behavioral therapy techniques, such as relaxation and coping and communication strategies, have a small but positive effect on parental depression and anxiety symptoms.[55] Interventions for infants with CP typically do involve and seek to educate parents but may not necessarily target parental mental health. It is recommended that parents of infants at high risk of CP who are also experiencing depression or anxiety be offered evidence-based interventions because poor parental mental health can also have adverse consequences for infants.[56]

Most parents know that their child has CP before the diagnosis is officially given.[57] Receiving the news that their child has a permanent disability has been described as traumatizing and parents report experiencing grief and loss. Communicating the diagnosis to the family in a timely fashion is important, because late diagnosis is associated with higher rates of parental depression and parents are eager to find interventions that can help their child's development.[57] High-quality evidence from parent interviews recommends that a series of conversations are planned with both parents present; that adequate time for questions is provided; that the news is shared with the right blend of compassion, honesty, and hope; and that a plan for next steps is incorporated.[10,58]

One of the keys to effective communication of a diagnosis of CP or high risk of CP is understanding the clinical presentation of CP in children born preterm. Parents' concerns during the time of diagnosis is functional motor ability or whether their child will walk. Using evidence-based tools, such as the HINE, and triangulating these results with MRI results and assessment of motor development can give clinicians some indication of whether the child is likely to be ambulant or nonambulant. However, early prognostic information should be relayed with caution because severity of CP tends to become clearer after 2 years.[10] Because most children with hemiplegia and diplegia are eventually ambulatory there may well be instances where the likelihood of independent mobility is shared to reassure the family.[5,59]

There is strong evidence that involving and supporting parents as an integral part of EI is important and leads to better parent outcomes including reduced anxiety and depression.[60] Those programs that provided specific psychosocial support for parents rather than just education led to better outcomes.

COMORBIDITIES

Children with CP often have numerous comorbidities and co-occurring functional limitations, which are as disabling as the motor impairment itself.[3,59] A systematic review of international CP registers in high-income country contexts indicated that 75% (95% CI, 72–78) have chronic pain arising from multiple origins; 49% (95% CI, 34–64) have an intellectual disability (IQ <70); 35% (95% CI, 26–42) have epilepsy, which is active in 24%; 28% (95% CI, 21–34) have displaced hips (ie, migration >30%); 26% (95% CI, 24–28) have behavior problems; 24% (95% CI, incalculable) have bladder control problems; 23% (95% CI, 19–27) are nonverbal; 23% (95% CI, incalculable) have a pathologic sleep disorder; 22% (95% CI, incalculable) have sialorrhea; 11% (95% CI, 5–17) are functionally blind; 6% (95% CI, 3–9) require tube feeding; and 4% (95% CI, 2–6) have a severe hearing impairment.[59] Population CP data are more difficult to obtain in low-income country contexts, and the chance of survival after preterm birth is lower, meaning datasets are different. Best-available evidence indicates that children with CP in low-income country contexts have more severe physical disability and even higher rates of comorbidities.[61]

Other than chronic pain, comorbidities are more likely to occur in nonambulatory children with spastic quadriplegia and/or dyskinesia.[59,62] Children with CP following preterm birth have a greater proportion of children with milder forms of CP than those born at term, meaning their risk for comorbidities is slightly lower than the total CP population.[63,64] Regardless of risk, conventional evidence-based medical management of pain, epilepsy, sleep, vision, and hearing is strongly recommended to improve children's outcomes.[59] Early medical management requires attention to growth and nutrition monitoring weight gain; screening for silent aspiration where a child is having recurrent pneumonia; managing reactive airway disease especially in those with persistent pulmonary hypertension; measuring head growth among children requiring shunts using shunt protocol; and managing the child's pain to optimize learning in the neonatal period via facilitated flexed positions, massage, music, nonnutritive sucking, supervised time in prone, swaddling, and avoiding procedural pain where possible, and in infancy by detecting and managing reflux, constipation, and movement disorders causing pain.[65]

SUMMARY

Preterm birth is associated with an increased risk of CP. There are several perinatal risk factors, along with neuroimaging and clinical examination findings, that are used to assist in making the diagnosis of CP early in a preterm infant's life. Early diagnosis is not only beneficial to ensuring EI in a timely manner during maximal periods of brain plasticity but also for parental support and decreasing the severity of comorbidities.

Best Practices

What is the current practice?

Cerebral palsy in preterm is traditionally diagnosed late at 12 to 24 months.

Cerebral palsy in preterm infants is identified in the first 6 months of life using a combination of clinical history, neuroimaging, and neurologic examination findings.

What changes in current practice are likely to improve outcomes?

Early diagnosis of cerebral palsy ensures timely referral to early interventions services and parental support and reduces comorbidities.

Summary Statement

There is strong evidence the early detection of cerebral palsy in preterm infants is possible within first 6 months posterm.

There is moderate evidence that early intervention improves outcomes for infants born preterm with cerebral palsy.

REFERENCES

1. Stavsky M, Mor O, Mastrolia SA, et al. Cerebral palsy-trends in epidemiology and recent development in prenatal mechanisms of disease, treatment, and prevention. Front Pediatr 2017;5:21.
2. McIntyre S, Morgan C, Walker K, et al. Cerebral palsy–don't delay. Dev Disabil Res Rev 2011;17(2):114–29.
3. Rosenbaum P, Paneth N, Leviton A, et al. A report: the definition and classification of cerebral palsy April 2006. Dev Med Child Neurol Suppl 2007;109:8–14.
4. Himpens E, Van den Broeck C, Oostra A, et al. Prevalence, type, distribution, and severity of cerebral palsy in relation to gestational age: a meta-analytic review. Dev Med Child Neurol 2008;50(5):334–40.
5. Oskoui M, Coutinho F, Dykeman J, et al. An update on the prevalence of cerebral palsy: a systematic review and meta-analysis. Dev Med Child Neurol 2013;55(6):509–19.
6. Himpens E, Oostra A, Franki I, et al. Predictability of cerebral palsy in a high-risk NICU population. Early Hum Dev 2010;86(7):413–7.
7. Australia Cerebral Palsy Register. Australian Cerebral Palsy Register Report 2016. Sydney (Australia): Cerebral Palsy Alliance; 2016.
8. Tronnes H, Wilcox AJ, Lie RT, et al. Risk of cerebral palsy in relation to pregnancy disorders and preterm birth: a national cohort study. Dev Med Child Neurol 2014;56(8):779–85.
9. Spittle AJ, Orton J. Cerebral palsy and developmental coordination disorder in children born preterm. Semin Fetal Neonatal Med 2014;19(2):84–9.
10. Novak I, Morgan C, Adde L, et al. Early, accurate diagnosis and early intervention in cerebral palsy: advances in diagnosis and treatment. JAMA Pediatr 2017. https://doi.org/10.1001/jamapediatrics.2017.1689.
11. Linsell L, Malouf R, Morris J, et al. Prognostic factors for cerebral palsy and motor impairment in children born very preterm or very low birthweight: a systematic review. Dev Med Child Neurol 2016;58(6):554–69.
12. Zhao M, Dai H, Deng Y, et al. SGA as a risk factor for cerebral palsy in moderate to late preterm infants: a system review and meta-analysis. Sci Rep 2016;6:38853.
13. Wu YW, Colford JM Jr. Chorioamnionitis as a risk factor for cerebral palsy: a meta-analysis. JAMA 2000;284(11):1417–24.

14. Doyle LW, Ehrenkranz RA, Halliday HL. Early (< 8 days) postnatal corticosteroids for preventing chronic lung disease in preterm infants. Cochrane Database Syst Rev 2014;(5):CD001146.
15. Hunt RW, Hickey LM, Burnett AC, et al. Early surgery and neurodevelopmental outcomes of children born extremely preterm. Arch Dis Child Fetal Neonatal Ed 2017. https://doi.org/10.1136/archdischild-2017-313161.
16. Shepherd E, Salam RA, Middleton P, et al. Antenatal and intrapartum interventions for preventing cerebral palsy: an overview of Cochrane systematic reviews. Cochrane Database Syst Rev 2017;(8):CD012077.
17. Pierrat V, Marchand-Martin L, Arnaud C, et al. Neurodevelopmental outcome at 2 years for preterm children born at 22 to 34 weeks' gestation in France in 2011: EPIPAGE-2 cohort study. BMJ 2017;358:j3448.
18. Doyle LW, Crowther CA, Middleton P, et al. Magnesium sulphate for women at risk of preterm birth for neuroprotection of the fetus. Cochrane Database Syst Rev 2009;(1):CD004661.
19. Schmidt B, Roberts RS, Davis P, et al. Long-term effects of caffeine therapy for apnea of prematurity. N Engl J Med 2007;357(19):1893–902.
20. de Vries LS, Groenendaal F. Neuroimaging in the preterm infant. Ment Retard Dev Disabil Res Rev 2002;8(4):273–80.
21. Bosanquet M, Copeland L, Ware R, et al. A systematic review of tests to predict cerebral palsy in young children. Dev Med Child Neurol 2013;55(5):418–26.
22. Sherlock RL, Anderson PJ, Doyle LW, et al. Neurodevelopmental sequelae of intraventricular haemorrhage at 8 years of age in a regional cohort of ELBW/very preterm infants. Early Hum Dev 2005;81(11):909–16.
23. Nongena P, Ederies A, Azzopardi DV, et al. Confidence in the prediction of neurodevelopmental outcome by cranial ultrasound and MRI in preterm infants. Arch Dis Child Fetal Neonatal Ed 2010;95(6):F388–90.
24. Bassan H, Limperopoulos C, Visconti K, et al. Neurodevelopmental outcome in survivors of periventricular hemorrhagic infarction. Pediatrics 2007;120(4): 785–92.
25. van Haastert IC, de Vries LS, Eijsermans MJ, et al. Gross motor functional abilities in preterm-born children with cerebral palsy due to periventricular leukomalacia. Dev Med Child Neurol 2008;50(9):684–9.
26. Kitai Y, Hirai S, Ohmura K, et al. Cerebellar injury in preterm children with cerebral palsy after intraventricular hemorrhage: prevalence and relationship to functional outcomes. Brain Dev 2015;37(8):758–63.
27. Zayek MM, Benjamin JT, Maertens P, et al. Cerebellar hemorrhage: a major morbidity in extremely preterm infants. J Perinatol 2012;32(9):699–704.
28. Woodward LJ, Anderson PJ, Austin NC, et al. Neonatal MRI to predict neurodevelopmental outcomes in preterm infants. N Engl J Med 2006;355(7):685–94.
29. Miller SP, Ferriero DM, Leonard C, et al. Early brain injury in premature newborns detected with magnetic resonance imaging is associated with adverse early neurodevelopmental outcome. J Pediatr 2005;147(5):609–16.
30. De Bruine FT, Van Wezel-Meijler G, Leijser LM, et al. Tractography of white-matter tracts in very preterm infants: a 2-year follow-up study. Dev Med Child Neurol 2013;55(5):427–33.
31. Spittle AJ, Doyle LW, Boyd RN. A systematic review of the clinimetric properties of neuromotor assessments for preterm infants during the first year of life. Dev Med Child Neurol 2008;50(4):254–66.
32. Spittle AJ, Boyd RN, Inder TE, et al. Predicting motor development in very preterm infants at 12 months' corrected age: the role of qualitative magnetic

resonance imaging and general movements assessments. Pediatrics 2009;
123(2):512–7.

33. Ferrari F, Cioni G, Einspieler C, et al. Cramped synchronized general movements
in preterm infants as an early marker for cerebral palsy. Arch Pediatr Adolesc
Med 2002;156(5):460–7.

34. Guzzetta A, Belmonti V, Battini R, et al. Does the assessment of general movements without video observation reliably predict neurological outcome? Eur J
Paediatr Neurol 2007;11(6):362–7.

35. Einspieler C, Prechtl HFR. Prechtl's assessment of general movements: a diagnostic tool for the functional assessment of the young nervous system. Ment
Retard Dev Disabil Res Rev 2005;11(1):61–7.

36. Cioni G, Ferrari F, Einspieler C, et al. Comparison between observation of spontaneous movements and neurologic examination in preterm infants. J Pediatr
1997;130(5):704–11.

37. Ferrari F, Frassoldati R, Berardi A, et al. The ontogeny of fidgety movements from
4 to 20 weeks post-term age in healthy full-term infants. Early Hum Dev 2016;103:
219–24.

38. Morgan C, Crowle C, Goyen TA, et al. Sensitivity and specificity of general movements assessment for diagnostic accuracy of detecting cerebral palsy early in an
Australian context. J Paediatr Child Health 2015. https://doi.org/10.1111/jpc.12995.

39. Spittle AJ, Olsen J, Kwong A, et al. The Baby Moves prospective cohort study
protocol: using a smartphone application with the General Movements Assessment to predict neurodevelopmental outcomes at age 2 years for extremely preterm or extremely low birthweight infants. BMJ Open 2016;6(10):e013446.

40. Sæther R, Støen R, Vik T, et al. A change in temporal organization of fidgety
movements during the fidgety movement period is common among high risk infants. Eur J Paediatr Neurol 2016. https://doi.org/10.1016/j.ejpn.2016.04.016.

41. Haataja L, Mercuri E, Regev R, et al. Optimality score for the neurologic examination of the infant at 12 and 18 months of age. J Pediatr 1999;135(2 Pt 1):153–61.

42. Haataja L, Mercuri E, Guzzetta A, et al. Neurologic examination in infants with
hypoxic-ischemic encephalopathy at age 9 to 14 months: use of optimality scores
and correlation with magnetic resonance imaging findings. J Pediatr 2001;138(3):
332–7.

43. Romeo DM, Cioni M, Scoto M, et al. Prognostic value of a scorable neurological
examination from 3 to 12 months post-term age in very preterm infants: a longitudinal study. Early Hum Dev 2009;85(6):405–8.

44. Romeo DM, Cioni M, Palermo F, et al. Neurological assessment in infants discharged
from a neonatal intensive care unit. Eur J Paediatr Neurol 2013;17(2):192–8.

45. Frisone MF, Mercuri E, Laroche S, et al. Prognostic value of the neurologic optimality score at 9 and 18 months in preterm infants born before 31 weeks' gestation. J Pediatr 2002;140(1):57–60.

46. Romeo DM, Guzzetta A, Scoto M, et al. Early neurologic assessment in preterm-
infants: integration of traditional neurologic examination and observation of general movements. Eur J Paediatr Neurol 2008;12(3):183–9.

47. Kolb B, Muhammad A, Gibb R. Searching for factors underlying cerebral plasticity in the normal and injured brain. J Commun Disord 2011;44(5):503–14.

48. Shonkoff JP, Meidels SJ. Handbook of early childhood intervention. Cambridge
(England): Cambridge University Press; 2000.

49. Morgan C, Darrah J, Gordon AM, et al. Effectiveness of motor interventions in infants with cerebral palsy: a systematic review. Dev Med Child Neurol 2016;58(9):
900–9.

50. Spittle A, Orton J, Anderson PJ, et al. Early developmental intervention programmes provided post hospital discharge to prevent motor and cognitive impairment in preterm infants. Cochrane Database Syst Rev 2015;(11):CD005495.

51. Novak I, McIntyre S, Morgan C, et al. A systematic review of interventions for children with cerebral palsy: state of the evidence. Dev Med Child Neurol 2013; 55(10):885–910.

52. Palmer FB, Shapiro BK, Wachtel RC, et al. The effects of physical therapy on cerebral palsy. A controlled trial in infants with spastic diplegia. N Engl J Med 1988; 318(13):803–8.

53. Hadders-Algra M, Boxum AG, Hielkema T, et al. Effect of early intervention in infants at very high risk of cerebral palsy: a systematic review. Dev Med Child Neurol 2017;59(3):246–58.

54. Nordstrand L, Holmdfure M, Kits A, et al. Improvements in bimanual hand function after baby-CIMT in two-year old children with unilateral cerebral palsy: a retrospective study. Res Dev Disabil 2015;41:86–93.

55. Kraljevic M, Warnock FF. Early educational and behavioral RCT interventions to reduce maternal symptoms of psychological trauma following preterm birth: a systematic review. J Perinat Neonatal Nurs 2013;27(4):311–27.

56. Spittle A, Treyvaud K. The role of early developmental intervention to influence neurobehavioral outcomes of children born preterm. Semin Perinatol 2016; 40(8):542–8.

57. Baird G, McConachie H, Scrutton D. Parents' perceptions of disclosure of the diagnosis of cerebral palsy. Arch Dis Child 2000;83(6):475–80.

58. Novak I, Thornton M, Morgan M, et al. Truth with hope: ethical challenges in disclosing 'bad' diagnostic, prognostic and intervention information. In: Rosenbaum P, Ronen GM, Racine E, et al, editors. Ethics in child health: principles and cases in neurodisability. London: MacKeith Press; 2016.

59. Novak I, Hines M, Goldsmith S, et al. Clinical prognostic messages from a systematic review on cerebral palsy. Pediatrics 2012;130(5):e1285–312.

60. Benzies KM, Magill-Evans JE, Hayden KA, et al. Key components of early intervention programs for preterm infants and their parents: a systematic review and meta-analysis. BMC Pregnancy Childbirth 2013;13(Suppl 1):S10.

61. Khandaker G, Smithers-Sheedy H, Islam J, et al. Bangladesh Cerebral Palsy Register (BCPR): a pilot study to develop a national cerebral palsy (CP) register with surveillance of children for CP. BMC Neurol 2015;15:173.

62. Venkateswaran S, Shevell MI. Comorbidities and clinical determinants of outcome in children with spastic quadriplegic cerebral palsy. Dev Med Child Neurol 2008;50(3):216–22.

63. McIntyre S, Badawi N, Brown C, et al. Population case-control study of cerebral palsy: neonatal predictors for low-risk term singletons. Pediatrics 2011;127(3): e667–73.

64. ACPR Group. Australian cerebral palsy register report 2016, birth years 1993-2009. Sydney (Australia): Cerebral Palsy Alliance; 2016.

65. Novak I, Msall M. Beyond the NICU: comprehensive care of the high-risk infant. In: Malcom WF, editor. Cerebral palsy. McGraw Hill Professional; 2014.

66. Henderson-Smart DJ, De Paoli AG. Prophylactic methylxanthine for prevention of apnoea in preterm infants. Cochrane Database Syst Rev 2010;(12):CD000432.

Neuroimaging for Neurodevelopmental Prognostication in High-Risk Neonates

Elizabeth K. Sewell, MD, MPH[a],*, Nickie N. Andescavage, MD[b]

KEYWORDS

- Neonate • Brain injury • Neurodevelopmental outcome
- Magnetic resonance imaging • Cranial ultrasound • Prematurity-related brain injury
- Hypoxic-ischemic encephalopathy • Extracorporeal membrane oxygenation

KEY POINTS

- Neuroimaging is a promising biomarker of neurodevelopmental outcomes in high-risk neonates.
- Various neuroimaging modalities exist for the detection and delineation of brain injury and maldevelopment in high-risk neonates.
- Additional knowledge on the benefits and limitations of these studies is needed to appropriately counsel families regarding neurodevelopmental outcomes.
- Advances in neuroimaging may improve neurodevelopmental outcome prediction in neonates.

INTRODUCTION

Brain injury in neonates and subsequent neurodevelopmental delays remain a significant source of morbidity despite many advances in obstetric and neonatal care. Early diagnosis of brain injury is important for prognostication as well as decision making and early treatment.[1,2] Advances in neuroimaging have improved our ability to detail and classify neonatal brain injury, although the relative value of each modality in predicting outcome remains controversial. This review discusses existing data relating neuroimaging with neurodevelopmental outcomes (NDO), specifically cranial ultrasound (CUS) imaging and brain MRI (**Table 1**).

Disclosure Statement: The authors have nothing to disclose.
[a] Department of Pediatrics, Emory University School of Medicine, Children's Healthcare of Atlanta, 2015 Uppergate Drive, Room 318, Atlanta, GA 30322, USA; [b] Department of Pediatrics, George Washington University, Children's National Medical Center, 111 Michigan Avenue Northwest, Washington, DC 20010, USA
* Corresponding author. 901 Adair Avenue, Atlanta, GA 30306.
E-mail address: elizabeth.sewell@emory.edu

Clin Perinatol 45 (2018) 421–437
https://doi.org/10.1016/j.clp.2018.05.004
0095-5108/18/© 2018 Elsevier Inc. All rights reserved.

Table 1
Overview of neuroimaging techniques

Technique	Advantages	Disadvantages	Clinical Application
CUS			
• Coronal and sagittal views of the brain are obtained using the anterior fontanelle as an acoustic window for the transducer • Additional views of posterior fossa using posterior and mastoid fontanelles[1,2,20,108]	• Inexpensive • Noninvasive • Performed at beside without sedation • Accurately diagnose IVH, cystic WMI, ventriculomegaly, and large strokes[1,2,20,108]	• Interoperator variability • Interreader variability, especially for small lesions • Less accurate at detecting diffuse non-cystic WMI, posterior fossa lesions, myelination, or metabolic disturbances[1,2,20,108]	• Traditional neuroimaging technique that is most widely used • Ideal for screening and serial imaging, especially in sick neonates[1,2,20,108]
MRI			
• Standard T1- and T2-weighted imaging used as qualitative assessment that can evaluate abnormalities in anatomy or myelination • Variety of advanced MR techniques that use quantitative analysis[109]	• Markedly improved structural evaluation, with better visualization of peripheral cerebrum, delineation of cerebral white and gray matter, and visualization of posterior fossa.[1,110]	• Expense • Necessary technical and clinical expertise • Availability, especially in resource limited settings, as well as specialized equipment • Limited feasibility in very ill neonates • Need for transport and at times sedation[109,110]	• More commonly used in high-risk neonates • Development of MRI compatible equipment and protocols, along with technological advances, now allow for safe feasible imaging with proper thermoregulation and cardiorespiratory monitoring[109,110]

Abbreviations: IVH, intraventricular hemorrhage; WMI, white matter injury.

PREMATURITY-RELATED BRAIN INJURY

Prematurity-related brain injury (PRBI) remains a significant cause of morbidity and mortality in preterm infants. PRBI includes cerebral and cerebellar hemorrhages, post-hemorrhagic hydrocephalus (PHH), and white matter injury (WMI). Some are primary destructive lesions that occur early in the neonatal period; others are consequences of these early injuries or sequelae of ongoing disruption of brain development.[3] Therefore, predicting NDO for this population depends on both the time point of assessment as well as the mode of neuroimaging.

Intraventricular Hemorrhage

Many studies have demonstrated the reliability of early screening CUS examination in the identification of intraventricular hemorrhage (IVH; **Fig. 1**).[1] The relationship of high-grade IVH with neuromotor deficits including cerebral palsy is well-established; Nongena and colleagues[4] estimated the pooled probability of abnormal 2-year motor development to be 26% with grade III IVH and 53% with periventricular hemorrhagic infarct (PVHI; also referred to as grade IV IVH), although both had wide confidence intervals. A recent meta-analysis by Mukerji and colleagues[5] assessed the association of IVH with death or moderate to severe neurodevelopmental impairment at 18 to

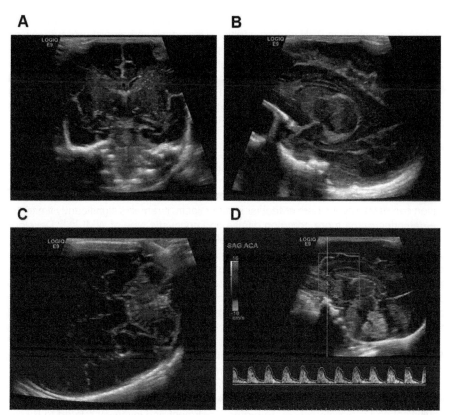

Fig. 1. Cranial ultrasound depicting coronal (*A*) and sagittal (*B*) images of brain through anterior fontanelle, view of posterior fossa using mastoid window (*C*), and Doppler waveform through the middle cerebral artery (*D*).

24 months of age, defined as moderate to severe cerebral palsy, moderate to severe cognitive delay, or severe visual or hearing impairment. Infants with large grade III IVH or PVHI on CUS examination had 4 times the odds of adverse outcome than those without IVH. The relationship of mild IVH with NDO is more controversial, with mixed results relating to short-term neurodevelopmental impairment at 18 to 36 months of age.[6,7] Unlike the earliest reports suggesting little to no impairment with mild IVH, the most recent studies report that infants with mild IVH have almost 1.5 times the odds of adverse outcome than infants without IVH, including neurosensory impairments, developmental delays, and cerebral palsy.[5,6] However, these results must be interpreted with caution because many of these odd ratios remain unadjusted for confounders and other clinical and neuroimaging findings known to further influence NDO.[3]

Posthemorrhagic Ventricular Dilation and Hydrocephalus

CUS examination is also routinely used to detect and monitor the evolution of posthemorrhagic ventricular dilation and PHH over time. Infants with higher grades of IVH are more likely to develop posthemorrhagic ventricular dilation and PHH; of these, infants with additional parenchymal lesions, as well as infants who require cerebrospinal fluid diversion, are at greatest risk for adverse NDO, particularly cerebral palsy.[8–10]

It has been suggested that posthemorrhagic ventricular dilation may reflect white matter loss alone, whereas PHH implies additional increased intracranial pressure, which may result in ongoing injury to the developing white matter.[11] Other studies have demonstrated that parenchymal injury might be more prognostic of NDO than the extent of ventricular dilation alone.[12,13] These distinctions, however, remain difficult to isolate in clinical practice. Although it has been proposed that the addition of Doppler ultrasound imaging can better detect increased intracranial pressure and compliance in PHH,[14] data relating Doppler measures in PHH and NDO are lacking.

White Matter Injury

WMI is the most common type of brain injury in premature infants, often associated with or a direct consequence of IVH, but also seen in the absence of IVH. WMI includes both cystic and diffuse periventricular leukomalacia and PVHI. Although CUS examination can detect cystic periventricular leukomalacia, it remains significantly limited in the detection of the more common diffuse and noncystic type of WMI.[15,16] Developmental outcomes for infants with WMI are related to the degree and location of parenchymal involvement, with larger and bilateral injuries associated with worse outcomes.[17,18] Specifically, there is a strong association between cystic periventricular leukomalacia on CUS examination and adverse motor outcomes, including cerebral palsy.[9,19–22] Less frequently, cognitive, hearing, and visual deficits have also been associated with WMI on CUS imaging in some studies.[9,22,23] It is possible that these nonmotor outcomes are more often related to noncystic WMI, which is less commonly diagnosed on CUS examination, especially in the early neonatal period.[15] As such, it is not surprising that many infants with normal CUS examination are later diagnosed with neurodevelopmental abnormalities.[20,21,24–26]

In contrast, structural MRI is widely accepted to be very sensitive for detecting WMI in preterm infants. Many studies have demonstrated that WMI on MRI at term-equivalent age is directly related to motor impairment and inversely related to Bayley scores.[2,16,27–29] These findings are supported even after controlling for a variety of clinical factors, particularly gestational age and postnatal infection.[16,28,29] According to a recent review, presence of WMI on term-equivalent age MRI can significantly increase the risk for motor and cognitive impairment (odds ratios of 10.0 and 8.3, respectively, defined as an IQ of <70 at 9 years of age for the latter).[30,31] These deficiencies seem to persist at least through school age.[32–36] Conversely, mild WMI including punctate lesions or diffuse excessive high signal intensity, do not seem be significantly associated with NDO in the first few years of life.[29,37]

Although MRI seems to be more sensitive in detecting WMI, some controversy remains as to whether these differences are clinically significant when MRI is used in addition to CUS alone. This is particularly true in the prognostication of motor delays, given the high specificity of both early CUS and TEA MRI in the detection of injury and subsequent cerebral palsy.[26] However, more recent studies that report cognition and motor delays in both the short- and long-term suggest that MRI may outperform CUS in predicting global neurodevelopmental outcome than CUS alone.[29,38]

Cerebellar Injury

In additional to the widely acknowledged risk of supratentorial bleeding and WMI, cerebellar hemorrhages are increasingly recognized as an early and important complication of preterm birth (see **Fig. 1**).[39,40] Although cerebellar hemorrhages are often seen in conjunction with severe IVH/PVHI, even isolated cerebellar injury is associated with cognitive, learning, and behavioral deficits, including functional limitations in day-to-day activities.[41] Limperopoulos and colleagues[41] demonstrated that up to two-thirds of preterm infants with large cerebellar hemorrhages diagnosed by CUS had neurologic abnormalities at 2.5 years of age compared with only 5% of infants without cerebellar injury; abnormalities in the injured group always included hypertonia, but also frequently included abnormal deep tendon reflexes, gait patterns, and ophthalmologic findings.

However, even with the additional of specific posterior fossa windows, CUS examination remains inferior to MRI for detecting cerebellar injury in the preterm infant.[2,40,42] Although large cerebellar lesions readily seen on both CUS imaging and MRI have the most worrisome outcomes, Tam and colleagues[40] demonstrated that cerebellar lesions only detected by MRI had 5 times the odds of abnormal neurologic examination at 3 to 6 years of age than those without cerebellar hemorrhage. In addition, cerebellar injury detected by MRI is associated with increased rates of impaired cognition, poor attention, and decreased learning capacity that persist through school age.[35,36,40,43,44]

Relationship Between Timing of Neuroimaging and Prediction of Neurodevelopmental Outcome

Early injury to the premature brain contributes to ongoing disturbances in brain growth and maturation, such as the loss of precursor cells important for subsequent myelination and neuronal–axon development that may not fully manifest until later in development.[3] Additional factors in an infant's postnatal course, including subsequent medical comorbidities, may lead to further damage. Thus, there has been a recent effort to obtain neuroimaging at term-equivalent age to better capture ongoing injury that may not be apparent soon after birth to improve neurodevelopmental prognostication.

Several publications suggest that studies at term-equivalent age might have additional prognostic value when added to early neuroimaging. Brouwer and colleagues[45] reported that the prognostic value of CUS imaging at term-equivalent age with ex vacuo ventriculomegaly was independently associated with worse cognitive and motor performance at 2 years of age. A more recent study by Hintz and colleagues[42] demonstrated that term-equivalent age CUS imaging improved prognostication of 18- to 22-month neurodevelopment when compared with perinatal–neonatal risk factors or early CUS alone (odds ratio, 9.8; 95% confidence interval, 2.8–35.0). Nonetheless, many infants with abnormal term-equivalent age CUS examinations had normal developmental outcomes, and some infants with normal term-equivalent age CUS examinations had abnormal developmental outcomes.[21,24,26,42,46] These studies emphasize the existing limitations of term-equivalent CUS alone in predicting NDO.

In contrast, numerous studies have associated term-equivalent age MRI results with both motor and cognitive outcomes.[26,27,29,31,47,48] Mirmiran and colleagues[26] found that term-equivalent age MRI had a greater sensitivity than term-equivalent age CUS for predicting cerebral palsy at 20 to 32 months of age, although both modalities were highly specific for motor outcomes. Woodward and colleagues[28] found that term-equivalent age MRI was predictive of cognitive delay, motor delay, cerebral palsy, and neurosensory impairment at 2 years, even after controlling for early CUS findings. Both Woodward and colleagues[32] and Iwata and colleagues[31] demonstrated that abnormal white matter appearance on term-equivalent age MRI was associated with cognitive impairments at school age. Hintz and colleagues[42] found that the predictive capability was best in models that included both CUS examination and MRI; however, the improvement with MRI added was small. Similarly, Edwards and colleagues[49] randomized 511 patients born before 33 weeks of gestation to receive either CUS examination or MRI at term-equivalent age. They found MRI slightly better predicted adverse motor outcomes than CUS imaging, and that both were inaccurate at predicting cognitive outcomes at 18 to 24 months of age.[49] MRI slightly reduces maternal anxiety more than CUS examination, but neither test led to improvement in health-related quality of life and MRI costs were greater than serial CUS examinations.[49] As with term-equivalent age CUS examinations, up to one-third of infants (2%–33%) with normal or mild abnormalities on MRI went on to develop cerebral palsy.[26,28,29,50]

Advanced Imaging

Given the limitations in both term-equivalent age CUS imaging and standard MRI, researchers are evaluating advanced MRI modalities as predictors of NDO. Decreased total and regional brain volumes using quantitative MRI are associated with worse memory, mental, and motor short-term outcomes at 6 to 24 months of age.[44,51–53] Diffusion tensor imaging (DTI), a specific, quantitative measure of white matter microstructural development, has also been studied in preterm infants. Early studies have demonstrated that DTI in preterm infants is associated with worse short- and long-term outcomes, including motor performance at 2 years, as well as memory, mathematics, and attention abilities at 7 years of age.[54–56] Studies of MR spectroscopy (MRS) measure specific cerebral metabolites in premature infants. N-Acetyl aspartate, a marker of neuronal development and health, has been studied relative to 18- to 24-month Bayley II and III scores, but with mixed results to date.[44,57] Other modalities of advanced MRI, including quantitative studies of global and regional perfusion and functional connectivity, in relation to short- and long-term NDO, have not been well-established. More recently, investigators have explored preterm MRI, obtained before 35 weeks of corrected gestational age, to predicted NDO.[58] These studies suggest that significant WMI and cerebellar injury, as well as white matter volume loss, are associated with NDO in the first few years of life; however, given the relatively few studies and small sample sizes for early MRI, it is not clear if earlier imaging confers significant advantage to the more common, term-equivalent age evaluations.[50,58] Perhaps a combination of preterm and term-equivalent imaging provides the most complete picture by documenting the evolution of brain injury over time.[59]

HYPOXIC–ISCHEMIC ENCEPHALOPATHY

Before the widespread use of therapeutic hypothermia for hypoxic ischemic encephalopathy (HIE), CUS abnormalities were associated with adverse outcomes in neonatal encephalopathy in many, but not all, studies.[60–63] Siegel and colleagues[60] found that 50% of infants with CUS abnormalities, most commonly periventricular hyperechogenicities, died by 15 days of life and, of the survivors, 80% had residual neurologic deficits. Another study by Babcock and Ball[62] found that CUS abnormalities such as cerebral atrophy or cystic encephalomalacia had high specificity for motor or developmental delay at 4 months of age. Several studies also demonstrated that abnormally low or high resistive indices on Doppler ultrasound imaging with CUS examination (see **Fig. 1**) were predictors for poor outcome.[64–66] In contrast, a larger prospective study did not find any association with CUS examination and abnormal outcomes at 1 year in infants with HIE.[63] The application of these studies in current practice where therapeutic hypothermia is now standard of care is limited, especially given the lack of association with long-term outcomes.

MRI is now recognized as the preferred neuroimaging modality to identify cerebral injury in neonatal encephalopathy (**Fig. 2**).[67] Numerous studies have linked severe injury detected by MRI to adverse NDO in infants presenting with HIE.[68,69] Reports from both the National Institute of Child Health and Human Development and Infant Cooling Evaluation trials further showed that severity and pattern of brain injury on

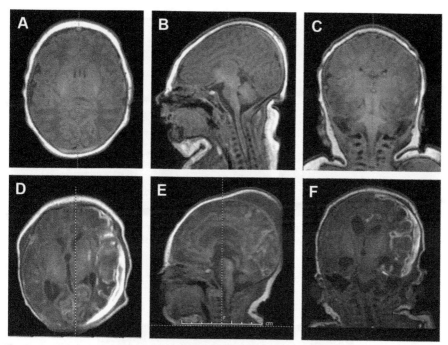

Fig. 2. T1-weighted spoiled gradient recalled MRI in neonatal encephalopathy for infant with moderate hypoxic–ischemic encephalopathy and normal imaging (*top*) and severe encephalopathy with abnormal findings (*bottom*), including extensive subdural and subarachnoid hemorrhages, bilateral necrosis of cerebral cortex and deep gray structures, and hydrocephalus with midline shift; image from the axial (*A*, *D*), sagittal (*B*, *E*), and coronal (*C*, *F*) planes.

MRI are predictive of adverse outcome (death or IQ of <70 and death or major disability, respectively) at 18 to 24 months of age with hypothermia treatment, and that these disabilities persist through school age.[70–72]

Researchers have begun to evaluate the predictive ability of a variety of advanced MR techniques to predict outcome in term infants with HIE, including measures of acute injury and edema (DWI), microstructural integrity (DTI), perfusion anomalies, and metabolic disturbances (MRS). Because DWI reflects early cellular injury, this modality has been recommended to identify injured areas before radiographic evidence of necrosis (**Fig. 3**A).[73,74] Several studies have demonstrated that DWI, including DTI, is predictive of NDO in the early neonatal period and may add prognostic value to standard MRI alone.[74–76] However, these studies also demonstrate that qualitative and quantitative results of DWI evolve during the first 2 weeks after injury, with periods of pseudonormalization that can influence interpretation and prognostication of injury.[73]

Cerebral perfusion studies using MRI can evaluate for regional hypoperfusion and hyperperfusion (**Fig. 3**B). Early studies suggest that global and regional hyperperfusion may be seen in areas with subsequent injury on standard MRI and hyperperfusion of the basal ganglia and thalamus may be predictive of death or cerebral palsy at 9 to 18 months of age, particularly when combined with MRS.[77,78] Additional spectroscopy studies (**Fig. 4**) suggest that both measures of lactate, as well as N-acetyl aspartate, may be the best predictor of death or moderate to severe disability at less than 12 months of age in this population, even when compared with both standard and advanced MRI.[68,78,79]

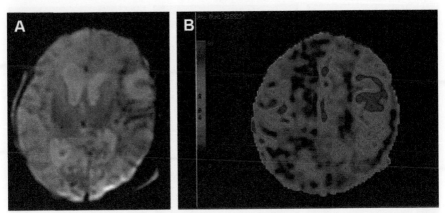

Fig. 3. Restricted diffusion on diffusion-weighted imaging for infants with severe hypoxic–ischemic encephalopathy on day of life 10 (A) and regional hyperperfusion of the left cortex on arterial spin labeling (B).

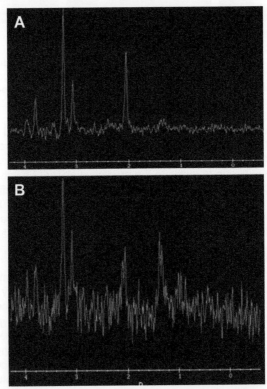

Fig. 4. MR spectroscopy of the left basal ganglia (long TE 288 ms) from infant with moderate hypoxic–ischemic encephalopathy and normal MR findings (A) and a severe hypoxic–ischemic encephalopathy (B). In (B), the decreased N-acetyl aspartate peak and elevated lactate suggest severe injury.

CONGENITAL HEART DISEASE

Neurodevelopmental delays in survivors of critical congenital heart disease (CHD) remain a major morbidity, owing to both the risk for perioperative brain injury with open heart surgery, but also from inherent abnormalities in cerebral perfusion and oxygenation in the fetal and postnatal periods before definitive repair. The risk of brain injury varies depending on the complexity of heart disease, but averages up to 49% in left-sided heart disease in a recent meta-analysis.[80] Brain injury and abnormalities in CHD have been well-described, and numerous clinical and demographic risk factors for neurodevelopmental delays have been identified.[81] Neuroimaging biomarkers in CHD in the prediction of NDO, however, remain difficult to identify, given that there are multiple and prolonged periods of susceptibility to the developing brain. Deviations from normal brain development have been described in the fetal, postnatal, and postoperative periods.[82–85] In the fetal period, abnormalities of fetal perfusion on Doppler ultrasound examination revealed mixed results with NDO outcomes, whereas fetal MRI and MRS revealed an association with delayed cerebral development and anaerobic metabolism (increased cerebral lactate) and NDO.[86] Similarly, in the immediate postnatal, but preoperative period, CUS examination was not associated with NDO, whereas injury detected by MRI was associated with lower language and motor scores.[86] Ongoing studies are not only needed to evaluate the long-term prognostic ability of neuroimaging in CHD, but also to determine the optimal timing of neuroimaging, to fully capture the extent of injury and provide the most meaningful prognostication.

RESPIRATORY FAILURE REQUIRING EXTRACORPOREAL MEMBRANE OXYGENATION

Several studies have used a combination of neuroimaging modalities to evaluate NDO after neonatal extracorporeal membrane oxygenation (ECMO) for acute respiratory failure, although the results are mixed. Although CUS examination can detect hemorrhagic lesions and is frequently used as a screening tool for intracranial hemorrhage, it is less accurate for ischemic lesions.[87,88] Two large cohort studies found that abnormalities on CUS examinations and computed tomography scans in infants after neonatal ECMO were associated with adverse NDO.[89,90] Although there are mixed data regarding the association of MRI abnormalities after neonatal outcome and short-term outcomes,[91,92] in the only prospective cohort study to date, 190 infants with respiratory failure requiring ECMO found that neonates with moderate or severe neuroimaging abnormalities on a combination of CUS, computed tomography, or MRI examinations at discharge were more likely to have adverse NDO at 12 to 20 months, defined as a mental or motor developmental index of less than 70, visual or auditory deficits, or cerebral palsy (odds ratio, 6.4; 95% confidence interval, 1.9–21.9).[93] Similarly, normal MRI findings after neonatal ECMO have also been associated with normal NDO at 24 months.[94]

The variety of diagnoses included and limited sample sizes make it difficult to interpret these results; larger, prospective, multicenter studies are needed to determine if NDO varies by type of brain injury, underlying disease process, or mode of ECMO. Additionally, research linking neuroimaging with long-term NDO in neonatal ECMO survivors has yet to be established.

FOCAL ISCHEMIC STROKE

MRI has been shown to be superior to CUS in diagnosing focal ischemic stroke.[95] The most common location of focal ischemic injury in the neonate is the territory perfused by the left middle cerebral artery, which is associated with motor asymmetry and contralateral hemiplegia.[96–99] Visual deficits at school age, such as abnormal acuity, visual field deficits, and stereopsis, are not uncommon in middle cerebral artery strokes and seem to be associated with hemiplegia and more extensive lesions.[100] The impact of focal ischemic stroke on cognitive development is less clear.[101–104] However, quantitative assessments of stroke, specifically volumetric delineation of injury may be more predictive of cognitive outcome.[105] Additionally, studies using DWI to evaluate neonatal stroke suggest that quantitative assessments of the corticospinal tracts may provide additional information on short-term motor outcomes, including mild motor disabilities.[106,107]

SUMMARY

Neurodevelopmental disabilities remain a significant morbidity for many high-risk neonates; however, the full impact of these high-risk conditions may not become fully evident until months or years after discharge from the neonatal intensive care unit. Developing early and accurate biomarkers of significant neurologic injury is necessary to accurately identify the infants at greatest risk for neurodevelopmental delays, as well as those most likely to benefit from novel therapeutics and interventions. CUS examination and MRI can improve neurodevelopmental outcome prediction in many high-risk neonates. Evidence linking neonatal neuroimaging with short- and long-term outcomes is most robust for infants with PRBI, HIE, and ischemic stroke. MRI may offer improved prognostication to CUS examination in some circumstances such as HIE, ischemic stroke, and term-equivalent imaging in PRBI. However, given the associated cost, resources, and needed expertise for the accurate execution and interpretation of these studies, the added benefits must be balanced with these limitations. Although neuroimaging can be useful as adjunctive prognostication tool, current studies suggest caution when counseling families. Advances in neuroimaging, including multimodal MRI and automated preprocessing and postprocessing methods for rapid, objective, and quantitative interpretations may improve diagnostics, clarify mechanisms of injury, and, in turn, also improve prognostication in many of these high-risk conditions.

Best Practices

What is the current practice?

Prematurity-related brain injury frequently includes early cranial ultrasound screening; some centers also obtain late neuroimaging but this is not currently standard practice. MRI is the preferred neuroimaging modality to identify and categorize brain injury in hypoxic ischemic encephalopathy and focal ischemic stroke.

What changes in current practice are likely to improve outcomes?

Late neuroimaging in prematurity-related brain imaging, either cranial ultrasound or MRI, improves outcome prediction. Posterior fossa windows on cranial ultrasound improve the detection of cerebellar injury, which is associated with worse neurodevelopmental outcome. Advanced MRI techniques may improve prognostication in high-risk neonates.

Is there a clinical algorithm? If so, please include.

Major recommendations
  Individual centers have neuroimaging protocols for specific types of neonatal brain injury, but algorithms vary by center. Clinical algorithms using neuroimaging for prognostication should be developed with consensus based on available evidence and updated as future studies become available.

Rating for the strength of the evidence

Neonatal neuroimaging prognostication varies by disease type; evidence is the most robust in prematurity-related brain injury, hypoxic–ischemic encephalopathy, and focal ischemic stroke.

Summary statement

Neuroimaging is a promising biomarker for neurodevelopmental outcomes in high-risk neonates, although limitations still exist and caution should be used when counseling families. Advances in neuroimaging may improve future prognostication.

REFERENCES

1. van Wezel-Meijler G, Steggerda SJ, Leijser LM. Cranial ultrasonography in neonates: role and limitations. Semin Perinatol 2010;34(1):28–38.
2. Plaisier A, Raets MM, Ecury-Goossen GM, et al. Serial cranial ultrasonography or early MRI for detecting preterm brain injury? Arch Dis Child Fetal Neonatal Ed 2015;100(4):F293–300.
3. Volpe JJ. Impaired neurodevelopmental outcome after mild germinal matrix-intraventricular hemorrhage. Pediatrics 2015;136(6):1185–7.
4. Nongena P, Ederies A, Azzopardi D, et al. Confidence in the prediction of neurodevelopmental outcome by cranial ultrasound and MRI in preterm infants. Arch Dis Child Fetal Neonatal Ed 2010;95(6):F388–90.
5. Mukerji A, Shah V, Shah PS. Periventricular/intraventricular hemorrhage and neurodevelopmental outcomes: a meta-analysis. Pediatrics 2015;136(6):1132–43.
6. Bolisetty S, Dhawan A, Abdel-Latif M, et al, New South Wales and Australian Capital Territory Neonatal Intensive Care Units' Data Collection. Intraventricular hemorrhage and neurodevelopmental outcomes in extreme preterm infants. Pediatrics 2014;133(1):55–62.
7. Payne AH, Hintz SR, Hibbs AM, et al. Neurodevelopmental outcomes of extremely low-gestational-age neonates with low-grade periventricular-intraventricular hemorrhage. JAMA Pediatr 2013;167(5):451–9.
8. Adams-Chapman I, Hansen NI, Stoll BJ, et al. Neurodevelopmental outcome of extremely low birth weight infants with posthemorrhagic hydrocephalus requiring shunt insertion. Pediatrics 2008;121(5):e1167–77.
9. O'Shea TM, Kuban KC, Allred EN, et al. Neonatal cranial ultrasound lesions and developmental delays at 2 years of age among extremely low gestational age children. Pediatrics 2008;122(3):e662–9.
10. Brouwer A, Groenendaal F, van Haastert I-L, et al. Neurodevelopmental outcome of preterm infants with severe intraventricular hemorrhage and therapy for post-hemorrhagic ventricular dilatation. J Pediatr 2008;152(5):648–54.
11. Robinson S. Neonatal posthemorrhagic hydrocephalus from prematurity: pathophysiology and current treatment concepts: a review. J Neurosurg Pediatr 2012;9(3):242–58.
12. Brouwer AJ, van Stam C, Uniken Venema M, et al. Cognitive and neurological outcome at the age of 5-8 years of preterm infants with post-hemorrhagic ventricular dilatation requiring neurosurgical intervention. Neonatology 2012;101(3):210–6.
13. Jary S, Kmita G, Wroblewska J, et al. Quantitative cranial ultrasound prediction of severity of disability in premature infants with post-haemorrhagic ventricular dilatation. Arch Dis Child 2012;97(11):955–9.

14. Taylor GA. Sonographic assessment of posthemorrhagic ventricular dilation. Radiol Clin North Am 2001;39(3):541–51.

15. Inder TE, Anderson NJ, Spencer C, et al. White matter injury in the premature infant: a comparison between serial cranial sonographic and MR findings at term. AJNR Am J Neuroradiol 2003;24(5):805–9.

16. Miller SP, Ferriero DM, Leonard C, et al. Early brain injury in premature newborns detected with magnetic resonance imaging is associated with adverse early neurodevelopmental outcome. J Pediatr 2005;147(5):609–16.

17. Maitre NL, Marshall DD, Price WA, et al. Neurodevelopmental outcome of infants with unilateral or bilateral periventricular hemorrhagic infarction. Pediatrics 2009;124(6):e1153–60.

18. McMenamin JB, Shcackelford GD, Volpe JJ. Outcome of neonatal intraventricular hemorrhage with periventricular echodense lesions. Ann Neurol 1984;15(3): 285–90.

19. Pinto-Martin JA, Whitaker AH, Feldman JF, et al. Relation of cranial ultrasound abnormalities in low-birthweight infants to motor or cognitive performance at ages 2, 6, and 9 years. Dev Med Child Neurol 1999;41(12):826–33.

20. Ancel PY, Livinec F, Larroque B, et al. Cerebral palsy among very preterm children in relation to gestational age and neonatal ultrasound abnormalities: the EPIPAGE cohort study. Pediatrics 2006;117(3):828–35.

21. Beaino G, Khoshnood B, Kaminski M, et al. Predictors of cerebral palsy in very preterm infants: the EPIPAGE prospective population-based cohort study. Dev Med Child Neurol 2010;52(6):e119–25.

22. O'Shea TM, Allred EN, Kuban KC, et al. Intraventricular hemorrhage and developmental outcomes at 24 months of age in extremely preterm infants. J Child Neurol 2012;27(1):22–9.

23. Bassan H, Limperopoulos C, Visconti K, et al. Neurodevelopmental outcome in survivors of periventricular hemorrhagic infarction. Pediatrics 2007;120(4): 785–92.

24. Laptook AR, O'Shea TM, Shankaran S, et al. Adverse neurodevelopmental outcomes among extremely low birth weight infants with a normal head ultrasound: prevalence and antecedents. Pediatrics 2005;115(3):673–80.

25. De Vries LS, Van Haastert IL, Rademaker KJ, et al. Ultrasound abnormalities preceding cerebral palsy in high-risk preterm infants. J Pediatr 2004;144(6): 815–20.

26. Mirmiran M, Barnes PD, Keller K, et al. Neonatal brain magnetic resonance imaging before discharge is better than serial cranial ultrasound in predicting cerebral palsy in very low birth weight preterm infants. Pediatrics 2004;114(4): 992–8.

27. Dyet LE, Kennea N, Counsell SJ, et al. Natural history of brain lesions in extremely preterm infants studied with serial magnetic resonance imaging from birth and neurodevelopmental assessment. Pediatrics 2006;118(2): 536–48.

28. Woodward LJ, Anderson PJ, Austin NC, et al. Neonatal MRI to predict neurodevelopmental outcomes in preterm infants. N Engl J Med 2006;355(7):685–94.

29. Skiold B, Vollmer B, Bohm B, et al. Neonatal magnetic resonance imaging and outcome at age 30 months in extremely preterm infants. J Pediatr 2012;160(4): 559–66.e1.

30. Plaisier A, Govaert P, Lequin MH, et al. Optimal timing of cerebral MRI in preterm infants to predict long-term neurodevelopmental outcome: a systematic review. AJNR Am J Neuroradiol 2014;35(5):841–7.

31. Iwata S, Nakamura T, Hizume E, et al. Qualitative brain MRI at term and cognitive outcomes at 9 years after very preterm birth. Pediatrics 2012;129(5): e1138–47.
32. Woodward LJ, Clark CA, Bora S, et al. Neonatal white matter abnormalities an important predictor of neurocognitive outcome for very preterm children. PLoS One 2012;7(12):e51879.
33. Spittle AJ, Cheong J, Doyle LW, et al. Neonatal white matter abnormality predicts childhood motor impairment in very preterm children. Dev Med Child Neurol 2011;53(11):1000–6.
34. Murray AL, Scratch SE, Thompson DK, et al. Neonatal brain pathology predicts adverse attention and processing speed outcomes in very preterm and/or very low birth weight children. Neuropsychology 2014;28(4):552.
35. Omizzolo C, Scratch SE, Stargatt R, et al. Neonatal brain abnormalities and memory and learning outcomes at 7 years in children born very preterm. Memory 2014;22(6):605–15.
36. Reidy N, Morgan A, Thompson DK, et al. Impaired language abilities and white matter abnormalities in children born very preterm and/or very low birth weight. J Pediatr 2013;162(4):719–24.
37. Kidokoro H, Anderson P, Doyle L, et al. High signal intensity on T2-weighted MR imaging at term-equivalent age in preterm infants does not predict 2-year neurodevelopmental outcomes. AJNR Am J Neuroradiol 2011;32(11):2005–10.
38. Anderson PJ, Treyvaud K, Neil JJ, et al. Associations of newborn brain magnetic resonance imaging with long-term neurodevelopmental impairments in very preterm children. J Pediatr 2017;187:58–65.e1.
39. Benders MJ, Kersbergen KJ, de Vries LS. Neuroimaging of white matter injury, intraventricular and cerebellar hemorrhage. Clin Perinatol 2014;41(1):69–82.
40. Tam EW, Rosenbluth G, Rogers EE, et al. Cerebellar hemorrhage on magnetic resonance imaging in preterm newborns associated with abnormal neurologic outcome. J Pediatr 2011;158(2):245–50.
41. Limperopoulos C, Bassan H, Gauvreau K, et al. Does cerebellar injury in premature infants contribute to the high prevalence of long-term cognitive, learning, and behavioral disability in survivors? Pediatrics 2007;120(3):584–93.
42. Hintz SR, Barnes PD, Bulas D, et al. Neuroimaging and neurodevelopmental outcome in extremely preterm infants. Pediatrics 2015;135(1):e32–42.
43. Keunen K, Išgum I, van Kooij BJ, et al. Brain volumes at term-equivalent age in preterm infants: imaging biomarkers for neurodevelopmental outcome through early school age. J Pediatr 2016;172:88–95.
44. Van Kooij BJ, Benders MJ, Anbeek P, et al. Cerebellar volume and proton magnetic resonance spectroscopy at term, and neurodevelopment at 2 years of age in preterm infants. Dev Med Child Neurol 2012;54(3):260–6.
45. Brouwer MJ, van Kooij BJ, van Haastert IC, et al. Sequential cranial ultrasound and cerebellar diffusion weighted imaging contribute to the early prognosis of neurodevelopmental outcome in preterm infants. PloS One 2014;9(10):e109556.
46. Broitman E, Ambalavanan N, Higgins RD, et al. Clinical data predict neurodevelopmental outcome better than head ultrasound in extremely low birth weight infants. J Pediatr 2007;151(5):500–5, 505.e1–2.
47. Kidokoro H, Anderson PJ, Doyle LW, et al. Brain injury and altered brain growth in preterm infants: predictors and prognosis. Pediatrics 2014;134(2):e444–53.
48. Setänen S, Haataja L, Parkkola R, et al. Predictive value of neonatal brain MRI on the neurodevelopmental outcome of preterm infants by 5 years of age. Acta Paediatr 2013;102(5):492–7.

49. Edwards AD, Redshaw ME, Kennea N, et al. Effect of MRI on preterm infants and their families: a randomised trial with nested diagnostic and economic evaluation. Arch Dis Child Fetal Neonatal Ed 2018. https://doi.org/10.1136/archdischild-2017-313102.

50. Badr LK, Bookheimer S, Purdy I, et al. Predictors of neurodevelopmental outcome for preterm infants with brain injury: MRI, medical and environmental factors. Early Hum Dev 2009;85(5):279–84.

51. Woodward LJ, Edgin JO, Thompson D, et al. Object working memory deficits predicted by early brain injury and development in the preterm infant. Brain 2005;128(Pt 11):2578–87.

52. Inder TE, Warfield SK, Wang H, et al. Abnormal cerebral structure is present at term in premature infants. Pediatrics 2005;115(2):286–94.

53. Gadin E, Lobo M, Paul DA, et al. Volumetric MRI and MRS and early motor development of infants born preterm. Pediatr Phys Ther 2012;24(1):38–44.

54. Rogers CE, Smyser T, Smyser CD, et al. Regional white matter development in very preterm infants: perinatal predictors and early developmental outcomes. Pediatr Res 2016;79(1–1):87–95.

55. Ullman H, Spencer-Smith M, Thompson DK, et al. Neonatal MRI is associated with future cognition and academic achievement in preterm children. Brain 2015;138(Pt 11):3251–62.

56. Murray AL, Thompson DK, Pascoe L, et al. White matter abnormalities and impaired attention abilities in children born very preterm. Neuroimage 2016; 124(Pt A):75–84.

57. Augustine EM, Spielman DM, Barnes PD, et al. Can magnetic resonance spectroscopy predict neurodevelopmental outcome in very low birth weight preterm infants? J Perinatol 2008;28(9):611–8.

58. Cornette L, Tanner S, Ramenghi L, et al. Magnetic resonance imaging of the infant brain: anatomical characteristics and clinical significance of punctate lesions. Arch Dis Child Fetal Neonatal Ed 2002;86(3):F171–7.

59. Martinez-Biarge M, Groenendaal F, Kersbergen KJ, et al. MRI based preterm white matter injury classification: the importance of sequential imaging in determining severity of injury. PloS One 2016;11(6):e0156245.

60. Siegel M, Shackelford G, Perlman J, et al. Hypoxic-ischemic encephalopathy in term infants: diagnosis and prognosis evaluated by ultrasound. Radiology 1984; 152(2):395–9.

61. Rutherford MA, Pennock JM, Dubowitz L. Cranial ultrasound and magnetic resonance imaging in hypoxic-ischaemic encephalopathy: a comparison with outcome. Dev Med Child Neurol 1994;36(9):813–25.

62. Babcock D, Ball W Jr. Postasphyxial encephalopathy in full-term infants: ultrasound diagnosis. Radiology 1983;148(2):417–23.

63. Boo N, Chandran V, Zulfiqar M, et al. Early cranial ultrasound changes as predictors of outcome during first year of life in term infants with perinatal asphyxia. J Paediatr Child Health 2000;36(4):363–9.

64. Liao H-T, Hung K-L. Anterior cerebral artery Doppler ultrasonography for prediction of outcome after perinatal asphyxia. Zhonghua Min Guo Xiao Er Ke Yi Xue Hui Za Zhi 1997;38(3):208–12.

65. Archer L, Levene M, Evans D. Cerebral artery Doppler ultrasonography for prediction of outcome after perinatal asphyxia. Lancet 1986;328(8516):1116–8.

66. Kumar AS, Chandrasekaran A, Asokan R, et al. Prognostic value of resistive index in neonates with hypoxic ischemic encephalopathy. Indian Pediatr 2016; 53(12):1079–82.

67. American Association of Pediatrics. Neonatal encephalopathy and neurologic outcome. Pediatrics 2014;133(5):e1482–8.
68. Thayyil S, Chandrasekaran M, Taylor A, et al. Cerebral magnetic resonance biomarkers in neonatal encephalopathy: a meta-analysis. Pediatrics 2010. https://doi.org/10.1542/peds.2009-1046.
69. van Laerhoven H, de Haan TR, Offringa M, et al. Prognostic tests in term neonates with hypoxic-ischemic encephalopathy: a systematic review. Pediatrics 2013;131(1):88–98.
70. Shankaran S, Barnes PD, Hintz SR, et al. Brain injury following trial of hypothermia for neonatal hypoxic–ischaemic encephalopathy. Arch Dis Child Fetal Neonatal Ed 2012;97(6):F398–404.
71. Cheong JL, Coleman L, Hunt RW, et al. Prognostic utility of magnetic resonance imaging in neonatal hypoxic-ischemic encephalopathy: substudy of a randomized trial. Arch Pediatr Adolesc Med 2012;166(7):634–40.
72. Shankaran S, McDonald SA, Laptook AR, et al. Neonatal magnetic resonance imaging pattern of brain injury as a biomarker of childhood outcomes following a trial of hypothermia for neonatal hypoxic-ischemic encephalopathy. J Pediatr 2015;167(5):987–93.e3.
73. Rutherford M, Counsell S, Allsop J, et al. Diffusion-weighted magnetic resonance imaging in term perinatal brain injury: a comparison with site of lesion and time from birth. Pediatrics 2004;114(4):1004–14.
74. Barkovich A, Miller S, Bartha A, et al. MR imaging, MR spectroscopy, and diffusion tensor imaging of sequential studies in neonates with encephalopathy. AJNR Am J Neuroradiol 2006;27(3):533–47.
75. Massaro AN, Evangelou I, Fatemi A, et al. White matter tract integrity and developmental outcome in newborn infants with hypoxic-ischemic encephalopathy treated with hypothermia. Dev Med Child Neurol 2015;57(5):441–8.
76. Tusor N, Wusthoff C, Smee N, et al. Prediction of neurodevelopmental outcome after hypoxic-ischemic encephalopathy treated with hypothermia by diffusion tensor imaging analyzed using tract-based spatial statistics. Pediatr Res 2012;72(1):63–9.
77. Wintermark P, Moessinger AC, Gudinchet F, et al. Temporal evolution of MR perfusion in neonatal hypoxic-ischemic encephalopathy. J Magn Reson Imaging 2008;27(6):1229–34.
78. De Vis JB, Hendrikse J, Petersen ET, et al. Arterial spin-labelling perfusion MRI and outcome in neonates with hypoxic-ischemic encephalopathy. Eur Radiol 2015;25(1):113–21.
79. Goergen S, Ang H, Wong F, et al. Early MRI in term infants with perinatal hypoxic–ischaemic brain injury: interobserver agreement and MRI predictors of outcome at 2 years. Clin Radiol 2014;69(1):72–81.
80. Khalil A, Suff N, Thilaganathan B, et al. Brain abnormalities and neurodevelopmental delay in congenital heart disease: systematic review and meta-analysis. Ultrasound Obstet Gynecol 2014;43(1):14–24.
81. Gaynor JW, Stopp C, Wypij D, et al. Neurodevelopmental outcomes after cardiac surgery in infancy. Pediatrics 2015. https://doi.org/10.1542/peds.2014-3825.
82. Dimitropoulos A, McQuillen PS, Sethi V, et al. Brain injury and development in newborns with critical congenital heart disease. Neurology 2013;81(3):241–8.
83. Li Y, Yin S, Fang J, et al. Neurodevelopmental delay with critical congenital heart disease is mainly from prenatal injury not infant cardiac surgery: current

evidence based on a meta-analysis of functional magnetic resonance imaging. Ultrasound Obstet Gynecol 2015;45(6):639–48.

84. Wong A, Chavez T, O'Neil S, et al. Synchronous aberrant cerebellar and opercular development in fetuses and neonates with congenital heart disease: correlation with early communicative neurodevelopmental outcomes, initial experience. AJP Rep 2017;7(01):e17–27.

85. Limperopoulos C, Tworetzky W, McElhinney DB, et al. Brain volume and metabolism in fetuses with congenital heart disease. Circulation 2010;121(1):26–33.

86. Mebius MJ, Kooi EM, Bilardo CM, et al. Brain injury and neurodevelopmental outcome in congenital heart disease: a systematic review. Pediatrics 2017. https://doi.org/10.1542/peds.2016-4055.

87. van Heijst AF, de Mol AC, Ijsselstijn H. ECMO in neonates: neuroimaging findings and outcome. Semin Perinatol 2014;38(2):104–13.

88. Bulas D, Glass P. Neonatal ECMO: neuroimaging and neurodevelopmental outcome. Semin Perinatol 2005;29(1):58–65.

89. Bulas DI, Glass P, O'Donnell RM, et al. Neonates treated with ECMO: predictive value of early CT and US neuroimaging findings on short-term neurodevelopmental outcome. Radiology 1995;195(2):407–12.

90. Taylor GA, Fitz CR, Miller MK, et al. Intracranial abnormalities in infants treated with extracorporeal membrane oxygenation: imaging with US and CT. Radiology 1987;165(3):675–8.

91. Lago P, Rebsamen S, Clancy RR, et al. MRI, MRA, and neurodevelopmental outcome following neonatal ECMO. Pediatr Neurol 1995;12(4):294–304.

92. Rollins MD, Yoder BA, Moore KR, et al. Utility of neuroradiographic imaging in predicting outcomes after neonatal extracorporeal membrane oxygenation. J Pediatr Surg 2012;47(1):76–80.

93. Vaucher YE, Dudell GG, Bejar R, et al. Predictors of early childhood outcome in candidates for extracorporeal membrane oxygenation. J Pediatr 1996;128(1):109–17.

94. Griffin MP, Minifee PK, Landry SH, et al. Neurodevelopmental outcome in neonates after extracorporeal membrane oxygenation: cranial magnetic resonance imaging and ultrasonography correlation. J Pediatr Surg 1992;27(1):33–5.

95. Cowan F, Mercuri E, Groenendaal F, et al. Does cranial ultrasound imaging identify arterial cerebral infarction in term neonates? Arch Dis Child Fetal Neonatal Ed 2005;90(3):F252–6.

96. Mercuri E, Barnett A, Rutherford M, et al. Neonatal cerebral infarction and neuromotor outcome at school age. Pediatrics 2004;113(1):95–100.

97. Mercuri E, Rutherford M, Cowan F, et al. Early prognostic indicators of outcome in infants with neonatal cerebral infarction: a clinical, electroencephalogram, and magnetic resonance imaging study. Pediatrics 1999;103(1):39–46.

98. Boardman JP, Ganesan V, Rutherford MA, et al. Magnetic resonance image correlates of hemiparesis after neonatal and childhood middle cerebral artery stroke. Pediatrics 2005;115(2):321–6.

99. De Vries L, Groenendaal F, Eken P, et al. Infarcts in the vascular distribution of the middle cerebral artery in preterm and fullterm infants. Neuropediatrics 1997;28(02):88–96.

100. Mercuri E, Anker S, Guzzetta A, et al. Neonatal cerebral infarction and visual function at school age. Arch Dis Child Fetal Neonatal Ed 2003;88(6):F487–91.

101. Ricci D, Mercuri E, Barnett A, et al. Cognitive outcome at early school age in term-born children with perinatally acquired middle cerebral artery territory infarction. Stroke 2008;39(2):403–10.

102. Westmacott R, Askalan R, MacGregor D, et al. Cognitive outcome following unilateral arterial ischaemic stroke in childhood: effects of age at stroke and lesion location. Dev Med Child Neurol 2010;52(4):386–93.
103. Westmacott R, MacGregor D, Askalan R. Late emergence of cognitive deficits after unilateral neonatal stroke. Stroke 2009;40(6):2012–9.
104. Chabrier S, Peyric E, Drutel L, et al. Multimodal outcome at 7 years of age after neonatal arterial ischemic stroke. J Pediatr 2016;172:156–61.e3.
105. Hajek CA, Yeates KO, Anderson V, et al. Cognitive outcomes following arterial ischemic stroke in infants and children. J Child Neurol 2014;29(7):887–94.
106. Kirton A, Shroff M, Visvanathan T, et al. Quantified corticospinal tract diffusion restriction predicts neonatal stroke outcome. Stroke 2007;38(3):974–80.
107. Roze E, Harris PA, Ball G, et al. Tractography of the corticospinal tracts in infants with focal perinatal injury: comparison with normal controls and to motor development. Neuroradiology 2012;54(5):507–16.
108. Fanaroff AAM, Fanaroff RJAA, Martin RJ. Neonatal-perinatal medicine: diseases of the fetus and infant. Philadelphia: Mosby; 2002.
109. Kwon SH, Vasung L, Ment LR, et al. The role of neuroimaging in predicting neurodevelopmental outcomes of preterm neonates. Clin Perinatol 2014;41(1):257–83.
110. Tocchio S, Kline-Fath B, Kanal E, et al. MRI evaluation and safety in the developing brain. Semin Perinatol 2015;39(2):73–104.

The Impact of Bronchopulmonary Dysplasia on Childhood Outcomes

Sara B. DeMauro, MD, MSCE

KEYWORDS

- Bronchopulmonary dysplasia • Chronic lung disease • Prematurity • Development
- Outcomes

KEY POINTS

- As mortality rates after extremely premature birth decrease, rates of survival with bronchopulmonary dysplasia (BPD) are increasing.
- BPD is associated with adverse health outcomes throughout early childhood and until school age; these include rehospitalizations, respiratory symptoms, and poor lung function.
- Preterm-born children with BPD have worse developmental outcomes in early childhood than both preterm-born and full-term peers. At school age, they often have lower intelligence quotient and worse performance on tests of academic achievement.
- Many interventions to decrease BPD and the sequelae of BPD have been studied; few to date have been proven to decrease both BPD and later disability.

INTRODUCTION

Worldwide, 5% to 18% of infants are born early (before 37 weeks) and, despite a slight decline in recent years, 10% of infants born in the United States each year are premature.[1,2] Modern practices have led to improved survival to discharge for preterm infants throughout the world, with the most significant improvements among the smallest and most immature infants. Mortality and both the incidence and severity of morbidities of prematurity increase with decreasing gestational age.[3] Lung diseases, namely respiratory distress syndrome (RDS) and bronchopulmonary dysplasia (BPD), remain leading causes of mortality among premature infants. Although

Disclosure Statement: The author has no relevant conflicts of interest to declare.
Division of Neonatology, The Children's Hospital of Philadelphia, 2nd Floor Main Building, 3401 Civic Center Boulevard, Philadelphia, PA 19104, USA
E-mail address: demauro@email.chop.edu

Clin Perinatol 45 (2018) 439–452
https://doi.org/10.1016/j.clp.2018.05.006

historically BPD was caused by a combination of barotrauma and oxygen toxicity, BPD in modern neonatology refers primarily to an arrest of lung development that is unique to the most extremely prematurely born children.[4] Although the optimal definition of BPD is under debate, it is most commonly defined as a need for supplemental oxygen at 36 weeks postmenstrual age (PMA) (**Fig. 1**).[5] The literature suggests that mortality from BPD and RDS in the United States has fallen in recent years, from 83 deaths per 1000 live births 22 to 28 6/7 weeks in 2000 to 2003 to 68 per 1000 live births in 2008 to 2011 ($P = .002$).[6] However, this also corresponds with significantly increasing rates of BPD among the same immature infants, from 32% in 1993 to 47% in 2012 (**Fig. 2**).[3] This trend reflects, at least in part, improved survival of the most extremely premature infants.[3] This article explores what is currently known about the effects of survival with BPD on respiratory and developmental outcomes during early and middle childhood. The article then discusses the impact of efforts to reduce BPD on these outcomes. Lastly, the article briefly presents an agenda for future research to improve the outcomes of infants and children in this high-risk population.

THE IMPACT OF BRONCHOPULMONARY DYSPLASIA ON MEDICAL OUTCOMES IN EARLY CHILDHOOD

In the early years, after discharge from the hospital, BPD is associated with increased hospital readmissions as well as increased utilization of medical resources.[7-9] Smith and colleagues[7] demonstrated that among infants born less than 33 weeks and discharged from 6 level 3 neonatal intensive care units in Northern California, 49% of those with BPD and 23% of those without BPD were rehospitalized in the first year of life. In addition, children with BPD had significantly more and longer rehospitalizations.[7] The inverse is also true. Extremely preterm infants who were rehospitalized between initial discharge and 18 to 22 months were more likely to have BPD, were more likely to have received postnatal steroids for prevention or treatment of BPD, and had a longer average duration of mechanical ventilation and supplemental oxygen exposure while in the hospital.[10] Furthermore, infants who were rehospitalized were more likely to have been discharged on supplemental oxygen or diuretics.[10] Importantly, excess hospitalizations among infants with BPD are not exclusively due to

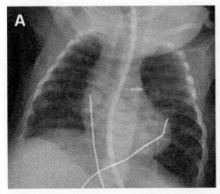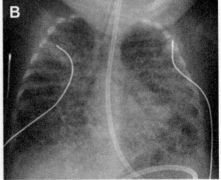

Fig. 1. Chest radiographs of infants born at 23 weeks gestation (*A*) and 26 weeks gestation (*B*), both obtained at 36 weeks PMA. Infant A remained on noninvasive positive pressure ventilation and less than 30% Fio_2, whereas infant B remained intubated with 40% to 50% Fio_2. Therefore, both met criteria for severe BPD. (*Data from* Jobe AH, Bancalari E. Bronchopulmonary dysplasia. Am J Respir Crit Care Med 2001;163(7):1723–9.)

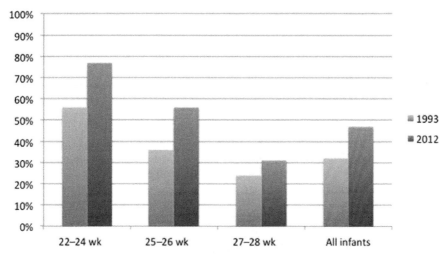

Fig. 2. BPD rates in infants who were born at 22 to 28 6/7 weeks of gestation and survived to 36 weeks postmenstrual age in 1993 and 2012. (*Data from* Stoll BJ, Hansen NI, Bell EF, et al. Trends in care practices, morbidity, and mortality of extremely preterm neonates, 1993-2012. JAMA 2015;314(10):1039–51.)

respiratory causes, highlighting the fact that children with BPD suffer from chronic illness that may affect many body systems.

Beyond hospitalizations, parents of children with BPD are far more likely to endorse respiratory symptoms and bring their children to the emergency room or doctor for these symptoms during the first 2 years of life. In the Breathing Outcomes Study conducted by the NICHD Neonatal Research Network, 48% of 918 extreme low birth weight (ELBW) study participants experienced wheezing more than twice per week during at least one 2-week period and 31% experienced more than 3 days of coughing without a cold before 18 to 22 months of age.[11] In the same cohort, 26% used inhaled steroids, 9% used systemic steroids, 63% went to the doctor, 47% went to the emergency room, and 31% were hospitalized for breathing problems.[11] Nearly all of these outcomes were significantly more common among children with BPD than among those without BPD. Furthermore, families of children with BPD were more likely to have to alter plans because of the child's breathing problems (41% vs 32%, $P<.05$).[11]

Lastly, growth failure is common among infants with BPD. This failure is concerning because both developmental outcomes and lung recovery are correlated with growth in extremely preterm infants.[12,13] Importantly, the cohort of infants with BPD who require supplemental oxygen after discharge may be at highest risk for poor growth after discharge and the associated sequelae.[9]

THE IMPACT OF BRONCHOPULMONARY DYSPLASIA ON DEVELOPMENTAL OUTCOMES IN EARLY CHILDHOOD

Several large trials and cohort studies have demonstrated increased risk for delays in development during early childhood in preterm-born children with BPD, when compared with preterms without BPD.[13–18] In a single-center cohort of ELBW infants born in the mid-1990s, Hack and colleagues[16] reported that BPD significantly increased odds of both scoring less than 70 (2 standard deviations below the expected population mean of 100) on the Bayley Scales of Infant Development: 2nd Edition Mental Development Index (MDI) (adjusted odds ratio [aOR] 2.18) and being diagnosed with a neurologic abnormality (aOR 2.46) at 20 months corrected age. In a multicenter cohort from the same era, Vohr reported that BPD was an independent risk factor for Bayley MDI less than 70, Bayley Psychomotor Development Index (PDI) <70, failure to walk independently, and failure to feed independently by 18 to 22 months corrected age.[17] In a large cohort of 3-year-olds with and without BPD, BPD was significantly associated with increased risk for both mild and severe neurodevelopmental disability.[13] In a longitudinal study, Singer and colleagues[18] compared preterm-born children with BPD to very low birth weight (VLBW) and full-term controls at 8, 12, 24, and 36 months. At all time points, the children with BPD had lower MDI and PDI scores than both control groups. In multivariable models, BPD was strongly and independently predictive of motor development (PDI) at 3 years.[18] Furthermore, in 2 separate multicenter trial cohorts, Schmidt demonstrated that BPD is independently predictive of death or developmental impairment at both 18 to 21 months corrected age and 5 years.[19,20] In these studies, the impact of BPD is similar in magnitude to, and independent of, the impact of severe brain injury or severe retinopathy of prematurity on neurodevelopmental impairment.

However, the consistency of results across these studies of early childhood assessments belies the complexity of the relationship between lung disease and outcomes. Not all infants with "BPD" have the same severity of respiratory illness or the same risk for adverse developmental outcomes over time; in fact, not all infants with BPD have poor outcomes. To date, no one characteristic or combination of characteristics have yet been identified that are sufficient to predict with certainty which infants with BPD will go on to have developmental problems. Two studies have demonstrated that infants with BPD who are discharged on supplemental oxygen do not have a specific developmental disadvantage at 1.5 to 3 years when compared with infants with BPD who are not discharged on oxygen.[13,21] On the other hand, the adjusted odds of death or developmental impairment at 18 to 22 months in preterm infants with tracheostomies are 3.3 (95% confidence interval [CI] 2.4–4.6) times higher than in those without tracheostomies.[22]

Nearly all prior studies define BPD as a dichotomous outcome, diagnosed after either 28 days of oxygen exposure or supplemental oxygen use at greater than 36 weeks postmenstrual age. Few have used more nuanced approaches to categorize children based on severity of lung disease. One study compared developmental quotient among preterm-born children with less than 28 days of oxygen, more than 28 days of oxygen, and oxygen until older than 36 weeks postmenstrual age.[23] Although there were no differences between groups based on these categorical outcomes, duration of mechanical ventilation (in days) was strongly and independently correlated with developmental quotient. Similarly, using observational data from the NICHD Neonatal Research Network, Walsh and colleagues[14] found that total duration of invasive respiratory support was correlated with risk for death or developmental impairment at 2 years in ELBW infants (**Fig. 3**). Thus, as compared with dichotomous outcomes, use of more detailed categorization schemes may allow for improved understanding of the impact of severity of neonatal lung disease on longer-term outcomes.

Given the frequency of BPD among preterm infants and the clear impact of lung disease on over the first few years of life, it is essential to also describe the longer-term impact of BPD as children grow. School age assessments are critical for understanding how medical status evolves over time. In addition, many cognitive and functional outcomes cannot be assessed until early school age.

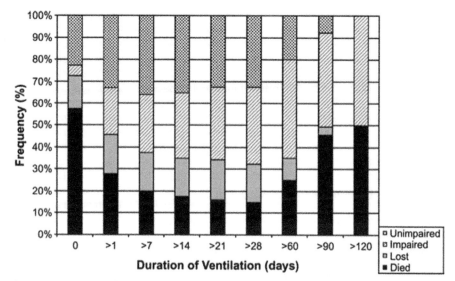

Fig. 3. Distribution of survival to 18 to 22 months corrected age with and without impairment, defined as Bayley-2 MDI less than 70, PDI less than 70, moderate or severe cerebral palsy, bilateral blindness, or deafness, among 3782 infants in the NICHD Neonatal Research Network. (*From* Walsh MC, Morris BH, Wrage LA, et al. Extremely low birthweight neonates with protracted ventilation: mortality and 18-month neurodevelopmental outcomes. J Pediatr 2005;146(6):801; with permission.)

THE IMPACT OF BRONCHOPULMONARY DYSPLASIA ON MEDICAL OUTCOMES AT SCHOOL AGE

BPD increases risk for rehospitalization during childhood. In a recent Israeli population-based study, VLBW children with BPD had significantly increased risk of rehospitalization at least through age 10 years, when compared with VLBW children without BPD.[24] In a population-based study in Washington State, teens (aged 12–20 years) with history of low or very low birth weight had increased risk of respiratory rehospitalizations; this was mediated in part by history of BPD.[25] School-age children with a history of BPD also continue to have frequent doctor visits and at least a quarter still require frequent use of bronchodilators to prevent or relieve cough or wheeze.[26,27]

School-age children with a history of prematurity have worse lung function on spirometry than term comparisons; these outcomes are even worse in the preterm-born children with BPD.[27–31] For example, in a regional follow-up study of school-age children born in Australia in the early 1990s, full-term/normal birth weight children (n = 208) had FEV_1 97.9 $\pm$ 11.8; ELBW or very preterm infants without BPD (n = 151) had FEV_1 87.1 $\pm$ 11.5; and ELBW/very preterm infants with BPD (n = 89) had FEV_1 81.1 $\pm$ 13.7.[29] Several subsequent studies have demonstrated findings consistent with these results.[27,30,31] In a systematic review of 59 studies that reported $\%FEV_1$ during childhood for preterm-born children, those who received supplemental oxygen at 36 weeks PMA had $\%FEV_1$ 18.9% lower than term-born controls.[32] These abnormal pulmonary mechanics translate into more frequent respiratory symptoms and more frequent need for respiratory medication at school age.[27] In the EPICure cohort of infants born before 26 weeks gestational age, 25% carried a diagnosis of asthma at 11 years.[27]

It has recently become apparent that adult survivors of BPD have limited exercise tolerance and increased sedentary behavior when compared with healthy adults.[33–35] Far less is known about how BPD affects functional respiratory outcomes such as exercise tolerance, health-related quality of life, and age-appropriate participation at school age. However, abnormal respiratory mechanics and frequent respiratory symptoms are likely to have important functional impact on school-age children. In a cohort of 126 10-year-old children with a history of preterm birth compared with 34 controls, the preterm-born children had significantly worse performance on some (but not all) measures of exercise capacity in addition to significantly worse lung function on spirometry.[36] Exercise capacity was reduced by more than half in the 20-meter shuttle run, although submaximal exercise capacity as measured by the 6-minute walk test was not significantly decreased in the children with BPD. Children with BPD had lower predicted peak oxygen consumption than preterms without BPD; however, similar to data from spirometry, even "healthy" preterms had predicted peak oxygen consumption far below normative data for their age. More recently, in a cohort of Canadian children born extremely preterm with and without BPD, the children with moderate or severe BPD again had significantly lower oxygen uptake during exercise capacity testing.[31] In a study of 18 children aged 8 to 9 years with a history of BPD, pulmonary function testing, 6-minute walk test distance, and quadriceps strength were significantly lower and exercise heart rate was significantly higher than full-term controls.[37] Yet, not all studies have demonstrated the same association.[38,39] Among 38 children born less than 25 weeks in the United Kingdom and Ireland and matched controls, the preterm infants had lower peak oxygen consumption.[39] In addition, the preterm-born children perceived that physical activity was harder and that they had more difficulty with breathing during exercise when compared with their friends. However, in this small sample with high rates of BPD (71% BPD), these outcomes were not different between preterm children with and without BPD. Because of the lingering uncertainties about the impact of BPD on exercise tolerance and participation at school age, future research focused on these patient-centered outcomes and, if appropriate, strategies to mitigate these effects are essential.

THE IMPACT OF BRONCHOPULMONARY DYSPLASIA ON COGNITIVE AND FUNCTIONAL OUTCOMES AT SCHOOL AGE

Adjusted odds of death or survival with disability at 5 years are 2.3 (95% CI 1.8–3.0) times higher among children with BPD than among those without BPD.[20] Understanding this association, it is critical to look beyond composite outcomes of disability to evaluate the relationships between BPD and specific aspects of development and then to assess the functional impact of these outcomes on the child and family at school age.

BPD is likely to have significant impact on school-age motor outcomes, which may have important functional implications.[40–42] For example, developmental coordination disorder (DCD) is an impairment of fine and gross motor coordination abilities that significantly interferes with performance of daily activities or academic achievement. DCD generally cannot be diagnosed until children are at least 5 years old, and the most severe form is recognized in about 25% of 5- to 14-year-old former very preterm or VLBW children.[43] BPD is a strong predictor of poor performance on the Movement-ABC assessment, the test which is most commonly used to diagnose DCD.[40] Similarly, in a small (n = 27) study of infants with severe BPD and matched preterm-born controls without BPD at 10 years, infants with BPD had significantly increased rates of abnormal neurologic outcomes, including both fine and gross motor skills, postural stability, and behavioral problems.[42]

Reports of cognitive outcomes at school age are conflicting, and many are from smaller and older cohorts with varying definitions of BPD. However, most suggest that BPD is associated with decreased intelligence quotient (IQ) when compared with both preterm controls without BPD and full-term controls (**Table 1**).[41,44–48] In a 2003 study, Short reported that 8-year-old children with BPD had worse motor, academic, attention, and cognitive skills than both preterm peers without BPD and full-term controls.[41] Furthermore, even when only children without severe neurologic injury were evaluated, both BPD and severity of BPD were associated with worse outcomes across domains and more need for therapy.[41]

On the other hand, a study of 31 infants with BPD and matched preterm controls in North Carolina reported no difference in IQ at 4 to 5 years.[49] Another study of cognitive development and visual-motor skills among 60 very preterm-born children with and without BPD reported no differences when all children with lung disease were grouped together.[50] However, those with the most severe lung disease had the worst developmental outcomes at 5.5 years. Similarly, in a small follow-up study of 11-year-old preterm-born children with and without BPD and full-term controls, Vohr and colleagues[47] reported no difference in full-scale IQ (see **Table 1**), but some children with BPD could not be tested and were therefore excluded from the analyses. They also reported significant increase in need for special assistance in the classroom and abnormal neurologic examination among the children with a history of BPD. Thus, definitions of BPD and classification of children who cannot be tested or scored have significant impact on the results of studies of school-age children with BPD.

Two single-center studies (n <100 children in each) have evaluated the impact of BPD based on the NIH consensus definition of mild, moderate, and severe disease on school-age developmental outcomes, with conflicting results.[5,51,52] In the first, children with severe BPD performed more poorly on the Bayley-2 MDI and PDI at 3 years and had lower full-scale IQ on the Wechsler Intelligence Scale for Children, third edition (WISC-III) at 8 years than those with mild or moderate BPD.[51] A second study found no differences in cognitive, motor, or language outcomes of 3- to 6-year-olds based on severity of BPD.[52]

In parallel, children with BPD have been reported in multiple studies to have worse performance on tests of educational skills than both preterm and full-term controls.[41,44,45,48,53] Those with severe BPD may have the lowest performance on

Table 1			
Full-scale intelligence quotient of school-age preterm-born children with and without BPD and full-term controls			
First Author and Publication Year	Preterm or VLBW with BPD	Preterm or VLBW Without BPD	Full-Term Controls
Vohr et al,[47] 1991	n = 13 93 ± 21	n = 15 94 ± 13	n = 15 108 ± 11
Robertson et al,[44] 1992	n = 21[a] 88 ± 21	n = 21 97 ± 20	n = 21 115 ± 10
Hughes et al,[45] 1999	n = 95 86 ± 18	n = 311 96 ± 18	n = 188 100 ± 17
Short et al,[41] 2003	n = 98 87 ± 20	n = 75 95 ± 16	n = 99 102 ± 15

[a] Born less than 32 weeks gestation with oxygen dependence at 36 weeks postmenstrual age.

language tests and most measures of academic skills.[51] Children with BPD are more likely to require speech-language services and special assistance in the classroom.[41,47] Importantly, academic success depends on far more than IQ alone; children must integrate executive function, attention, memory, and visual-spatial perception skills. To date, few of these essential aspects of neurocognitive performance have been thoroughly evaluated in large populations of children with BPD.[53,54] Furthermore, it remains unknown how lower IQ and poor academic performance at school age translate into longer-term participation and functional outcomes such as wage earning, social competency, and quality of life in adolescents and adults with BPD.

STRATEGIES TO IMPROVE OUTCOMES

Countless randomized trials have attempted to rigorously evaluate interventions or strategies to decrease the incidence of BPD and thereby improve both short- and long-term outcomes of preterm infants. The international "Caffeine for Apnea of Prematurity" trial demonstrated that neonatal treatment with caffeine reduces BPD, improves developmental outcomes at 2 years, and is associated with improved respiratory mechanics and reduced risk of motor impairment at least until 11 years.[55–58] On the other hand, although treatment with vitamin A reduces BPD, it does not improve developmental outcomes at 2 years.[10] Similarly, surfactant therapy reduces mortality and early morbidities but does not seem to improve longer-term developmental outcomes.[59]

Corticosteroids have been used antenatally, immediately postnatally, and up to several weeks after preterm birth in an effort to reduce lung inflammation and injury. Antenatal steroids reduce mortality and early respiratory distress syndrome and improve developmental outcomes at least until 2 years.[60,61] This effect is evident even down to at least 23 weeks of gestation.[61] However, antenatal steroids do not seem to reduce rates of BPD, especially in the youngest infants. In fact, infants born at 22 to 25 weeks of gestation after antenatal steroid exposure are more likely to survive with BPD than unexposed infants.[61] Postnatal treatment with dexamethasone has been repeatedly demonstrated to reduce BPD; however, use in the first week is associated with increased risk for cerebral palsy and abnormal neurologic outcomes and is therefore not recommended.[62–64] Given these concerns, a recent trial of early prophylactic hydrocortisone demonstrated that this strategy reduced BPD without increasing rates of neurodevelopmental impairment at 2 years.[65,66] Unfortunately, the reduction in BPD also did not translate into improved outcomes at 2 years.

Based on clear observational data that exposure to mechanical ventilation is associated with risk for BPD and adverse outcomes, several trials attempted to decrease rates of intubation and use of mechanical ventilation after birth in extremely preterm infants. These individual trials have failed to demonstrate improved rates of death or BPD.[67,68] However, a meta-analysis of these trials reports a relative risk of death or BPD of 0.91 (95% CI 0.84–0.99) favoring CPAP over immediate intubation at birth for preterm infants less than 32 weeks of gestation.[69] With a 4% risk difference, this translates into a number-needed-to-treat of 25. In the SUPPORT trial, use of noninvasive support in the delivery room was associated with less use of postnatal steroids for treatment of BPD and shorter duration of ventilation during the neonatal hospitalization.[67] At 2 years, this was associated with fewer episodes of wheezing without a cold, respiratory illnesses, and physician or emergency room visits for breathing problems but no improvement in developmental outcomes.[11,70] In fact, recent work from the Victorian Infant Collaborative Study Group in Australia suggests that despite decreasing use of noninvasive respiratory support over time, respiratory and developmental outcomes in school-age children who were born extremely premature may actually be getting worse.[71,72]

The optimal approach to management of children with BPD after discharge from the hospital is unknown. Little published data are available to guide clinical decision-making for those infants discharged on supplemental oxygen; therefore, oxygen saturation targets, rate of supplemental oxygen titration, and criteria for discontinuation vary widely.[73,74] Management of medication, including diuretics, bronchodilators, inhaled steroids, and many others, is at times performed by general practitioners, pediatricians, developmental follow-up clinics, or pulmonologists. Although early aggressive and goal-directed therapies are increasingly recognized as integral for children at risk for motor disorders, these have not yet been studied specifically in the context of BPD.[75]

Perhaps most importantly, pulmonary function and exercise capacity are linked with cognitive function throughout the lifespan.[76,77] Physical activity interventions improve outcomes of children with attention and behavior problems and improve executive functioning.[78–80] In parallel, increased sedentary behavior is negatively associated with some cognitive outcomes.[81] One study even reported an association between motor development during infancy and cognitive performance at an average age of 64 years.[82] Exercise training or rehabilitation programs improve quality of life and respiratory symptoms for adults with chronic obstructive pulmonary disease; whether the same is true for children with BPD is not known.[83]

SUMMARY AND FUTURE DIRECTIONS

BPD is associated with adverse developmental and medical outcomes both in early childhood and at least through school age. Therefore, BPD imposes a significant burden on infants and children, their families, and society. Whether and how strongly BPD influences trajectories of disease and health over the lifespan remains largely unexplored. Lung function worsens over the lifespan in normal, healthy people. It remains unknown whether lung function deteriorates more quickly in people with a history of BPD and whether this or even a normal trajectory of decline will position adult survivors of BPD for earlier onset of respiratory failure or even mortality.[84]

The current research predominantly uses dichotomous outcomes of "BPD," most recently leaning heavily on the National Institutes of Health consensus definition of supplemental oxygen use at 36 weeks postmenstrual age.[5] However, this definition has been questioned because it is not consistently predictive of longer-term clinically important outcomes and is based on treatment decisions rather than physiology.[85,86] As described earlier, duration of ventilation is independently predictive of developmental outcomes at least until 2 years. Such a graded relationship between severity of lung disease and outcomes has not yet been clearly demonstrated beyond 2 years. It is possible that in future research, more nuanced description of the spectrum of neonatal lung disease will allow investigators to draw stronger associations with specific adverse neurocognitive and respiratory outcomes.

Few therapies have definitively improved both BPD and the longer-term outcomes that are associated with BPD. In future work, it will be essential for neonatologists to continue to pursue therapies that limit damage to the preterm lung and reduce BPD as aggressively as possible. This must include evaluation of treatments and management strategies both in the neonatal intensive care unit and after discharge. Beneficial strategies may include not only modifications of current care such as different approaches to ventilation but also novel therapeutics in the neonatal period, including stem cell therapy, liquid ventilation, and use of the artificial womb and aggressive pulmonary rehabilitation and exercise training for children with BPD. Long-term follow-up will be critical for understanding the influence of these new interventions on functional outcomes of children with BPD over the lifespan.

REFERENCES

1. Blencowe H, Cousens S, Oestergaard MZ, et al. National, regional, and worldwide estimates of preterm birth rates in the year 2010 with time trends since 1990 for selected countries: a systematic analysis and implications. Lancet 2012;379(9832):2162–72.
2. March of Dimes Peristats. Available at: www.marchofdimes.org/peristats. Accessed October 1, 2017.
3. Stoll BJ, Hansen NI, Bell EF, et al. Trends in care practices, morbidity, and mortality of extremely preterm neonates, 1993-2012. JAMA 2015;314(10):1039–51.
4. Jobe AJ. The new BPD: an arrest of lung development. Pediatr Res 1999;46(6): 641–3.
5. Jobe AH, Bancalari E. Bronchopulmonary dysplasia. Am J Respir Crit Care Med 2001;163(7):1723–9.
6. Patel RM, Kandefer S, Walsh MC, et al. Causes and timing of death in extremely premature infants from 2000 through 2011. N Engl J Med 2015;372(4):331–40.
7. Smith VC, Zupancic JAF, McCormick MC, et al. Rehospitalization in the first year of life among infants with bronchopulmonary dysplasia. J Pediatr 2004;144(6): 799–803.
8. Gross SJ, Iannuzzi DM, Kveselis DA, et al. Effect of preterm birth on pulmonary function at school age: a prospective controlled study. J Pediatr 1998;133(2): 188–92.
9. Chye JK, Gray PH. Rehospitalization and growth of infants with bronchopulmonary dysplasia: a matched control study. J Paediatr Child Health 1995;31(2): 105–11.
10. Ambalavanan N, Carlo WA, McDonald SA, et al. Identification of extremely premature infants at high risk of rehospitalization. Pediatrics 2011;128(5):e1216–25.
11. Stevens TP, Finer NN, Carlo WA, et al. Respiratory outcomes of the surfactant positive pressure and oximetry randomized trial (SUPPORT). J Pediatr 2014; 165(2):240–9.e4.
12. Ehrenkranz RA, Dusick AM, Vohr BR, et al. Growth in the neonatal intensive care unit influences neurodevelopmental and growth outcomes of extremely low birth weight infants. Pediatrics 2006;117(4):1253–61.
13. Lodha A, Sauvé R, Bhandari V, et al. Need for supplemental oxygen at discharge in infants with bronchopulmonary dysplasia is not associated with worse neurodevelopmental outcomes at 3 years corrected age. PLoS One 2014;9(3):e90843.
14. Walsh MC, Morris BH, Wrage LA, et al. Extremely low birthweight neonates with protracted ventilation: mortality and 18-month neurodevelopmental outcomes. J Pediatr 2005;146(6):798–804.
15. Lifschitz MH, Seilheimer DK, Wilson GS, et al. Neurodevelopmental status of low birth weight infants with bronchopulmonary dysplasia requiring prolonged oxygen supplementation. J Perinatol 1987;7(2):127–32.
16. Hack M, Wilson-Costello D, Friedman H, et al. Neurodevelopment and predictors of outcomes of children with birth weights of less than 1000 g: 1992-1995. Arch Pediatr Adolesc Med 2000;154(7):725–31.

17. Vohr BR, Wright LL, Dusick AM, et al. Neurodevelopmental and functional outcomes of extremely low birth weight infants in the National Institute of Child Health and Human Development Neonatal Research Network, 1993-1994. Pediatrics 2000;105(6):1216–26.
18. Singer L, Yamashita T, Lilien L, et al. A longitudinal study of developmental outcome of infants with bronchopulmonary dysplasia and very low birth weight. Pediatrics 1997;100(6):987–93.
19. Schmidt B, Asztalos EV, Roberts RS, et al. Impact of bronchopulmonary dysplasia, brain injury, and severe retinopathy on the outcome of extremely low-birth-weight infants at 18 months: results from the trial of indomethacin prophylaxis in preterms. JAMA 2003;289(9):1124–9.
20. Schmidt B, Roberts RS, Davis PG, et al. Prediction of late death or disability at age 5 years using a count of 3 neonatal morbidities in very low birth weight infants. J Pediatr 2015;167(5):982–6.e2.
21. Trittmann JK, Nelin LD, Klebanoff MA. Bronchopulmonary dysplasia and neurodevelopmental outcome in extremely preterm neonates. Eur J Pediatr 2013; 172(9):1173–80.
22. DeMauro SB, D'Agostino JA, Bann C, et al. Developmental outcomes of very preterm infants with tracheostomies. J Pediatr 2014;164(6):1303–10.e2.
23. Grégoire MC, Lefebvre F, Glorieux J. Health and developmental outcomes at 18 months in very preterm infants with bronchopulmonary dysplasia. Pediatrics 1998;101(5):856–60.
24. Kuint J, Lerner-Geva L, Chodick G, et al. Rehospitalization through childhood and adolescence: association with neonatal morbidities in infants of very low birth weight. J Pediatr 2017;188:135–41.e2.
25. Walter EC, Koepsell TD, Chien JW. Low birth weight and respiratory hospitalizations in adolescence. Pediatr Pulmonol 2011;46(5):473–82.
26. Greenough A, Alexander J, Boorman J, et al. Respiratory morbidity, healthcare utilisation and cost of care at school age related to home oxygen status. Eur J Pediatr 2011;170(8):969–75.
27. Fawke J, Lum S, Kirkby J, et al. Lung function and respiratory symptoms at 11 years in children born extremely preterm: the EPICure study. Am J Respir Crit Care Med 2010;182(2):237–45.
28. Pelkonen AS, Hakulinen AL, Turpeinen M. Bronchial lability and responsiveness in school children born very preterm. Am J Respir Crit Care Med 1997;156(4 Pt 1): 1178–84.
29. Doyle LW, Victorian Infant Collaborative Study Group. Respiratory function at age 8-9 years in extremely low birthweight/very preterm children born in Victoria in 1991-1992. Pediatr Pulmonol 2006;41(6):570–6.
30. Hove Vom M, Prenzel F, Uhlig HH, et al. Pulmonary outcome in former preterm, very low birth weight children with bronchopulmonary dysplasia: a case-control follow-up at school age. J Pediatr 2014;164(1):40–5.e4.
31. MacLean JE, DeHaan K, Fuhr D, et al. Altered breathing mechanics and ventilatory response during exercise in children born extremely preterm. Thorax 2016; 71(11):1012–9.
32. Kotecha SJ, Edwards MO, Watkins WJ, et al. Effect of preterm birth on later FEV1: a systematic review and meta-analysis. Thorax 2013;68(8):760–6.
33. Landry JS, Tremblay GM, Li PZ, et al. Lung function and bronchial hyperresponsiveness in adults born prematurely. a cohort study. Ann Am Thorac Soc 2016; 13(1):17–24.

34. Lovering AT, Elliott JE, Laurie SS, et al. Ventilatory and sensory responses in adult survivors of preterm birth and bronchopulmonary dysplasia with reduced exercise capacity. Ann Am Thorac Soc 2014;11(10):1528–37.

35. Malleske DT, Chorna O, Maitre NL. Pulmonary sequelae and functional limitations in children and adults with bronchopulmonary dysplasia. Paediatr Respir Rev 2018;26:55–9.

36. Smith LJ, van Asperen PP, McKay KO, et al. Reduced exercise capacity in children born very preterm. Pediatrics 2008;122(2):e287–93.

37. Vardar-Yagli N, Inal-Ince D, Saglam M, et al. Pulmonary and extrapulmonary features in bronchopulmonary dysplasia: a comparison with healthy children. J Phys Ther Sci 2015;27(6):1761–5.

38. Bader D, Ramos AD, Lew CD, et al. Childhood sequelae of infant lung disease: exercise and pulmonary function abnormalities after bronchopulmonary dysplasia. J Pediatr 1987;110(5):693–9.

39. Welsh L, Kirkby J, Lum S, et al. The EPICure study: maximal exercise and physical activity in school children born extremely preterm. Thorax 2010;65(2):165–72.

40. Dewey D, Creighton DE, Heath JA, et al. Assessment of developmental coordination disorder in children born with extremely low birth weights. Dev Neuropsychol 2011;36(1):42–56.

41. Short EJ, Klein NK, Lewis BA, et al. Cognitive and academic consequences of bronchopulmonary dysplasia and very low birth weight: 8-year-old outcomes. Pediatrics 2003;112(5):e359.

42. Majnemer A, Riley P, Shevell M, et al. Severe bronchopulmonary dysplasia increases risk for later neurological and motor sequelae in preterm survivors. Dev Med Child Neurol 2000;42(1):53–60.

43. Edwards J, Berube M, Erlandson K, et al. Developmental coordination disorder in school-aged children born very preterm and/or at very low birth weight: a systematic review. J Dev Behav Pediatr 2011;32(9):678–87.

44. Robertson CM, Etches PC, Goldson E, et al. Eight-year school performance, neurodevelopmental, and growth outcome of neonates with bronchopulmonary dysplasia: a comparative study. Pediatrics 1992;89(3):365–72.

45. Hughes CA, O'Gorman LA, Shyr Y, et al. Cognitive performance at school age of very low birth weight infants with bronchopulmonary dysplasia. J Dev Behav Pediatr 1999;20(1):1–8.

46. Taylor HG, Klein N, Schatschneider C, et al. Predictors of early school age outcomes in very low birth weight children. J Dev Behav Pediatr 1998;19(4):235–43.

47. Vohr BR, Coll CG, Lobato D, et al. Neurodevelopmental and medical status of low-birthweight survivors of bronchopulmonary dysplasia at 10 to 12 years of age. Dev Med Child Neurol 1991;33(8):690–7.

48. Gray PH, O'Callaghan MJ, Rogers YM. Psychoeducational outcome at school age of preterm infants with bronchopulmonary dysplasia. J Paediatr Child Health 2004;40(3):114–20.

49. O'Shea TM, Goldstein DJ, deRegnier RA, et al. Outcome at 4 to 5 years of age in children recovered from neonatal chronic lung disease. Dev Med Child Neurol 1996;38(9):830–9.

50. Böhm B, Katz-Salamon M. Cognitive development at 5.5 years of children with chronic lung disease of prematurity. Arch Dis Child Fetal Neonatal Ed 2003; 88(2):F101–5.

51. Short EJ, Kirchner HL, Asaad GR, et al. Developmental sequelae in preterm infants having a diagnosis of bronchopulmonary dysplasia: analysis using a

severity-based classification system. Arch Pediatr Adolesc Med 2007;161(11):
1082–7.

52. Newman JB, Debastos AG, Batton D, et al. Neonatal respiratory dysfunction and
neuropsychological performance at the preschool age: a study of very preterm
infants with bronchopulmonary dysplasia. Neuropsychology 2011;25(5):666–78.

53. Farel AM, Hooper SR, Teplin SW, et al. Very-low-birthweight infants at seven
years: an assessment of the health and neurodevelopmental risk conveyed by
chronic lung disease. J Learn Disabil 1998;31(2):118–26.

54. Anderson PJ, Doyle LW. Neurodevelopmental outcome of bronchopulmonary
dysplasia. Semin Perinatol 2006;30(4):227–32.

55. Doyle LW, Ranganathan S, Cheong JLY. Neonatal caffeine treatment and respiratory function at 11 years in children <1251 g birth weight. Am J Respir Crit Care
Med 2017;196:1318–24.

56. Schmidt B, Roberts RS, Davis P, et al. Caffeine therapy for apnea of prematurity.
N Engl J Med 2006;354(20):2112–21.

57. Schmidt B, Roberts RS, Davis P, et al. Long-term effects of caffeine therapy for
apnea of prematurity. N Engl J Med 2007;357(19):1893–902.

58. Schmidt B, Roberts RS, Anderson PJ, et al. Academic performance, motor function, and behavior 11 years after neonatal caffeine citrate therapy for apnea of
prematurity: an 11-year follow-up of the CAP randomized clinical trial. JAMA Pediatr 2017;171(6):564–72.

59. Sinn JKH, Ward MC, Henderson-Smart DJ. Developmental outcome of preterm
infants after surfactant therapy: systematic review of randomized controlled trials.
J Paediatr Child Health 2002;38(6):597–600.

60. Roberts D, Dalziel S. Antenatal corticosteroids for accelerating fetal lung
maturation for women at risk of preterm birth. Cochrane Database Syst Rev
2006;(3):CD004454.

61. Carlo WA, McDonald SA, Fanaroff AA, et al. Association of antenatal corticosteroids with mortality and neurodevelopmental outcomes among infants born at 22
to 25 weeks' gestation. JAMA 2011;306(21):2348–58.

62. Halliday HL, Ehrenkranz RA, Doyle LW. Delayed (>3 weeks) postnatal corticosteroids for chronic lung disease in preterm infants. Cochrane Database Syst Rev
2003;(1):CD001145.

63. Halliday HL, Ehrenkranz RA, Doyle LW. Early postnatal (<96 hours) corticosteroids for preventing chronic lung disease in preterm infants. Cochrane Database
Syst Rev 2003;(1):CD001146.

64. Halliday HL, Ehrenkranz RA, Doyle LW. Moderately early (7-14 days) postnatal
corticosteroids for preventing chronic lung disease in preterm infants. Cochrane
Database Syst Rev 2003;(1):CD001144.

65. Baud O, Maury L, Lebail F, et al. Effect of early low-dose hydrocortisone on survival without bronchopulmonary dysplasia in extremely preterm infants (PREMI-
LOC): a double-blind, placebo-controlled, multicentre, randomised trial. Lancet
2016;387(10030):1827–36.

66. Baud O, Trousson C, Biran V, et al. Association between early low-dose hydrocortisone therapy in extremely preterm neonates and neurodevelopmental outcomes
at 2 years of age. JAMA 2017;317(13):1329–37.

67. Finer NN. Early CPAP versus surfactant in extremely preterm infants (vol 362, pg
1970, 2010). N Engl J Med 2010;362(23):2235.

68. Morley CJ, Davis PG, Doyle LW, et al. Nasal CPAP or intubation at birth for very
preterm infants. N Engl J Med 2008;358(7):700–8.

69. Schmölzer GM, Kumar M, Pichler G, et al. Non-invasive versus invasive respiratory support in preterm infants at birth: systematic review and meta-analysis. BMJ 2013;347:f5980.
70. Vaucher YE, Peralta-Carcelen M, Finer NN, et al. Neurodevelopmental outcomes in the early CPAP and pulse oximetry trial. N Engl J Med 2012;367(26):2495–504.
71. Doyle LW, Carse E, Adams A-M, et al. Ventilation in extremely preterm infants and respiratory function at 8 years. N Engl J Med 2017;377(4):329–37.
72. Cheong JLY, Anderson PJ, Burnett AC, et al. Changing neurodevelopment at 8 years in children born extremely preterm since the 1990s. Pediatrics 2017; 139(6):e20164086.
73. Ellsbury DL, Acarregui MJ, McGuinness GA, et al. Controversy surrounding the use of home oxygen for premature infants with bronchopulmonary dysplasia. J Perinatol 2004;24(1):36–40.
74. Palm K, Simoneau T, Sawicki G, et al. Assessment of current strategies for weaning premature infants from supplemental oxygen in the outpatient setting. Adv Neonatal Care 2011;11(5):349–56.
75. Novak I, Morgan C, Adde L, et al. Early, accurate diagnosis and early intervention in cerebral palsy: advances in diagnosis and treatment. JAMA Pediatr 2017; 171(9):897–907.
76. Carroll D, Batty GD, Mortensen LH, et al. Low cognitive ability in early adulthood is associated with reduced lung function in middle age: the Vietnam experience study. Thorax 2011;66(10):884–8.
77. Svedenkrans J, Kowalski J, Norman M, et al. Low exercise capacity increases the risk of low cognitive function in healthy young men born preterm: a population-based cohort study. PLoS One 2016;11(8):e0161314.
78. Tomporowski PD, Lambourne K, Okumura MS. Physical activity interventions and children's mental function: an introduction and overview. Prev Med 2011; 52(Suppl 1):S3–9.
79. Heijer Den AE, Groen Y, Tucha L, et al. Sweat it out? The effects of physical exercise on cognition and behavior in children and adults with ADHD: a systematic literature review. J Neural Transm (Vienna) 2017;124(Suppl 1):3–26.
80. Bowling A, Slavet J, Miller DP, et al. Cybercycling effects on classroom behavior in children with behavioral health disorders: an RCT. Pediatrics 2017;139(2): e20161985.
81. Carson V, Kuzik N, Hunter S, et al. Systematic review of sedentary behavior and cognitive development in early childhood. Prev Med 2015;78:115–22.
82. Poranen-Clark T, Bonsdorff von MB, Lahti J, et al. Infant motor development and cognitive performance in early old age: the Helsinki Birth Cohort Study. Age (Dordr) 2015;37(3):9785.
83. McCarthy B, Casey D, Devane D, et al. Pulmonary rehabilitation for chronic obstructive pulmonary disease. Cochrane Database Syst Rev 2015;(2):CD003793.
84. Doyle LW, Faber B, Callanan C, et al. Bronchopulmonary dysplasia in very low birth weight subjects and lung function in late adolescence. Pediatrics 2006; 118(1):108–13.
85. Poindexter BB, Feng R, Schmidt B, et al. Comparisons and limitations of current definitions of bronchopulmonary dysplasia for the prematurity and respiratory outcomes program. Ann Am Thorac Soc 2015;12(12):1822–30.
86. Isayama T, Lee SK, Yang J, et al. Revisiting the definition of bronchopulmonary dysplasia: effect of changing panoply of respiratory support for preterm neonates. JAMA Pediatr 2017;171(3):271–9.

Necrotizing Enterocolitis and Neurodevelopmental Outcome

Ira Adams-Chapman, MD, MPH

KEYWORDS

• Necrotizing enterocolitis • Neurodevelopment • Sepsis • Follow-up

KEY POINTS

- Surgical necrotizing enterocolitis (NEC) is associated with adverse neurodevelopmental outcome.
- Morbidities associated with NEC increase the risk for central nervous system injury in preterm infants.
- Additional data are needed to determine whether surgical drain or laparotomy is associated with the best neurocognitive outcome in preterm infants.

INTRODUCTION

Necrotizing enterocolitis (NEC) is a devastating complication of prematurity affecting 3% to 9% of prematurely born infants.[1–3] Although the etiology is poorly understood, it is most likely multifactorial, including a combination of factors, such as immaturity of the developing gastrointestinal (GI) tract, imbalance of immune mediators in the GI tract, inflammatory response to tissue injury, and bacterial invasion. This diseases manifests clinically on a spectrum from mild clinical disease associated with feeding intolerance to bowel perforation and tissue necrosis. The risk for NEC is clearly inversely associated with gestational age, but neonates of all gestational ages can be affected, including term infants. Those who require surgical intervention are known to have an increased risk for adverse neurodevelopmental (ND) outcome, including an increased risk for cerebral palsy and cognitive impairment. Limited data are available on the ND outcome of affected term infants. In this review, we highlight various factors that are likely contributors to the increased risk for adverse ND outcome in preterm infants with a history of NEC.

Disclosure Statement: The author has no commercial or financial conflicts of interests or any funding sources.
Department of Pediatrics, Division of Neonatology, Emory University School of Medicine, Children's Healthcare of Atlanta, 2015 Uppergate Drive, Atlanta, GA 30303, USA
E-mail address: iadamsc@emory.edu

PATHOGENESIS OF NECROTIZING ENTEROCOLITIS

Despite decades of research and prevention strategies to prevent NEC, the etiology of this disease remains elusive. Limited understanding has been learned from animal studies, but these models are considered by many to be poorly representative of neonatal disease.[4] NEC is a disease that primarily affects preterm infants. Thus, the immaturity of the preterm GI tract has long been considered a contributing factor. Researchers have identified various factors in the immature GI tract that may predispose to the development of this disease, including innate gut immaturity, immature immune response, bacterial colonization patterns in the preterm infant, and regulation of blood flow to the GI tract.[2,3] It is beyond the scope of this review to discuss these factors in detail. However, they have been outlined by other investigators[3,5] and the schematic in **Fig. 1** provides an overview of the possible mechanisms involved (see **Fig. 1**).[5]

The risk for both disease and the need for surgical intervention varies inversely with gestational age.[6,7] In a review by Stoll and colleagues[7] in the Neonatal Research Network (NRN) evaluating trends in neonatal morbidity over the past 20 years for

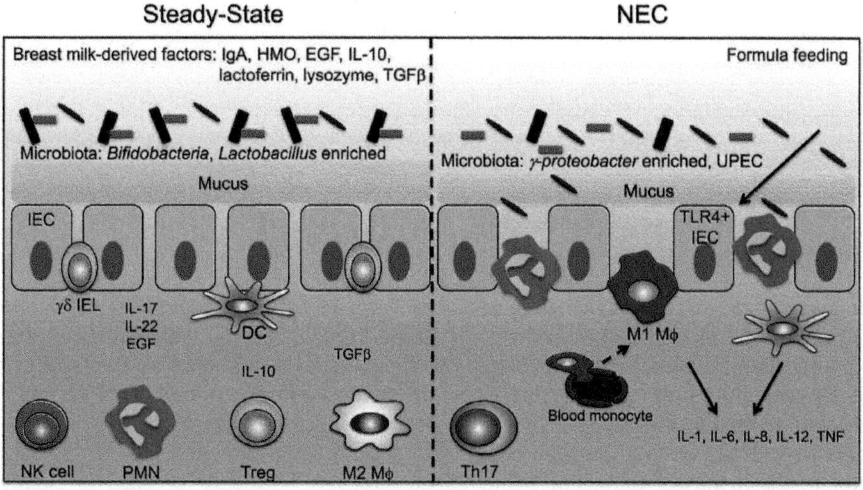

Fig. 1. Premature infant gut in the steady state and during NEC. In the steady state, homeostasis is promoted by beneficial bacteria (*Bifidobacteria* and *Lactobacillus*) and breast milk components (immunoglobulin A, human milk oligosaccharides [HMO], epidermal growth factor [EGF], IL-10, lactoferrin, lysozyme, TGF-β). In the preterm gut, γδ intraepithelial lymphocytes (IELs) are among the first intestinal-resident immune cells contributing to the maintenance of epithelial integrity via IL-17A and EGF. Natural killer (NK) cells also protect against and repair barrier damage. Neutrophils (PMN) may be important during initial colonization in the neonatal gut, providing transient barrier protection in response to threats from potentially pathogenic bacteria, via IL-22 production. Resident macrophages (Mφ) and dendritic cells (DCs) maintain tolerance toward the intestinal microbiota via the production of IL-10, which, in combination with TGF-β, induce regulatory T (Treg) cells. During NEC, lack of breast milk protective components and dysbiotic flora (eg, Gammaproteobacter) may allow barrier breakdown and bacterial translocation. This leads to innate signaling via Toll-like receptor 4 (TLR-4) (in response to PAF and LPS), which in turn causes recruitment of neutrophils and monocytes into the intestine, where they, along with resident DCs, drive proinflammatory cytokine production, including IL-1β, TNF, IL-8, and IL-12, which can promote pathogenic Th1 and Th17 responses. UPEC, uropathogenic E. Coli. (*From* Denning TL, Bhatia AM, Kane AF, et al. Pathogenesis of NEC: role of the innate and adaptive immune response. Semin Perinatol 2017;41(1):22; with permission.)

34,636 very low birth weight infants of <1500 g, after an increase in the NEC prevalence rate from 7% to 13% between 1993 and 2008, there was a statistically significant decrease between 2009 and 2012 to 9%. Similarly, the associated mortality rate ranges from 15% to 35%, with the greatest risk being among those of lowest birth weight.[7] Overall mortality for surgically treated NEC among very low birthweight infants is approximately 35% compared with 21% in those treated medically.[8]

Most affected infants have received enteral feedings; therefore, the type of feeding and rate of feeding advancement are often discussed as critical variables in the causal pathway for this disease. Although data are limited, it does not appear that rate of feeding advancement is associated with an increased risk for NEC.[3,9] In a Cochrane Library meta-analysis published in 2017, slow feeding advancement did not affect the risk of NEC or all-cause mortality but may have delayed time to reach full feeds and increased the risk for invasive bloodstream infections.[9] Even so, most clinicians exercise caution as feeds are introduced into the immature GI tract of these medically fragile patients. Careful attention is needed to monitor for signs of feeding intolerance, ileus, or early clinical signs of NEC, which can often be nonspecific. This caution is balanced by the desire to decrease catheter days, which has been associated with an increased risk of nosocomial infections. Some investigators are evaluating the role of noninvasive near-infrared spectroscopy measurements to screen for changes in blood flow to the gastrointestinal tract as a potential early indicator of NEC.[10,11]

Spontaneous intestinal perforation (SIP) is a distinct clinical scenario affecting preterm infants that may be difficult to distinguish from NEC. It occurs in approximately 2% of extremely low birthweight (ELBW) infants.[12,13] This disease tends to present earlier and often occurs before the initiation of enteral feedings. The underlying pathophysiology is likely different from the etiology of NEC. The immature premature GI tract is at risk for ischemic injury, and isolated focal perforation can occur. These infants are noted to have a pneumoperitoneum but are often not clinically compromised and do not exhibit evidence of multisystem organ dysfunction. The associated inflammatory response is nonexistent or mild. Unlike classic NEC, these children often have not initiated enteral feedings and the event tends to occur at an earlier postnatal age. All of these variables suggest that the pathogenesis of SIP is likely different from what occurs in patients with NEC. The resultant cytokine response is muted, which may potentially result in a decreased risk for cytokine-mediated brain injury. The ability to distinguish the difference between a diagnosis of NEC and SIP can be difficult, particularly in those children who do not ultimately require surgical intervention.

MORBIDITIES ASSOCIATED WITH NECROTIZING ENTEROCOLITIS AND BRAIN INJURY

Children with surgical NEC have a higher risk of both short-term and long-term complications. The body generates a systemic inflammatory response when an infant develops NEC secondary to the bowel injury and necrosis. The upregulation of proinflammatory mediators is typically generalized and not localized to the site of bowel injury. Therefore, many of the downstream consequences of NEC, including the risk for central nervous system (CNS) injury, may be a result of this generalized systemic inflammatory response. Many of the same cytokines implicated in the pathogenesis of NEC have also been associated with cytotoxic injury to the premature brain.[14–16] In addition, many of these children develop cardiac compromise and hypotension, resulting in decreased perfusion to the CNS. The combination of ischemia and inflammation has deleterious effects on the developing brain. These children are at risk for sepsis associated with the primary insult or secondary to the need for prolonged parenteral nutrition requiring central venous access.[17,18] Sepsis is a known risk factor for adverse neurologic outcome in the preterm infants.[19] The long-term implications of compromised nutritional intake due to the disruption in enteral feed are concerning but yet unknown. However, as outlined by Fisher and colleagues,[13] the morbidity profile for children with either SIP or NEC is higher than a general preterm cohort, and those with NEC are at greatest risk for these complications. All of these morbidities are associated with an increased risk of adverse ND outcome (**Table 1**). The relationship between NEC and associated neonatal morbidities creates a complex web, which has an additive impact on the risk for adverse neurologic outcome.

NECROTIZING ENTEROCOLITIS, INFECTION, AND INFLAMMATION

NEC is an inflammatory condition that starts as a focal process but often progresses to involve more extensive segments of bowel resulting in necrosis and/or perforation. Many affected infants develop overwhelming sepsis or generate a systemic inflammatory response often associated with hypotension, respiratory failure, and disseminated intravascular coagulopathy. The resultant cytokinemia can potentially affect the developing brain and increase the risk for both intraventricular hemorrhage and white matter injury, both of which are associated with adverse neurodevelopmental outcome.

Although the pathophysiology resulting in NEC is most likely multifactorial, it appears clear from both clinical and animal research studies that inflammation of the GI tract is an important contributor. NEC appears to be a result of overactivation of the immune system in response to some type of insult (ischemia, infection, bacterial translocation, response to feeding stimulus) that involves the GI tract.[6] The resultant immune response results in disruption of the GI epithelial barrier and activation of secondary cytokines. The GI tract of the premature infant has decreased integrity of

Table 1
Comorbid conditions and exposures

Measure	Baseline (No NEC No SIP; n = 171,506)	Laparotomy-Confirmed SIP (n = 2036)	Laparotomy-Confirmed NEC (n = 4076)	P (SIP vs NEC)
PDA, %	38.4	72.4	56.9	<.001
IVH, %	24.1	49.1	37.5	<.001
Cystic PVL, %	2.7	8.2	7.7	.485
Early bacterial sepsis, %	1.7	2.8	2.9	.784
Late bacterial pathogen, %	8.4	27.1	34.3	<.001
Coagulase-negative staphylococci, %	9.0	25.9	25.8	.945
Fungal infection, %	1.2	7.4	6.0	.027
PDA ligation, %	8.7	36.2	21.4	<.001
Indomethacin, %	24.5	48.6	36.4	<.001
Antenatal steroids, %	78.0	76.0	76.9	.449
Steroids for CLD, %	8.4	21.3	15.5	<.001
Indomethacin and steroids for CLD, %	4.2	11.4	7.3	<.001

Abbreviations: CLD, chronic lung disease; IVH, intraventricular hemorrhage; NEC, necrotizing enterocolitis; PDA, patent ductus arteriosus; PVL, periventricular leukemia; SIP, spontaneous intestinal perforation.

From Fisher JG, Jones BA, Gutierrez IM, et al. Mortality associated with laparotomy-confirmed neonatal spontaneous intestinal perforation: a prospective 5-year multicenter analysis. J Pediatr Surg 2014;49(8):1217; with permission.

barrier protection and tight junctions, resulting in increased permeability and altered regeneration after injury. The premature gut may have limited ability to generate appropriate immune response to nosocomial bacteria or respond appropriately to colonization of commensal bacteria. Ischemia to the bowel wall has long been implicated as an essential role in the pathophysiology of NEC; however, reperfusion is required to stimulate the inflammatory cascade that is known in vitro to be deleterious to bowel wall integrity.[3]

The counterregulation of proinflammatory and anti-inflammatory mediators is likely a critical component of bowel injury in NEC. Nitric oxide (NO) produced in low levels results in vasodilatation in the GI tract during homeostasis. In the face of bowel injury and high levels of NO, this cytokine may be directly cytotoxic to enterocytes.[6] Platelet-activating factor (PAF) is considered an endogenous inflammatory mediator and causes direct bowel injury via production of oxygen free radicals. Elevated PAF levels have been reported in neonates with NEC.[6] Lipopolysaccharide (LPS) has long been implicated in the cytokine-mediated bowel injury associated with NEC. It disrupts intestinal barrier protection and also activates the production of other cytokine mediators that cause direct bowel injury. LPS also potentiates the deleterious effects of PAF.

Previous reports have shown that preterm neonates with a history of NEC have increased tissue and plasma levels of various inflammatory mediators, including tumor necrosis factor (TNF), interleukin (IL)-1β, IL-6, and IL-8. Lodha and colleagues[19] evaluated the relationship between cytokine levels in neonates with NEC and neurodevelopmental outcomes at 24 to 48 months. They evaluated 40 neonates of whom 13 were controls, 17 had feeding intolerance, and 10 had stage 2 or 3 NEC based on the Bell staging criteria. IL-6 levels were elevated in those with NEC. Developmental delay was more common among those with NEC compared with unaffected infants, and these children tended to have elevation of cytokines.

There is evidence that certain cytokines may be involved in the pathogenesis of NEC, including TNF, IL-1β, IL-6, and IL-8.[14,15,20] These cytokines are important because they also have the potential to disrupt the GI barrier and stimulate cytokine-mediated injury in the gut. Some researchers have shown that a deficiency of transforming growth factor (TGF)-β is associated with an increased risk of NEC. TGF-β typically downregulates the immune response from macrophages. However, in a state of deficiency, an exaggerated immune response results when the GI tract is exposed to an infectious stimulus. Some have postulated that this deficiency and resultant immune response results in additional bowel injury. Maheshwari and colleagues[16] evaluated cytokine levels in 104 infants with NEC and compared them with 893 infants who did not develop NEC. Serial cytokine measurements were obtained on day of life 1, 7, 14, and 21 and correlated with clinical symptoms.[16] They found that infants with NEC were more likely to have low TGF-β levels at all time points. NEC was associated with increased expression of IL-6, IL-8, chemokine ligand 8, IL-10, IL-18, CCL2, CCL3, neurotrophin-4, and C-reactive protein.[16] Other studies have implicated a similar profile of cytokine elevation in children with NEC. Mohan Kumar and colleagues[14] created an animal model to induce inflammatory intestinal injury in murine pups and found that LPS induced IL-1β, IL-6, TNF, and interferon-gamma. Activation of these agents results in upregulation of various other cytokines.[17] Variability in cytokine profile varies based on the half-life of the agent and disease severity and findings have not been consistent between studies.

Children who develop NEC are known to have an increased risk of late-onset sepsis (LOS) secondary to the need for prolonged parenteral nutrition requiring central intravascular access.[17,18] It is known that LOS is a risk factor for poor neurologic outcome in preterm infants.[19] Intestinal failure (defined as the need for parenteral nutrition for >6 weeks) and the need for prolonged parenteral nutrition are common in children who develop surgical NEC. Cole and colleagues[17] reported that among a cohort of preterm infants between 401 and 1500 g, those with a history of surgical NEC and intestinal failure were more likely to develop bloodstream infections compared with those with medical NEC and those who were unaffected. Cole and colleagues[17] reported that the percentage of infants with 1 to 3 bloodstream infections at the time of diagnosis of NEC was higher among those who developed intestinal failure compared with those with NEC without intestinal failure (45% vs 33%; $P = .04$) and those with medical NEC (45% vs 20%; $P = .01$).

NECROTIZING ENTEROCOLITIS AND INTESTINAL FAILURE

At the time of surgery, necrotic segments of the bowel are surgically resected. If bowel continuity is unable to be maintained, a diverting ostomy is typically created. From a nutritional perspective, this disruption of bowel continuity can result in malabsorption and difficulty obtaining enteral autonomy. If massive resection is required, the infant may develop short bowel syndrome because the infant has inadequate bowel length needed to absorb adequate amount of nutrition for growth. Loss of specific segments of the intestines, such as the ileocecal valve and terminal ileum may result in inability to absorb specific nutrients, such as bile salts and vitamin B12. Infants with surgical NEC are more likely to have intestinal failure and poor growth, both of which have been associated with adverse neurologic outcome.[17,18] The inability at attain enteral autonomy results in increased catheter days and dependence on parenteral nutrition. The risk for LOS is associated with increased number of catheter days and an increased risk for adverse ND outcome.

NUTRITION AND NEURODEVELOPMENTAL OUTCOME

Compared with infant formula preparations, human milk has been shown to decrease the risk for developing NEC.[3,21,22] In a multicenter randomized double-blind trial using either pasteurized donor milk or preterm infant formula whenever mother's milk was not available for the first 90 days of life, Unger and colleagues[23] sought to determine if donor milk was associated with improved neurologic outcome. Although there were no differences in neurodevelopmental outcome at 18 months between those receiving donor milk and those receiving infant formula, the donor milk group had a lower incidence of stage 2 or greater NEC (1.7% in donor milk group vs 6.6% in infant formula group). Another clinical trial is ongoing to evaluate this question through the National Institute of Child Health and Human Development (NICHD) NRN, entitled "Neurodevelopmental effects of donor breast milk versus preterm formula in ELBW infants—The MILK Trial," Clinical Trail NCT01534481(available at www.clinicaltrial.gov; accessed January 5, 2018). Recent data suggest that there are immunoprotective properties in human milk that partially explain the lower risk of NEC, including immunoglobulins, lactoferrin, cytokines, lysozyme, PAF-acetylhydrolase, and oligosaccharides. The protective effect of these and other substances found in breast milk on the developing brain are largely unknown.

Prolonged dependence on parenteral nutrition is associated with cholestasis and liver injury. NEC associated with intestinal failure is among the most common causes for liver-bowel organ transplantation in children.[24] Recently, there has been much interest in understanding how lipid minimization strategies or the use of alternative lipid sources may decrease the risk for liver disease in neonates. Additional research is needed to understand the impact that use of these products may have on somatic or brain growth or ND outcomes.

Hong and colleagues[25] from the Vermont Oxford Network evaluated growth outcomes in a cohort of 9171 extremely low birth weight preterm infants at hospital discharge and 18-month to 24-month follow-up. They defined severe growth failure as lower than the third percentile using Fenton and Centers for Disease Control and Prevention growth charts. Rates of severe growth impairment at discharge was higher among those with surgical NEC (61%) compared with those with medical NEC (56%) and those without NEC (36%). Interestingly, these differences were no longer present at the 18-month to 24-month follow-up visit (**Fig. 2**). Those with surgical NEC had the highest rate of sepsis, chronic lung disease, severe intraventricular hemorrhage (IVH), and periventricular leukemia (PVL), all of which are known to be associated with adverse ND outcome.

BRAIN INJURY AND NECROTIZING ENTEROCOLITIS

Limited data are available that compare the risk of CNS injury in neonates with NEC compared with unaffected preterm peers. Conclusions can be inferred from available data and other publications that include a significant number of infants with NEC. In most cohort studies of preterm infants, surgical NEC is associated with an increased risk for adverse neurodevelopmental outcome. Therefore, one would speculate that these children have an increased risk of structural brain injury.

In the cohort analysis of ND outcomes of preterms with NEC by Hintz and colleagues,[26] infants with surgical NEC had a similar risk for severe grade 3 or 4 IVH compared with those with medical NEC and those who were unaffected. However, the infants with surgical NEC were more likely to have cystic PVL on cranial ultrasound compared with those who had no NEC (14% vs 7%; $P<.05$).

Kidokoro and colleagues[27] evaluated 325 very preterm infants with term equivalent MRI and ND testing at 2 years of age using the Bayley Scales of Infant Development (BSID) II or BSID III to determine if severity of brain injury affected brain growth. Severe brain injury was more common in infants with a history of NEC and was associated with an increased risk of cerebral palsy and poor cognitive outcome. Infants with NEC stage II or greater were more likely to have IVH grade 3/4 or PVL (odds ratio

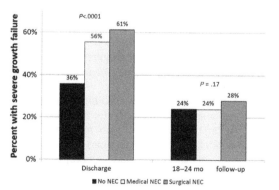

Fig. 2. Rates of severe growth failure among extremely low birth weight infants at 18 to 24 months compared on the basis of NEC status. Discharge: No NEC, n = 7300; Medical NEC, n = 326; Surgical NEC, n = 341; χ^2 135.6, df = 2, $P<.0001$. Eighteen to 24 months' follow-up: No NEC, n = 8972; Medical NEC, n = 408; Surgical NEC, n = 452; χ^2 = 3.6, df = 2, P = .17. (*From* Hong CR, Fullerton BS, Mercier CE, et al. Growth morbidity in extremely low birth weight survivors of necrotizing enterocolitis at discharge and 2-year follow-up. J Pediatr Surg 2018;53(6):1201; with permission.)

6.8 [1.68–28]; $P<.05$) defined by the presence of extensive cysts in the periventricular white matter. The risk for severe IVH was similar to preterms with a history of NEC. Shin and colleagues[28] reviewed term equivalent MRI of the brain of 33 preterm infants with a diagnosis of SIP or surgical NEC. The study was limited by small sample size but those with surgical NEC were more likely to demonstrate white matter abnormalities compared with those with SIP.

Improved understanding of the inherent vulnerability of the developing pre-oligodendroglia in the preterm brain has helped researchers explain the link between infection/inflammation and brain injury. The microglia represent 5% to 15% of the developing brain and are believed to play a critical role in the maturation of the white matter and the axonal crossroad resulting in the highly integrated network of neuronal fibers.[29] Microglia produce a variety of proinflammatory cytokines. Rochefort and others[30] postulate that the microglia regulate axonal bundles and transcallosal projections in the developing brain. These crossroads in white matter development are vulnerable to cytokine-mediated injury and are strongly correlated with focal or diffuse CNS injury.[29] In animal models, hypoxia-ischemia and infection activate the microglia to produce proinflammatory cytokines. Researchers have documented a temporal relationship between insult and subsequent influx of cytokines in the developing brain to substantiate the causal relationship. Subsequent injury to surrounding tissues potentially occurs through the so-called "gap junction mediated bystander effect" through connecting intercellular channels allowing passage of small molecules and ions. Recent data implicate hemi-channels or connexons, which reside of the cell membrane of the adjacent glial cell, in the pathogenesis of downstream injury.

NECROTIZING ENTEROCOLITIS, SURGERY, AND ADVERSE NEUROLOGIC OUTCOME

Historically, peritoneal drainage was used for neonates deemed too clinically unstable to tolerate an open laparotomy. Recently, some have used it as the primary procedure for children with NEC and only subsequently perform a laparotomy if the child does not clinically improve. The decision regarding surgical approach has been primarily based on clinical outcomes because neurodevelopmental follow-up was not systematically performed in many of these studies. At present, there is not a clear consensus about the most appropriate surgical approach to manage neonates with NEC. Often the decision is guided by gestational age, patient instability, and the overall clinical picture. Assessment of the underlying pathology (NEC vs SIP) may also factor into the decision-making process. In some clinical scenarios, there is overlap in presentation such that the primary diagnosis of NEC versus SIP is unclear, which makes it difficult to compare both clinical and ND outcomes.

For the purposes of this review, I have focused on large cohort studies of patients who required some type of surgical intervention for their disease process in an effort to avoid potential bias created by small sample size and attempts to draw conclusions from a small number of critically ill children who had surgically managed disease.

Limited data are currently available and, furthermore, these studies are limited in sample size and most are single-center studies. Nonetheless, trends in outcome from these published trials were used to inform design and decision-making for a larger randomized controlled trial.

In 2006, Blakely and colleagues[12] published an observational study comparing outcomes of ELBW infants <1000 g with a diagnosis of SIP or NEC. Mortality, short-term surgical outcomes, and ND outcomes at 18 to 22 months' adjusted age were reported. They reported that 5.2% of the ELBW infants from 16 centers in the United States developed NEC or SIP during the study period. In this study, 80 infants had a peritoneal drain placement and 76 infants had laparotomy as the initial surgical management. Sixty-two percent had a preoperative diagnosis of NEC and 38% had a presumed diagnosis of SIP. The mortality was high in this cohort, and 50% of the children had died before the 18-month follow-up evaluation. At follow-up, 72% had either died or had significant ND impairment. The composite outcome of ND impairment was reported in 49% of patients. Low cognitive scores with Mental Developmental Index (MDI) on the BSID-IIR were noted in 45% of patients, low motor scores reflective of Psychomotor Developmental Index (PDI) less than 70 was reported in 32%, and 24% had a diagnosis of moderate/severe cerebral palsy. Rates of sensory impairment were much lower, including 3% with blindness and 5% with deafness. The risk for adverse outcome was striking in this high-risk cohort. Among those with a primary diagnosis of NEC, 80% either died or survived with ND impairment (NDI) compared with 69% of those with a primary diagnosis of SIP[12] (**Fig. 3**).

In 2005, Hintz and colleagues[26] from the NICHD NRN compared growth and ND outcomes of ELBW infants with surgical NEC compared with those with medical NEC and those who were unaffected (**Fig. 4**). Children were evaluated at 18 months' adjusted age using the BSID-IIR and a standardized neurologic examination. Compared with those with medical NEC or no NEC, those with surgical NEC were more likely to have a diagnosis of cerebral palsy (surgical NEC 24% vs no NEC 15%; $P<.05$). Similarly, those with surgical NEC had significantly lower scores on both the cognitive and motor scales of the BSID-IIR and were more likely to have Bayley scores less than 70, which is considered significantly delayed (**Table 2**). Patients with medical NEC had similar outcomes to those with no NEC. These investigators also evaluated a composite outcome of NDI that included BSID II MDI or PDI score <70, moderate/severe cerebral palsy, deafness, or blindness between the groups. Rates of NDI were significantly higher in those with surgical NEC compared with the 2 other groups (surgical NEC 58.7% vs medical NEC 31.4% vs no NEC 29.4%; $P<.05$) The investigators postulated that the profound inflammatory response generated secondary to the infection and/or prior history of intrauterine infection, increased the risk for CNS injury. Interestingly, those with surgical NEC were also more likely to have compromised growth parameters at follow-up.

Fullerton and colleagues[31] evaluated rates of severe disability and health care outcomes of a cohort of preterm infants 401 to 1000 g cared for in centers

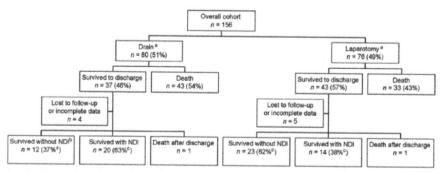

Fig. 3. Flow of patients through study. [a] Initial surgical management; [b] NDI at 18 to 22 months; [c] Percentage of survivors who had full follow-up assessment. (*From* Blakely ML, Tyson JE, Lally KP, et al. Laparotomy vs peritoneal drainage for necrotizing enterocolitis or isolated intestinal perforation in extremely low birth weight infants: outcomes through 18 months adjusted age. Pediatrics 2006;117(4):e680–7.)

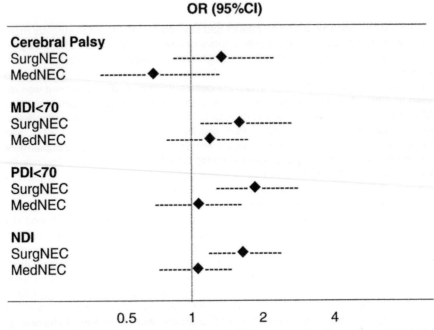

Fig. 4. Adjusted odds ratios (ORs) for CP, MDI less than 70, PDI less than 70, and NDI in Surgical NEC and Medical NEC compared with No NEC infants. (*From* Hintz SR, Kendrick DE, Stoll BJ, et al. Neurodevelopmental and growth outcomes of extremely low birth weight infants after necrotizing enterocolitis. Pediatrics 2005;115(3):696–703.)

participating in the Vermont Oxford Network between 1999 and 2012. Outcomes were evaluated between 18 and 24 months' adjusted age using the BSID. Severe disability was defined as bilateral blindness, hearing impairment requiring amplification, BSID II PDI or MDI less than 70/BSID III Cognitive or Motor less than 70,

Table 2
Bayley-II MDI and PDI and NDI at 18 to 22 months' corrected age

	SurgNEC	MedNEC	No NEC	SurgNEC vs No NEC	MedNEC vs No NEC
MDI					
Mean ± SD	72.0 ± 18.0	76.9 ± 16.0	79.5 ± 18.4	$P<.0001$	$P = .14$
<70, n (%)	52 (44)	41 (37)	772 (31)	$P = .003$	$P = .20$
N	118	112	2533	—	—
PDI					
Mean ± SD	74.0 ± 19.1	82.5 ± 20.7	82.6 ± 18.6	$P<.0001$	$P = .94$
<70, n (%)	44 (37)	28 (25)	556 (22)	$P = .0003$	$P = .53$
N	119	111	2500	—	—
NDI, n (%)	69 (57)	50 (44)	1014 (40)	$P = .0003$	$P = .43$
N	121	113	2531	—	—

Abbreviations: MDI, Mental Development Index; MedNEC, medical NEC; NDI, neurodevelopmental impairment; NEC, necrotizing enterocolitis; PDI, Psychomotor Developmental Index; SurgNEC, surgical NEC.

From Hintz SR, Kendrick DE, Stoll BJ, et al. Neurodevelopmental and growth outcomes of extremely low birth weight infants after necrotizing enterocolitis. Pediatrics 2005;115(3):700; with permission.

or moderate/severe cerebral palsy. Surgical NEC survivors were significantly more likely to have evidence of severe neurologic disability and require postdischarge surgery (P<.001).[31] In this cohort of 24,018 infants, survival to follow-up varied by diagnosis, with 62% of those with NEC/perforation surviving to discharge compared with 74% of those with medical NEC and 88% of those who were unaffected (P<.01.) Rates of associated morbidities were highest among those with surgical NEC for severe IVH/PVL, chronic lung disease, or severe retinopathy of prematurity. The ARR [Adjusted Risk Ratio] of severe ND disability for those with surgical NEC was 1.87 (95% confidence interval [CI] 1.58–2.20; P<.05) compared with the reference group of infants who were unaffected.

In a meta-analysis of available data using fixed effects models reporting ND outcome of neonates with NEC, Schulzke and colleagues[32] reported an increased risk of adverse ND outcome and NDI compared with unaffected infants (odds ratio 1.82; 95% CI 1.46–2.27).

In a meta-analysis by Rees and colleagues[33] in 2007, ND outcomes were compared between preterm infants with medically versus surgically treated NEC. ND outcomes were worse compared with unaffected children and those with surgical NEC had worse outcome than those with medical NEC. Those with surgical NEC had a 2.3-fold increased risk of NDI compared with those with medical NEC (**Fig. 5**). In the most recent Cochrane Library meta-analysis, no firm recommendations were offered regarding surgical management of NEC because mortality and ND outcome among survivors was similar in the 2 groups.[34]

The Eunice Shriver National Institute of Health and Human Services NRN is currently conducting a randomized clinical trial of neonates with NEC in which the children are randomized to either peritoneal drainage or exploratory laparotomy: the Laparotomy versus

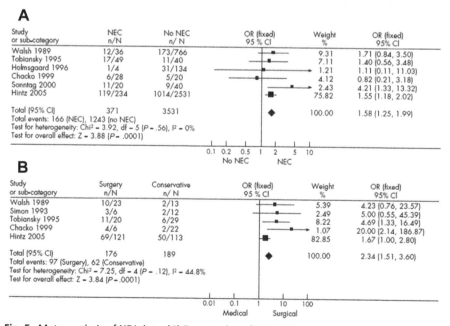

Fig. 5. Meta-analysis of NDI data. (*A*) Forrest plot of NDI NEC versus No NEC. (*B*) Forrest plot of NDI Surgical NEC versus Medical NEC. (*From* Rees CM, Pierro A, Eaton S. Neurodevelopmental outcomes of neonates with medically and surgically treated necrotizing enterocolitis. Arch Dis Child Fetal Neonatal Ed 2007;92(3):F196; with permission.)

Drainage for Infants with Necrotizing Enterocolitis, the NEST Trial (NCT01029353; available at www.clinicaltrials.gov; accessed January 5, 2018). Short-term outcomes, including surgical complications, will be evaluated, but the trial is powered to determine if the type of surgical intervention affects ND outcomes at 24 months' adjusted age. This is a long-anticipated trial of which neonatologists and surgeons are hopeful will provide better guidance about surgical intervention and outcomes in this high-risk population of infants.

From the available data, it is clear that neonates with surgical NEC are at increased risk for adverse ND outcome. Neonatologists and surgeons are awaiting the results of the NEST trial to determine which surgical approach (peritoneal drainage or laparotomy) is associated with improved ND outcome. Affected infants may be at risk for adverse outcome for a variety of reasons, including exposure to systemic cytokines and increased risk for associated morbidities, including sepsis, suboptimal nutrition, exposure to anesthesia, and increased exposure to narcotics. Ongoing clinical trials should help us better understand the relationship between surgical approach and the risk for various morbidities, including adverse ND outcome.

Best Practices

What is the current practice?

Necrotizing enterocolitis (NEC) is a potentially life-threatening disease that primarily affects prematurely born infants. Those requiring surgery are at greatest risk for adverse neurologic outcome and death. Prevention of the primary disease process and prevention of associated morbidity form the foundation of current practice. Studies are ongoing to guide recommendations for surgical management of NEC and its impact on neurodevelopmental outcomes.

Best Practice/Guideline/Care Path Objective(s)

Clinical practice guidelines focus on minimizing the risk of NEC through the use of human milk and the prevention of associated morbidities in those affected, including decreasing the risk of bloodstream infections and optimizing nutrition.

What changes in current practice are likely to improve outcomes?

1. Improved knowledge regarding impact of surgical management (drain vs laparotomy) on neurodevelopmental outcome will provide critically important information needed to improve neurodevelopmental outcomes of affected infants.

2. Strategies to prevent necrotizing enterocolitis are needed.

3. Improved nutritional management of affected patients may improve outcome.

Is there a Clinical Algorithm? No

Major Recommendations:
1. Neurodevelopmental follow-up evaluations are recommended for all infants with surgical necrotizing enterocolitis.
2. Parents should be informed of the risk for adverse neurodevelopmental outcome.

Clinical Algorithm(s)

Rating for the Strength of the Evidence

Bibliographic Source(s)

Summary Statement

Prematurely born children with a history of surgical NEC are at increased risk for adverse neurodevelopmental outcome. Secondary complications, including late-onset infection and suboptimal nutrition, contribute to these adverse outcomes. Research is ongoing to better understand the relationship between surgical management of the disease on neurodevelopmental outcomes.

REFERENCES

1. Stoll BJ, Hansen NI, Bell EF, et al. Neonatal outcomes of extremely preterm infants from the NICHD neonatal research network. Pediatrics 2010;126(3):443–56.
2. Lin PW, Nasr TR, Stoll BJ. Necrotizing enterocolitis: recent scientific advances in pathophysiology and prevention. Semin Perinatol 2008;32(2):70–82.
3. Caplan MS, Fanaroff A. Necrotizing: a historical perspective. Semin Perinatol 2017;41(1):2–6.
4. Neu J, Walker WA. Necrotizing enterocolitis. N Engl J Med 2011;364(3):255–64.
5. Denning TL, Bhatia AM, Kane AF, et al. Pathogenesis of NEC: role of the innate and adaptive immune response. Semin Perinatol 2017;41(1):15–28.
6. Berman L, Moss RL. Necrotizing enterocolitis: an update. Semin Fetal Neonatal Med 2011;16(3):145–50.
7. Stoll BJ, Hansen NI, Bell EF, et al. Trends in care practices, morbidity, and mortality of extremely preterm neonates, 1993-2012. JAMA 2015;314(10):1039–51.
8. Hull MA, Fisher JG, Gutierrez IM, et al. Mortality and management of surgical necrotizing enterocolitis in very low birth weight neonates: a prospective cohort study. J Am Coll Surg 2014;218(6):1148–55.
9. Oddie SJ, Young L, McGuire W. Slow advancement of enteral feed volumes to prevent necrotising enterocolitis in very low birth weight infants. Cochrane Database Syst Rev 2017;(8):CD001241.
10. Gay AN, Lazar DA, Stoll B, et al. Near-infrared spectroscopy measurement of abdominal tissue oxygenation is a useful indicator of intestinal blood flow and necrotizing enterocolitis in premature piglets. J Pediatr Surg 2011;46(6):1034–40.
11. Schat TE, Schurink M, van der Laan ME, et al. Near-infrared spectroscopy to predict the course of necrotizing enterocolitis. PLoS One 2016;11(5):e0154710.
12. Blakely ML, Tyson JE, Lally KP, et al. Laparotomy versus peritoneal drainage for necrotizing enterocolitis or isolated intestinal perforation in extremely low birth weight infants: outcomes through 18 months adjusted age. Pediatrics 2006;117(4):e680–7.
13. Fisher JG, Jones BA, Gutierrez IM, et al. Mortality associated with laparotomy-confirmed neonatal spontaneous intestinal perforation: a prospective 5-year multicenter analysis. J Pediatr Surg 2014;49(8):1215–9.
14. MohanKumar K, Namachivayam K, Ho TTB, et al. Cytokines and growth factors in the developing intestine and during necrotizing enterocolitis. Semin Perinatol 2017;41(1):52–60.
15. Carlo WA, McDonald SA, Tyson JE, et al. Cytokines and neurodevelopmental outcomes in extremely low birth weight infants. J Pediatr 2011;159(6):919–25.e3.
16. Maheshwari A, Schelonka RL, Dimmitt RA, et al. Cytokines associated with necrotizing enterocolitis in extremely low birth weight infants. Pediatr Res 2014;76(1):100–8.
17. Cole CR, Hansen NI, Higgins RD, et al. Bloodstream infections in very low birth weight infants with intestinal failure. J Pediatr 2012;160(1):54–9.e52.
18. Cole CR, Hansen NI, Higgins RD, et al. Very low birth weight preterm infants with surgical short bowel syndrome: incidence, morbidity and mortality, and growth outcomes at 18 to 22 months. Pediatrics 2008;122(3):e573–82.
19. Stoll BJ, Hansen N, Fanaroff AA, et al. Late-onset sepsis in very low birth weight neonates: the experience of the NICHD Neonatal Research Network. Pediatrics 2002;110(2 Pt 1):285–91.

20. Lodha A, Asztalos E, Moore AM. Cytokine levels in neonatal necrotizing enterocolitis and long-term growth and neurodevelopment. Acta Paediatr 2010;99(3): 338–43.
21. Lucas A, Cole TJ. Breast milk and neonatal necrotising enterocolitis. Lancet 1990; 336(8730):1519–23.
22. Meinzen-Derr J, Poindexter B, Wrage L, et al. Role of human milk in extremely low birth weight infants' risk of necrotizing enterocolitis or death. J Perinatol 2009; 29(1):57–62.
23. Unger S, Gibbins S, Zupancic J, et al. DoMINO: donor milk for improved neurodevelopmental outcomes. BMC Pediatr 2014;14:123.
24. Kaufman SS, Atkinson JB, Bianchi A, et al. Indications for pediatric intestinal transplantation: a position paper of the American Society of Transplantation. Pediatr Transplant 2001;5(2):80–7.
25. Hong CR, Fullerton BS, Mercier CE, et al. Growth morbidity in extremely low birth weight survivors of necrotizing enterocolitis at discharge and two-year follow-up. J Pediatr Surg 2018. [Epub ahead of print].
26. Hintz SR, Kendrick DE, Stoll BJ, et al. Neurodevelopmental and growth outcomes of extremely low birth weight infants after necrotizing enterocolitis. Pediatrics 2005;115(3):696–703.
27. Kidokoro H, Anderson PJ, Doyle LW, et al. Brain injury and altered brain growth in preterm infants: predictors and prognosis. Pediatrics 2014;134(2):e444–53.
28. Shin SH, Kim EK, Yoo H, et al. Surgical necrotizing enterocolitis versus spontaneous intestinal perforation in white matter injury on brain magnetic resonance imaging. Neonatology 2016;110(2):148–54.
29. Mallard C, Davidson JO, Tan S, et al. Astrocytes and microglia in acute cerebral injury underlying cerebral palsy associated with preterm birth. Pediatr Res 2013; 75:234.
30. Rochefort N, Quenech'du N, Watroba L, et al. Microglia and astrocytes may participate in the shaping of visual callosal projections during postnatal development. J Physiol Paris 2002;96(3):183–92.
31. Fullerton BS, Hong CR, Velazco CS, et al. Severe neurodevelopmental disability and healthcare needs among survivors of medical and surgical necrotizing enterocolitis: a prospective cohort study. J Pediatr Surg 2017;53(1):101–7.
32. Schulzke SM, Deshpande GC, Patole SK. Neurodevelopmental outcomes of very low-birth-weight infants with necrotizing enterocolitis: a systematic review of observational studies. Arch Pediatr Adolesc Med 2007;161(6):583–90.
33. Rees CM, Pierro A, Eaton S. Neurodevelopmental outcomes of neonates with medically and surgically treated necrotizing enterocolitis. Arch Dis Child Fetal Neonatal Ed 2007;92(3):F193–8.
34. Rao SC, Basani L, Simmer K, et al. Peritoneal drainage versus laparotomy as initial surgical treatment for perforated necrotizing enterocolitis or spontaneous intestinal perforation in preterm low birth weight infants. Cochrane Database Syst Rev 2011;(6):CD006182.

What Are We Measuring as Outcome? Looking Beyond Neurodevelopmental Impairment

Howard W. Kilbride, MD[a],*, Glen P. Aylward, PhD, ABPP[b],
Brian Carter, MD[a]

KEYWORDS

- Neonatal follow-up • Outcome measures • Neurodevelopmental impairment (NDI)
- Quality of life • NICU survivors • Very preterm infants

KEY POINTS

- Categorization of neurodevelopmental impairments allows quantification of severe problematic outcomes in early childhood but these may not reflect later more subtle, functional outcomes.
- More prevalent, less severe, neurobehavioral dysfunctions are often not identified in early childhood but are important predictors of later academic achievement and social outcomes.
- Extremely preterm and other high-risk neonatal intensive care unit graduates are at risk for lifelong health needs that are often underappreciated.
- Postnatal influences, including psychosocial factors, are important for resilience and quality-of-life outcomes for extreme preterms.

The primary outcomes of neonatal intensive care have generally been presented as rates of survival and neurodevelopmental impairment (NDI).[1] This approach provides a rather complex outcome that varies with regard to categorical cutoffs. Levels of impairment are defined based on thresholds of cognition, motor performance, and neurosensory function. Moderate to severe NDI, which includes major disabilities (intelligence quotient [IQ]/developmental quotient [DQ] <70, cerebral palsy [CP], or neurosensory [vision, hearing] impairments) have been reported for approximately

All authors have contributed to this article and declare no conflict of interest.
[a] Division of Neonatology, Department of Pediatrics, Children's Mercy-Kansas City, University of Missouri-Kansas City School of Medicine, 2401 Gillham Road, Kansas City, MO 64108, USA;
[b] Division of Developmental and Behavioral Pediatrics, Southern Illinois University School of Medicine, PO Box 19658, Springfield, IL 62794-9658, USA
* Corresponding author.
E-mail address: hkilbride@cmh.edu

Clin Perinatol 45 (2018) 467–484
https://doi.org/10.1016/j.clp.2018.05.008
0095-5108/18/© 2018 Elsevier Inc. All rights reserved.

20% to 25% of extremely preterm infants, based on follow-up evaluations at 2 years of age.[2] However, there are important outcomes that go beyond discharge and short-term morbidity/mortality endpoints. In fact, these should be considered the first of many endpoint outcome measurements.[3]

Understanding the risk for NDI in preterm survivors is important for public health decisions and as a metric for research initiatives designed to improve outcomes. However, recent criticisms challenge the assumptions on which this follow-up model is based.[4,5] More specifically, preschool developmental testing has limited value in predicting later cognitive performance. There are many other important variables that need to be identified so as to understand implications of NDI in terms of functional outcomes and quality of life (QoL). It is also important to recognize other, perhaps less severe, but significant dysfunctions that become apparent at older ages in NICU survivors. In this article, we briefly review limitations of early developmental testing of NDI, discuss other important areas of evaluation needed to better understand functional outcomes, and highlight medical outcomes that have ramifications on QoL. The focus is on outcomes of infants born prematurely, but many of these issues are also relevant to term gestation survivors following a difficult neonatal intensive care unit (NICU) course.[6–8]

EARLY DEVELOPMENTAL TESTING FOR NEURODEVELOPMENTAL IMPAIRMENT

Two-year follow-up data, including assessments in cognitive, motor, and neurosensory domains, have traditionally been considered "long-term outcomes" for neonatal studies, although that view is changing.[3] Findings in each of these areas have been used to define NDI as "mild," "moderate," or "severe," based on preset thresholds. Although a composite score may produce greater power than individual components,[1] there are concerns about overinterpretation of findings using this model. A "severe" finding in any of the domains would categorize the child as having "severe NDI" even with "normal" findings in the other areas; for example, a child with diplegia that interferes with ambulation would be classified as having severe NDI even if cognition is normal.[9] With regard to cognitive and motor function, the National Institute of Child Health and Human Development Neonatal Research Network has defined scores of less than 70 as severe and scores in the 70 to 84 range as moderate NDI.[10] The components of NDI are often interrelated: grossly one-half of those with CP have cognitive impairment, and sensory disabilities are associated with CP as well. Moreover, it is easier to assess whether an infant or young child has CP than it is to measure DQ in a severely impaired child because motor and speech impairments interfere with cognitive testing.[11]

The Bayley Scales are often used for infant assessments with categorization of findings based on reference standards. The Bayley was introduced as a developmental testing tool in 1969 and several versions have subsequently been introduced. Currently, the Bayley Scales of Infant and Toddler Development (Bayley III)[12] is used, particularly the cognitive, language (receptive, expressive), and motor (gross, fine) subscales. Although the DQ is often thought of as a measure of cognition, it is not, as only precursors of cognitive function are being tested. Predicting cognitive outcomes at school age from these early assessments has been called a "conundrum."[13] Changes to the Bayley Scales items and format over time (Bayley II compared with Bayley III), as well as alterations to the reference standards, have made longitudinal comparisons challenging.[14] In comparison studies the Cognitive Composite has been reported to be 6 to 10 points higher with the Bayley III compared to the Bayley II Mental Developmental Index (MDI).[12,15] These issues are particularly of concern because the differences in Bayley versions are greater at the lower end and low cognitive scores comprise the most frequent component of NDI. Moreover, these scores tend to be poorly predictive. Hack and colleagues,[16] using the Bayley II at 20 months, found that a DQ <70 had a positive predictive value (PPV) of only 0.37 for a low IQ at school age and the PPV was 0.20 for those with normal neurosensory status. Infant tests assess current developmental levels and may identify developmental lag, but not more long-term cognitive impairment.

Cheong and colleagues[17] evaluated severe disability in extremely preterm (EPT) cohorts born in 1991 to 1992, 1997, and 2005, at several time points, the last being 8 years of age. Although no change in severe disability rates were found in the 1991 to 1992 and 1997 comparisons, severe disability decreased significantly from 1997 to 2005 (15.4% to 3.7%). It should be underscored that the Bayley III was used with the 2005 cohort and this might have affected these findings. Bernardo and colleagues[18] compared 2 cohorts of extremely low birth weight (ELBW) children with neurologic impairments, born 1990 to 1999 and 2000 to 2005, using the original Bayley and Bayley II with a correction factor. Although there were decreased rates of neurologic impairment and a "suggestion" of improved motor function between the cohorts, cognitive function was unchanged.

Neurodevelopmental outcomes, particularly cognitive function, are influenced by important postnatal factors, many of which are not usually considered in predicting outcomes of preterm children. For children without structural brain injury following the NICU course, cognitive scores tend to improve from preschool to school age in high socioeconomic status (SES) homes, suggesting a protective environmental influence. Ment and colleagues[19] found higher IQ scores were associated with higher maternal education and early interventions. Similarly, Breslau and colleagues[20] reported IQs of urban children declined over school age, whereas those of suburban children did not, suggesting protective environmental effects in the latter milieu. Kilbride and colleagues[21] compared ELBW children with their full-term siblings and found ELBWs' IQs were on average 10 points lower than the full-term siblings. However, the average IQ for the low SES full-term children was equivalent to that of the high SES ELBW children, suggesting a comparable effect of SES and extreme prematurity on cognitive outcomes. Follow-up data from the "Caffeine for Apnea of Prematurity" study also showed increased cognitive scores from 18 months to 5 years in association with social advantages. Higher maternal education, higher paternal education, and caregiver employment had independent and additive effects on cognitive gain; for those with all 3 protective factors, cognitive scores improved on average by 10.9 points, compared with children without these advantages.[22]

Poverty has been linked to developmental differences in brain structure, that, in turn, are associated with lower scores on standardized tests.[23] Cumulative data suggest that the largest effect of SES on neurocognitive function is in language processing and executive functioning. Language complexity is reduced in low SES preschool children compared with those from higher SES households, and studies have suggested brain activation differs by SES during a language task and with reading.[24] SES effects on executive functions of working memory and inhibitory control have been seen as early at 6 to 14 months[25] and are consistently reported in older children and adolescents.[26] These effects may have greater impact on the more vulnerable preterm brain and could explain SES effects on educational outcomes for these children. Understanding these important postnatal, environmental effects of developmental outcome is critical for interpretation of follow-up outcome data for high-risk newborns.

COMPREHENSIVE ASSESSMENT OF THE HIGH-RISK NEONATE: BEYOND NEURODEVELOPMENTAL IMPAIRMENT

A recent review suggested 4 domains of child variables that would be important in a model of high-risk follow-up: learning and cognition, mental health, physical health, and QoL.[27] We briefly summarize issues that may be considered within each domain as part of a comprehensive plan for assessment and monitoring of long-term outcomes for those born extremely preterm and other high-risk NICU graduates (**Box 1**).

Box 1
Assessing outcomes for neonatal intensive care unit graduates: beyond neurodevelopmental impairment

Category of function/areas of concern that warrant monitoring

Learning and cognition
- High-prevalence/low-severity dysfunctions
  - Low average/borderline intelligence quotient
  - Learning disabilities (math, written expression, spelling, reading)
  - Attention-deficit/hyperactivity disorder
  - Executive dysfunction (working memory, planning/organizing, cognitive flexibility)
  - Visual motor integration problems/poor handwriting
- Simultaneous processing difficulties
- Poor academic achievement/need for special educational resources

Mental health
- Internalizing behaviors
- Anxiety
- Poor social interactions/withdrawal
- Autism spectrum disorder
- Family stress/parental coping

Physical health
- Motor function
  - Minor neurologic dysfunction, developmental coordination disorder
  - Poor visual-perceptual skills
- Pulmonary function
  - Persistent oxygen supplementation
  - Asthma, wheezing
  - Abnormal pulmonary function/early adult-onset chronic obstructive pulmonary disease
- Cardiovascular function
  - Low exercise tolerance/activity level
  - Persistent pulmonary hypertension
- Renal/Metabolic
  - Systemic hypertension
  - Metabolic syndrome
- Vision
  - Myopia of prematurity
  - Retinopathy of prematurity sequelae: peripheral field loss/late retinal detachment
  - Refractive errors/astigmatism/diminished visual acuity
  - Strabismus
- Growth/nutrition
  - Poor oral intake/persistent gastrostomy tube feeding
  - Metabolic bone disease
  - Poor growth/failure to thrive/short stature

Quality of life
- Functional status (physical, mental, social)
- Adaptive skills
- Community resources/psychosocial support
- Health-related quality of life

LEARNING AND COGNITION

Besides major disabilities that are usually considered in NDI, there is much interest in so-called "high-prevalence/low-severity dysfunctions" in NICU survivors.[28,29] These include low average to borderline IQ, learning disabilities, neuropsychological problems (eg, executive dysfunction, visual motor integration problems), attention-deficit/hyperactivity disorder (ADHD), and behavioral issues. These problems become more evident as the child grows older; they may not be apparent until school age, when specific performance demands are placed on the child that involve previously unidentified deficits. These more subtle problems differ from severe NDIs that have a greater probability of earlier identification.

The high-prevalence/low-severity dysfunctions also tend to cluster and not occur in isolation. For example, a child with borderline intellectual disability also may have a learning disability in math, visual motor integrative problems, and deficits in working memory. Children born EPT tend to plateau cognitively and with regard to neurosensory outcomes at school age, but academic skills may deteriorate further.[30] It is inferred that disruptions in brain development in conjunction with alterations in brain microstructure and neural connectivity due to conditions such as periventricular leukomalacia or intraventricular hemorrhage (IVH) produce these more subtle problems.[31,32] In children born EPT with a history of transient neurologic abnormalities (TNAs) that peak at age 6 to 7 months, there is increased risk for lower levels of cognitive and academic functioning during the first year of school, in comparison with those with normal neurologic findings.[33] Children with TNAs typically do not have neurologic abnormalities evident after 1 or 2 years of age, and therefore do not receive services until underlying problems again surface in school.

Many NICU graduates have normal IQ scores when tested in early childhood; however, even those without evidence of NDI or intellectual disability frequently experience difficulties with academic achievement compared with term children. In one study, 65% of EPT children met criteria for 1 or more learning disabilities compared with 13% of term children.[34] Problems in math, written expression, spelling, and reading, in that order of frequency, are found in ELBW children. With regard to grade retention, more than 50% of those born EPT, 25% to 40% of very preterm (VPT), and 20% to 30% of moderate preterm (MPT) children repeat a grade.[35] Moreover, 33% function a grade below their current placement. Heredity, gender, and environmental influences add further complexity to causal inferences.[5] However, Saigal and colleagues[36] reported 58% of teenagers born low birthweight (LBW), even in a middle-class, primarily white Canadian sample, had repeated a grade or received special education compared with 13% of controls.

Children born EPT whose date of birth and date of delivery cross the cutoff date for school entry, essentially begin school an academic year earlier, which may add to their academic disadvantage, including a twofold increase in the need for special education support. In a longitudinal study, Odd and colleagues[37] showed an association between early school entry (based on expected due date) for preterm children and increased risk for special education needs in later school years.

IQ subscales include verbal IQ, measuring reasoning and conceptual abilities, and Performance IQ (PIQ). Preterm children show more difficulty with PIQ, which measures nonverbal reasoning and spatial and perceptual tasks, than do full-term peers.[38,39] Comparable results were seen in studies that used the Kaufman Assessment Battery for Children to assess sequential and simultaneous information processing. VPT children had a discrepancy of more than 1 SD for simultaneous compared with sequential processing.[1] These findings suggest that nonverbal reasoning, visual-spatial skills, and simultaneous processing of stimuli are compromised in children born VPT. In addition, the mean full-scale IQ of children born EPT or VPT, although grossly "normal," typically falls in the low average to borderline range, being 0.5 to 1.0 SDs below peers.[40] For each week of gestational age less than 33 weeks, the average decline in mean IQ scores is 1.5 to 2.5 points. These cognitive differences correlate with academic, social, and behavioral difficulties seen in this population.[41,42]

Preterm children with normal IQ but with academic challenges often are identified having abnormalities in executive function (EF) after specific process testing in later childhood. EF refers to coordination of interrelated processes that involve planning, goal-directed behavior, and self-regulation.[43] Measures of EF, on average, are 0.3 to 0.6 SDs lower for VPT than full-term children, and may be even worse for those born EPT.[44] Children born VPT/EPT are 2 to 3 times more likely than those born full-term to have trouble starting activities, displaying problem-solving flexibility, and have problems in short-term memory and organizing information. Subtle deficits in EF interfere with ability to maintain high levels of efficiency when faced with increasingly complex tasks. Parent and teacher ratings also frequently reflect observations of poor emotional self-regulation. Preschoolers may show deficiency of inhibitory control; school-age preterm children exhibit impairment in working memory, cognitive switching, and complex planning.

Executive dysfunction continues to be a problem beyond early school age. In an Australian geographic cohort, EPT-born adolescents scored poorly on verbal processing, attentional control, and cognitive flexibility compared with controls, similar to findings obtained in early childhood.[45] Adults born preterm appear to use different neural pathways with less suppression of "default modes" based on neuroimaging studies.[46] Recently, in a longitudinal study of 180 individuals born EPT and evaluated at 8 and 18 years, EF was found to be stable and age appropriate for most, with persistent dysfunction for 15%, late-onset dysfunction in 19%, and remitting problems in 12%.[47] Those with persistent and late-onset problems displayed poorer academic performance. EF, and not IQ, is associated with behavior problems, specifically ADHD-inattentive type and increased difficulties with emotional control.[48] These findings suggest that routine screening for EF should be considered for children born EPT at their preschool assessment and throughout school-age years.

MENTAL HEALTH

Emotional and behavioral sequelae are usually assessed through self-report, and parent and teacher questionnaires; the Child Behavior Checklist is used most frequently.[49] Questions related to daily activities and behavioral interactions are grouped and scored to reflect problematic areas. Most studies have found that children born preterm have a higher prevalence of scores in the "clinically significant" range (T-scores 65 or greater), with both increased internalizing (withdrawn, depressed) and externalizing (aggressive, hyperactive) behaviors reported.[40,50] A recent meta-analysis concluded parents of preterms were most likely to identify internalizing behaviors at clinically significant levels.[51] An international comparison of former ELBW children at 10 years of age also found internalizing behaviors increased in one cohort, with none showing significant differences in externalizing behaviors.[52] However, the children had increased social, thought, and attention problems, consistent with other studies that indicate lower social competence for children born EPT.[53] Behavioral and emotional disturbances persist in adolescents and young adults who were born preterm.[54] Johnson and Marlow[55] reported a "preterm behavioral phenotype" that consists of inattention, anxiety, and social difficulties.

Autism spectrum disorders (ASDs) have been insufficiently investigated in this population, but there are several reports of higher scores on parent rating scales.[56,57] Studies have suggested that ASD is nearly 3 times more prevalent in EPTs and highest in those with NDI.[58,59] However, Pritchard and colleagues[60] reported an ASD prevalence of 1.8% in EPT children using the Autism Diagnostic Observable Schedule–Generic (ADOS-G) for confirmation, a rate lower than others. It has been suggested that many preterm children who fail autism screening do not have ASD but have a developmental communication disorder, which may improve over time.[61] Those with NDI more frequently are given the ASD diagnosis, raising the question as to whether the NDI, and not ASD, accounts for the symptoms. It is apparent that additional studies are needed to better understand implications of early behavioral patterns and ASD risk for EPT children.[58]

Psychiatric morbidity requiring hospitalization in adolescents and young adults was inversely related to gestational age in a Swedish national cohort study, with hazard ratio 1.68 for VPT, 1.21 MPT, and 1.08 for "early term."[62] Another large Scandinavian study found rates of schizophrenia in adults were inversely rated to birth weight, with increased risk for those less than 2500 g.[63]

There are multiple reports of increased stress in families of children born VPT. This is a bidirectional issue. Stress will be increased in those families with children having the greatest medical and developmental concerns. However, parental stress may have a negative impact on the child's emotional state and abilities to cope. Higher parental stress over the first 18 months of a preterm infant's life has been reported in a longitudinal study using the Parenting Stress Index questionnaire.[64] Stress was highest in families with children having lowest Bayley MDI scores. Wagner and colleagues[65] also reported parenting stress was highest for those families with children having worse EF. These studies suggest stress may result from realistic parent concerns regarding their child's development and academic performance. Maladaptive parent coping strategies may also contribute to parent stress in these settings.[66] Evaluation of family stress and provision of psychosocial support are important aspects of follow-up for high-risk NICU infants.[67]

PHYSICAL HEALTH
Motor Function

Although CP is a serious, but infrequent (<10%) consequence of extreme preterm birth, subtle motor and coordination difficulties are common, although often not recognized until school age. These findings may lead to a diagnosis of developmental coordination disorder (DCD).[68] DCD results in lower performance than would be expected for age and intellect for daily activities that require motor coordination. Children with DCD may have delayed motor milestones and demonstrate problems with routine activities, such as dressing, tying shoelaces, handwriting, and ball skills. Testing is often performed using the Movement Assessment Battery for Children (MABC)[69]; however, other screening tools and a DCD parent questionnaire are available.[70] The MABC involves 3 subsections for early school-age children: manual dexterity (eg, placing pegs into pegboard), ball skills (catch/bounce), and balance (jumping, balance on one foot). Multiple studies have shown that DCD is more prevalent in children born EPT and VPT compared with term controls. Depending on cutoff scores used, DCD has been identified in 30% to 50% of former EPT children.[71,72] A systematic review found increased odds ratio of 6.3 (95% confidence interval 4.4–9.1) for VPT compared with term-born children.[73] The etiology of DCD in most cases is unknown. No relationship was found to perinatal factors in one study[72]; however, DCD was associated with prolonged rupture of membranes and retinopathy of prematurity (ROP) in another,[74] suggesting the possibility of multiple pathways to the same end result. These subtle motor impairments may interfere with academic success, and increase the possibility of social isolation and diminished self-esteem with lifelong consequences.[75]

Pulmonary Outcomes

Respiratory distress is nearly universal for EPT newborns and approximately 50% to 60% will develop bronchopulmonary dysplasia (BPD). Nearly 40% of these infants will continue to need supplemental oxygen at home,[76] necessitating additional parent education and training as part of discharge planning, continuous home monitoring, and frequent outpatient medical visits. Children with BPD continue to have ongoing respiratory morbidity throughout childhood, including wheezing, increased diagnoses of asthma, and use of respiratory medications.[77-79] Thirty percent to 40% of EPT infants may be rehospitalized during the first years of life,[80,81] the percentage being highest for those with BPD.[82] Hospitalizations are often precipitated by a viral illness with complications, placing infants at risk for intensive medical care, mechanical ventilation, extracorporeal membrane oxygenation, and increased mortality, especially when accompanied by secondary pulmonary hypertension.[83] As adults, BPD survivors continue to be at greater risk for pulmonary morbidity compared with those born at term.[84]

EPT infants by definition are born during a period of critical lung development, before alveolar formation.[85] Abnormal postnatal lung growth results in a lung with fewer but larger alveoli and with abnormal airway elasticity.[86] Spirometry testing of young infants with BPD have shown decreased lung compliance, lower functional residual capacity, and abnormal forced expiratory flow.[87] Lung compliance appears to improve over the first 2 years, but airway dysfunction persists. In a recent meta-analysis, the percentage of predicted forced expiratory volume in 1 sec (%FEV1) was lower for VPT children compared with term children, with the greatest difference seen for those with BPD, showing a pooled average of only 79% of predicted ($\geq$80% is "normal").[88] Low %FEV1 is of significant concern because this metric has been used in adults to assess risk of chronic obstructive pulmonary disease, a major cause of early death and disability.[89] Disruption of normal lung angiogenesis, as may be seen with BPD, also appears to be associated with increased prevalence of pulmonary arterial hypertension into childhood, which could have additional concerning implications for adult survivors of BPD.[90]

There are reports that children born preterm tend to be less active and less likely to participate in organized sports.[91,92] Decreased physical activity could result from the cardiopulmonary limitations discussed previously or may relate to poor motor coordination and dysfunction, lower muscle mass, and low sports performance. Rogers and colleagues[91] found that former ELBW adolescents had lower aerobic fitness, lower muscle strength, and less endurance than term comparisons. They concluded the differences reflect an interaction of physiologic effects of preterm birth with less-active lifestyle. Decreased peak oxygen consumption has been reported for EPT children compared with term children,[93,94] but may not be associated with differences in activity levels.[94]

Further investigation of the effect of EPT birth on childhood exercise stamina is needed because this may have implications for early onset of cardiovascular disease, in addition to risks suggested by the Barker hypothesis. In 1989, Barker and colleagues[95] described an association of low birth weight with increased risk of hypertension, arteriosclerosis, and mortality from coronary heart disease. Longitudinal studies have shown an association between preterm birth and increased blood pressure in children and young adults.[96,97] Accelerated growth in the first 3 years of life has been associated with increased systolic and diastolic blood pressures in former VPT individuals,[98] which would be consistent with the Barker hypothesis. Investigations have found an increase in systolic blood pressure of 5 to 6 mm Hg for those born EPT, which has been interpreted as a possible 25% increased risk of cardiovascular death.[99] The pathogenesis of these findings could relate to impaired elastin synthesis resulting in arterial stiffness, impaired endothelium function, or abnormal glomerulogenesis and altered renal growth (see later in this article).[90] There are also data that suggest that the presence of persistent lung disease may be associated with arterial stiffness and cardiovascular risks, indicating BPD as another factor.[100]

This brief review of the cardiopulmonary outcomes in VPT children and theoretic adult consequences underscores the need to monitor such children closely for risk factors for cardiopulmonary dysfunction. Further studies regarding the unique impact of obesity, sedentary lifestyle, smoking, and other environmental risks are needed to better understand long-term implications.

Renal Outcomes

Renal function in VPT infants reflects the developmental stage of the newborn at birth, decreased renal size, number of glomeruli, immature cortical-medullary gradient, and the corresponding limited tubular function.[101] Additionally, the severity of illness experienced by the newborn (renal and nonrenal), the exposure to key nutritional components (protein), procedures (umbilical arterial catheterization), and medications (aminoglycosides, corticosteroids, indomethacin, diuretics) will impact both acute and chronic renal function.[102] Perhaps the most common long-term outcome that bears measurement is systemic hypertension, seen most frequently in the smallest and youngest preterm infants, and among those with BPD (0.2%–3.0%).[103] Of interest, the limited number of studies published to date suggest that neonatal hypertension usually does not require continuing medical management at the time of discharge from the NICU and for those infants with BPD who do continue to have systemic hypertension, the need for medical management largely resolves by 6 to 12 months of age. Nonetheless, there is a need for more robust and longitudinal neonatal follow-up studies to answer questions such as which renal tests, biomarkers, or metabolomic data may best indicate risk for the development of chronic kidney disease.[101] Finally, the contribution of prematurity, neonatal renal injury or toxicity, and subsequent nutritional, medical, or environmental influences on the development of adolescent, young adult, or adult "essential" hypertension remains to be elucidated.

Vision Outcomes

Infants born preterm are at significantly increased risk of visual impairment compared with those born at term.[104] ROP is the most recognized cause and is inversely related to gestational age and birth weight. Neonatal screening and intervention for severe ROP, including laser photocoagulation, and, more recently, anti–vascular endothelial growth factor agents, will decrease vision-impairing disease; however, long-term outcomes still may be suboptimal.[104] Following cryotherapy, infants are at risk for peripheral field loss, which could affect visual function. Late retinal hemorrhage or detachment are rare complications as well. However, preterm infants without ROP also remain at increased risk of ophthalmic sequelae, particularly for those with neurologic injury. On average, LBW infants have lower acuity at school age than those born at normal birth weight. These findings may be subtle and not identified by acuity evaluations in preschool years.[105] Strabismus is also more prevalent and the types of strabismus are more variable in the preterm population. Fewer than one-half of such cases may be identified in the first year and some not until 5 years of life.[105] The growth of the eye may be altered by early-gestation birth, resulting in an increase in refractive errors and astigmatism. "Myopia of prematurity" is well recognized as a mild condition with onset at the end of the first decade of life, but more severe myopia may be associated with ROP. Preterm birth also may result in arrest of retinal development, with reduction in rod and cone function.[106]

VPT infants with ROP and/or other NDI should have ongoing ophthalmologic follow-up based on current guidelines.[107] Although there are no similar guidelines for periodic ophthalmologic evaluations for VPT infants without ROP or for other high-risk NICU graduates, regular vision and ocular assessments at least to school age should be considered based on the increased risks as described.

GROWTH AND NUTRITION

EPT infants have reduced growth capacity throughout infancy and childhood. In a Swedish cohort of children born at 23 to 25 weeks' gestation, Farooqi and colleagues[108] demonstrated delays in weight, height, and head circumference through age 11 years in EPT infants without motor disorders. Weight and height catch-up growth were seen by age 11 years in EPT infants, but beyond 6 months corrected age there was no catch-up for head growth. In fact, a significant proportion (22%) of EPT infants had a head circumference greater than 2 SDs below the mean at age 11 years in the EPT group compared with controls (1%). The initially low body mass index in EPT infants is often followed by a period of rapid increase that might suggest a potential for insulin resistance. Data are conflicting on this issue, but there seems to be an association of preterm birth and increased risk for metabolic syndrome.[109]

In addition to assessment of baseline and longitudinal growth measurements in EPT infants, one must consider specific nutritional detriments, medication exposure, and neonatal pathologic conditions that can affect growth negatively. Decreased growth velocity has been seen in some infants with postnatal exposure to glucocorticoids and IVH, in many with BPD, and certainly in those with a history of necrotizing enterocolitis, that may endure for years.[110] Bone mineral content and growth is impaired in EPT infants who not only have missed out on in utero accretion, but may have increased renal wasting of calcium and poor intake of enteral phosphorous. Metabolic bone disease of prematurity was present in more than 15% of VPT individuals in a single institution study using bone density measurements before discharge.[111] Treatment of metabolic bone disease improves growth and avoids risk of fractures, but in one study there was delayed stature in pre-adolescents, even in those who had recovered.[112]

Nutritional concerns for EPT infants also frequently include difficulty with progression to full oral feeding, which may delay hospital discharge and complicate home care. Feeding problems continue to be a concern for parents after hospital discharge. Medical complications, particularly IVH and BPD, may be associated with requirement for prolonged tube feeding and oral aversion. A children's hospital consortium reported 24% of infants with serious chronic lung disease had a surgically placed gastrostomy tube (G-tube) before discharge.[113] In another single-center, retrospective study, prolonged duration of mechanical ventilation and placement of ventriculoperitoneal shunt were predictors of need for a G-tube.[114] Jadcherla and colleagues[115] reported that 40% of preterm infants evaluated for feeding disorders received a G-tube and nearly 80% of those continued to have full or partial G-tube feedings at 1 year of age. Failure to obtain full oral feedings by discharge was associated with NDI at follow-up assessment. Ensuring nutritional sufficiency in the first year of life is important for brain growth and neurodevelopmental outcome. Therefore, feeding difficulties increase long-term risks for VPT infants and increase stress for their care providers. To date, there has been insufficient evaluation of this aspect of follow-up care.

QUALITY OF LIFE

From the previous discussion it becomes apparent that children born EPT/VPT or ELBW/VLBW have different health and developmental trajectories that continue into adulthood than those born at term with normal weight. Functional status, defined as the ability to perform age-appropriate activities, may be assessed using tools such as WeeFIM,[116] Vineland Adaptive Behavior Scale (Vineland-3),[117] or the Pediatric Evaluation of Disability Inventory.[118] Children with similar impairments may display different levels of functional ability, depending on individual strengths, adaptive skills, and availability of support systems. Broad community resources are important for EPT/VPT children, even without identified NDI, to address and assist potential areas of concern.[119] Additional study of the impact of these interventions on functional status during childhood is needed to assist with public planning for optimal outcomes for these vulnerable children.

Functional outcomes need to be considered separately from QoL. When it is all said and done, QoL may arguably be one of the major benchmarks of outcome. QoL is an abstract concept involving assessment of the individual's perception of his or her physical, mental, and social characteristics.[120] "Health-related quality of life" (HRQL) relates to an individual's perception of the impact of the health status and treatments on personal well-being and ability to live a productive life. HRQL has been measured with disease-specific tools, but for preterm survivors, generic health-profile instruments generally have been used.[121] Individuals with the same health status may report very different levels of HRQL. Generally, QoL measures are viewed as being more problematic by general public or health care providers than by those who actually have the health condition.

Despite the apparent importance of understanding QoL outcomes, it is unusual for investigators to ask individual subjects to rate this variable. Utility measures, which are preference-based measures, may be used to provide a relative value for a given health state, reflecting the desirability or undesirability of specific states. Saigal and colleagues[122] used the "Standard Gamble" technique to reflect an individual's valuation of his or her health status. Using the Health Utility Index, these investigators found no statistical differences in HRQL between VPT and term-born adolescents, although functional status of those born preterm was lower. Studies that have used parents as proxies for child reports or have used health values based on general public preferences suggest lower QoL measures for former preterm children and adults.[121] As mentioned previously, although it would seem most important to understand survivors' perceptions and values of their health outcomes, currently this is primarily a research endeavor, because of the difficulty and expense incurred to obtain these unique follow-up data.

SUMMARY

The traditional approach to NICU follow-up has involved detection of NDI in the first years of life by serial examinations and standardized developmental testing, with categorization of levels of impairment, primarily used for research purposes. Such early childhood assessments do not consistently correlate with long-term outcome metrics, and may either underestimate or overestimate later functional concerns. Less severe, but more prevalent, neurobehavioral dysfunctions, which only may become evident in later childhood, often have greater impact on QoL issues, including academic success and social interactions. Ongoing health concerns for former preterm infants have been underappreciated, and the impact of these may not be fully addressed in routine follow-up protocols. Comprehensive NICU follow-up should include metrics related to physical and mental well-being, and ensure availability of environmental support and family factors necessary to promote resilience. Further investigation is needed to better define QoL assessments that could be incorporated into routine follow-up screening and potentially guide interventions to optimize outcomes.

REFERENCES

1. Marlow N, Wolke D, Bracewell M, et al. Neurologic and developmental disability at six years of age after extremely preterm birth. N Engl J Med 2005;352:9–19.
2. Rogers E, Hintz S. Early neurodevelopmental outcomes of extremely preterm infants. Semin Perinatol 2016;40:497–509.
3. Hintz S, Newman J, Vohr B. Changing definitions of long-term follow-up: should "long term" be even longer? Semin Perinatol 2016;40:398–409.
4. Kilbride H, Aylward G, Doyle L, et al. Prognostic neurodevelopmental testing of preterm infants: do we need to change the paradigm? J Perinatol 2017;37: 475–9.
5. McCormick M, Litt J. The outcomes of very preterm infants: is it time to ask different questions? Pediatrics 2017;139:1–3.
6. Hintz S. Defining outcomes for high-risk infants: problems and possibilities. Semin Perinatol 2016;40:495–6.
7. Martinez-Biarge M, Jowett V, Cowan F, et al. Neurodevelopmental outcome in children with congenital heart disease. Semin Fetal Neonatal Med 2013;8: 279–85.
8. Murthy K, Dykes F, Padula M, et al. The Children's Hospitals Neonatal Database: an overview of patient complexity, outcomes and variation in care. J Perinatol 2014;34:582–6.
9. Vohr B. Neurodevelopmental outcomes of extremely preterm infants. Clin Perinatol 2014;41:241–55.
10. Vohr B, Allan W, Westerveld M, et al. School-age outcomes of very low birth weight infants in the indomethacin intraventricular hemorrhage prevention trial. Pediatrics 2003;111:e340–6.
11. Hielkema T, Hadders-Algra M. Motor and cognitive outcome after specific early lesions of the brain—a systematic review. Dev Med Child Neurol 2016;58(Suppl 4):46–52.
12. Bayley N. Bayley scales of infant and toddler development. 3rd edition. San Antonio (TX): PsychCorp; 2006.
13. Aylward GP. The conundrum of prediction. Pediatrics 2005;116:491–2.
14. Aylward GP. Continuing issues with the Bayley-III: where to go from here. J Dev Behav Pediatr 2013;34:697–701.
15. Acton BV, Biggs W, Petrie JH, et al. Overestimating neurodevelopment using the Bayley-III after early complex cardiac surgery. Pediatrics 2011;128:794–800.
16. Hack M, Taylor H, Drotar D, et al. Poor predictive validity of the Bayley Scales of Infant Development for cognitive function of extremely low birth weight children at school age. Pediatrics 2005;116:333–41.
17. Cheong J, Anderson P, Burnett A, et al. Changing neurodevelopment at 8 years in children born extremely preterm since the 1990s. Pediatrics 2017;139:2–8.

18. Bernardo J, Friedman H, Minich N, et al. Cognitive and motor function of neurologically impaired extremely low birth weight children. Paediatr Child Health 2015;20:e33–7.
19. Ment L, Vohr B, Allan W, et al. Change in cognitive function over time in very low-birth-weight infants. JAMA 2003;289:705–11.
20. Breslau N, Chilcoat H, Susser E, et al. Stability and change in children's intelligence quotient scores: a comparison of two socioeconomically disparate communities. Am J Epidemiol 2001;154:711–7.
21. Kilbride H, Thorstad K, Daily D. Preschool outcome of less than 801-gram preterm infants compared with full-term siblings. Pediatrics 2004;113:742–7.
22. Manley B, Roberts R, Doyle L, et al. Social variables predict gains in cognitive scores across the preschool years in children with birth weights 500 to 1250 grams. J Pediatr 2015;166:870–6.
23. Hair N, Hanson J, Wolfe B, et al. Association of child poverty, brain development, and academic achievement. JAMA Pediatr 2015;169:822–9.
24. Hackman D, Farah M, Meaney M. Socioeconomic status and the brain: mechanistic insights from human and animal research. Nat Rev Neurosci 2010;11: 651–9.
25. Lipina S, Martelli M, Vuelta B, et al. Performance on the A-not-B task of Argentinian infants from unsatisfied and satisfied basic needs homes. Int J Psychol 2005;39:49–60.
26. Hackman D, Gallop R, Evan G, et al. Socioeconomic status and executive function: developmental trajectories and mediation. Dev Sci 2015;18:686–702.
27. Doyle L, Anderson P, Battin M, et al. Long term follow up of high risk children: who, why and how? BMC Pediatr 2014;14:279–93.
28. Aylward G. Cognitive and neuropsychological outcomes: more than IQ scores. Ment Retard Dev Disabil Res Rev 2002;8:234–40.
29. Aylward G. Neurodevelopmental outcomes of infants born prematurely. J Dev Behav Pediatr 2005;26:427–40.
30. Vohr B. Follow-up of extremely preterm infants: the long and short of it. Pediatrics 2017;139(6) [pii:e20170453].
31. Constable R, Ment L, Vohr B, et al. Prematurely born children demonstrate white matter microstructural differences at 12 years of age, relative to term control subjects: an investigation of group and gender effects. Pediatrics 2008;121: 458–63.
32. Lubson J, Vohr B, Myers E, et al. Microstructural and functional connectivity in the developing preterm brain. Semin Perinatol 2011;35:34–43.
33. Harmon H, Taylor H, Minich N, et al. Early school outcomes for extremely preterm infants with transient neurological abnormalities. Dev Med Child Neurol 2015;57:865–71.
34. Grunau R, Whitfield M, Davis C. Pattern of learning disabilities in children with extremely low birth weight and broadly average intelligence. Arch Pediatr Adolesc Med 2002;156:615–20.
35. Litt J, Taylor H, Klein N, et al. Learning disabilities in children with very low birthweight: prevalence, neuropsychological correlates, and educational interventions. J Learn Disabil 2005;38:130–41.
36. Saigal S, Hoult LA, Streiner DL, et al. School difficulties at adolescence in a regional cohort of children who were extremely low birth weight. Pediatrics 2000;105:325–31.
37. Odd D, Evans D, Emond A. Preterm birth, age at school entry and long term educational achievement. PLoS One 2016;11(5):e0155157.

38. Bohm B, Katz-Salamon M, Smedler A, et al. Developmental risks and protective factors for influencing cognitive outcome at 5½ years of age in very-low-birthweight children. Dev Med Child Neurol 2002;44:508–16.
39. Mikkola K, Ritari N, Tommiska V, et al. Neurodevelopmental outcome at 5 years of age of a national cohort of extremely low birth weight infants who were born in 1996-1997. Pediatrics 2005;116:1391–400.
40. Bhutta A, Cleves M, Casey P, et al. Cognitive and behavioral outcomes of school-aged children who were born preterm. A meta-analysis. JAMA 2002; 288:728–37.
41. Johnson S. Cognitive and behavioral outcomes following very preterm birth. Semin Fetal Neonatal Med 2007;12:363–73.
42. Huddy C. Preterm birth and the school years. Dev Med Child Neurol 2015;57: 502–3.
43. Taylor H, Clark C. Executive function in children born preterm: risk factors and implications for outcome. Semin Perinatol 2016;40:520–9.
44. Aarnoudse-Moens C, Smidts D, Oosterlassn J, et al. Executive function in very preterm children at early school age. J Abnorm Child Psychol 2009;37:981–93.
45. Burnett A, Scratch S, Lee K, et al. Executive function in adolescents born <1000 g or <28 weeks: a prospective cohort study. Pediatrics 2015;135: e826–34.
46. Lawrence E, Rubia K, Murray R, et al. The neural basis of response inhibition and attention allocation as mediated by gestational age. Hum Brain Mapp 2009;30:1038–50.
47. Costa D, Miranda D, Burnett A, et al. Executive function and academic outcomes in children who were extremely preterm. Pediatrics 2017;140 [pii: e20170257].
48. Scott M, Taylor H, Fristad M, et al. Behavior disorders in extremely preterm/ extremely low birth weight children in kindergarten. J Dev Behav Pediatr 2012;33:202–13.
49. Achenbach T. Manual for child behavior checklist; 4–18 and 1991 profile. Burlington (VT): University of Vermont Department of Psychiatry; 1991.
50. Grunau R, Whitfield M, Fay T. Psychosocial and academic characteristics of extremely low birth weight (<= 800 g) adolescents who are free of major impairment compared with term-born control subjects. Pediatrics 2004;114:725–32.
51. Aarnoudse-Moens C, Weisglas-Kuperus N, Van Goudoever J, et al. Meta-analysis of neurobehavioral outcomes in very preterm and/or very low birth weight children. Pediatrics 2009;124:717–28.
52. Hille E, den Ouden A, Saigal S, et al. Behavioral problems in children who weigh 1000 g or less at birth in four countries. Lancet 2001;357:1641–3.
53. Stjernqvist K, Svenningsen N. Ten-year follow-up of children born before 29 gestational weeks: health, cognitive development, behavior and school achievement. Acta Paediatr 1999;88:557–62.
54. Husby I, Stray K, Olsen A, et al. Long-term follow-up of mental health, health related quality of life and associations with motor skills in young adults born preterm with very low birth weight. Health Qual Life Outcomes 2016;14:56.
55. Johnson S, Marlow N. Preterm birth and childhood psychiatric disorders. Pediatr Res 2011;69:11R–8R.
56. Elgen I, Sommerfelt K, Markestad T. Population based, controlled study of behavioral problems and psychiatric disorders in low birthweight children at 11 years of age. Arch Dis Child Fetal Neonatal Ed 2002;87:F128–32.

57. Indredavik M, Vik T, Evensen K. Perinatal risk and psychiatric outcome in adolescents born preterm with very low birth weight or term small for gestational age. J Dev Behav Pediatr 2010;31:286–94.
58. Hofheimer J. Autism risk in very preterm infants—new answers, more questions. J Pediatr 2014;164:6–8.
59. Kuzniewicz M, Wi S, Qian Y, et al. Prevalence and neonatal factors associated with autism spectrum disorders in preterm infants. J Pediatr 2014;164:20–5.
60. Pritchard M, de Dassel T, Beller E, et al. Autism in toddlers born very preterm. Pediatrics 2016;137(2):e20151949.
61. Luu T, Vohr B, Allan W, et al. Evidence for catch-up in cognition and receptive vocabulary among adolescents born very preterm. Pediatrics 2011;128:313–22.
62. Lindstrom K, Lindblad F, Hjern A. Psychiatric morbidity in adolescents and young adults born preterm: a Swedish national cohort study. Pediatrics 2009; 123:47–53.
63. Abel K, Wicks S, Susser E, et al. Birth weight, schizophrenia, and adult mental disorder: is risk confined to the smallest babies? Arch Gen Psychiatry 2010;67: 923–30.
64. Brummelte S, Grunau R, Synnes A, et al. Declining cognitive development from 8 to 18 months in preterm children predicts persisting higher parenting stress. Early Hum Dev 2011;87:273–80.
65. Wagner S, Cepeda I, Krieger D, et al. Higher cortisol is associated with poorer executive functioning in preschool children: the role of parenting stress, parent coping and quality of daycare. Child Neuropsychol 2016;22:853–69.
66. Linden M, Cepeda I, Synnes A, et al. Stress in parents of children born very preterm is predicted by child externalizing behavior and parent coping at age 7 years. Arch Dis Child 2015;100:554–8.
67. Hynan M, Hall S. Psychosocial program standards for NICU parents. J Perinatol 2015;35(Suppl 1):S1–4.
68. American Psychiatric Association. Diagnostic and statistical manual of mental disorders. 5th edition. Arlington (VA): American Psychiatric Association; 2013.
69. Henderson S, Sugden D, Barnett A. Movement assessment battery for children—2 second edition. London: The Psychological Corporation; 2007.
70. Dewey D, Creighton D, Heath J, et al. Assessment of developmental coordination disorder in children born with extremely low birth weights. Dev Neuropsychol 2011;36:42–56.
71. Foulder-Hughes L, Cooke R. Motor, cognitive, and behavioral disorders in children born very preterm. Dev Med Child Neurol 2003;45:97–103.
72. Holsti L, Grunau R, Whitfield M. Developmental coordination disorder in extremely low birth weight children at nine years. J Dev Behav Pediatr 2002; 23:9–15.
73. Edwards J, Berube M, Erlandson K, et al. Developmental coordination disorder in school-aged children born very preterm and/or very low birth weight: a systematic review. J Dev Behav Pediatr 2011;32:678–87.
74. Goyen T, Liu K. Developmental coordination disorder in "apparently normal" schoolchildren born extremely preterm. Arch Dis Child 2009;94:298–302.
75. Missiuna C, Moll S, King S, et al. A trajectory of troubles: parents' impressions of the impact of developmental coordination disorder. Phys Occup Ther Pediatr 2009;27:98–101.
76. Yeh J, McGrath-Morrow S, Collaco J. Oxygen weaning after hospital discharge in children with bronchopulmonary dysplasia. Pediatr Pulmonol 2016;51: 1206–11.

77. Fawke J, Lum S, Kirby J, et al. Lung function and respiratory symptoms at 11 years in children born extremely preterm: the EPICure study. Am J Respir Crit Care Med 2010;182:237–45.

78. Hennessy E, Bracewell M, Wood N, et al. Respiratory health in pre-school and school age children following extremely preterm birth. Arch Dis Child 2008;93: 1037–43.

79. Vom H, Prenzel F, Uhlig H, et al. Pulmonary outcome in former preterm, very low birth weight children with bronchopulmonary dysplasia: a case-control follow-up at school age. J Pediatr 2014;164:40–5.

80. Gunville C, Sontag M, Stratton K, et al. Scope and impact of early and late preterm infants admitted to the PICU with respiratory illness. J Pediatr 2010;157: 209–14.

81. Underwood M, Danielson B, Gilbert W. Cost causes and rates of prehospitalization of preterm infants. J Perinatol 2007;27:614–9.

82. Greenough A. Long-term respiratory consequences of premature birth at less than 32 weeks of gestation. Early Hum Dev 2013;89:S25–7.

83. DeVries L, Heyne R, Ramaciotti C, et al. Mortality among infants with evolving bronchopulmonary dysplasia increases with major surgery and with pulmonary hypertension. J Perinatol 2017;37:1043–6.

84. Gough A, Linden M, Spence D, et al. Impaired lung function and health status in adult survivors of bronchopulmonary dysplasia. Eur Respir J 2014;43:808–16.

85. Joshi S, Kotecha S. Lung growth and development. Early Hum Dev 2007;83: 789–94.

86. Colin A, McEvoy C, Castille R. Respiratory morbidity and lung function in preterm infants of 32 to 36 weeks' gestational age. Pediatrics 2010;126:115–28.

87. McEvoy C, Aschner J. The natural history of bronchopulmonary dysplasia: the case for primary prevention. Clin Perinatol 2015;4:911–31.

88. Kotecha SJ, Edwards MO, Watkins WJ, et al. Effect of preterm birth on later FEV1: a systematic review and meta-analysis. Thorax 2013;68:760–6.

89. Lange P, Bartolome C, Agusti A, et al. Lung-function trajectories leading to chronic obstructive pulmonary disease. N Engl J Med 2015;373:111–22.

90. Poon C, Edwards M, Kotecha S. Long term cardiovascular consequences of chronic lung disease of prematurity. Paediatr Respir Rev 2013;14:242–9.

91. Rogers M, Fay T, Whitfield M, et al. Aerobic capacity, strength, flexibility, and activity level in unimpaired extremely low birth weight ($\leq$800 g) survivors at 17 years of age compared with term-born control subjects. Pediatrics 2005; 116(1):e58–65.

92. Lowe J, Watkins W, Kotecha S, et al. Physical activity and sedentary behavior in preterm-born 7-year old children. PLoS One 2016;11(5):e0155229.

93. Kilbride H, Gelatt M, Sabath R. Pulmonary function and exercise capacity for ELBW survivors in preadolescence: effect of neonatal chronic lung disease. J Pediatr 2003;143:488–93.

94. Welsh L, Kirkby J, Lum S, et al. The EPICure study: maximal exercise and physical activity in school children born extremely preterm. Thorax 2010;65: 165–72.

95. Barker D, Winter P, Osmond C, et al. Weight in infancy and death from ischaemic heart disease. Lancet 1989;2:577–80.

96. Doyle L, Faber B, Callanan C, et al. Blood pressure in late adolescence and very low birth weight. Pediatrics 2003;111:252–7.

97. Bonamy A, Kallen K, Norman M. High blood pressure in 2.5-year-old children born extremely preterm. Pediatrics 2012;129(5):e1199–204.

98. Vohr B, Allan W, Katz K, et al. Early predictors of hypertension in prematurely born adolescents. Acta Paediatr 2010;99:1812–8.

99. Norman M. Preterm birth—an emerging risk factor for adult hypertension. Semin Perinatol 2010;34:183–7.

100. Clarenbach C, Thurnheer R, Kohler M. Vascular dysfunction in chronic obstructive pulmonary disease: current evidence and perspectives. Expert Rev Respir Med 2012;6:37–43.

101. Askanazi D, Morgan C, Goldstein S, et al. Strategies to improve the understanding of long-term consequences after neonatal acute kidney injury. Pediatr Res 2016;79:502–8.

102. Vieux R, Gerard M, Roussel A, et al. Kidneys in 5-year-old preterm-born children: a longitudinal cohort monitoring of renal function. Pediatr Res 2017; 82(6):979–85.

103. Flynn J. Hypertension in the neonatal period. Curr Opin Pediatr 2012;24: 197–204.

104. Blencowe H, Lawn J, Vazquez T, et al. Preterm-associated visual impairment and estimates of retinopathy of prematurity at regional and global levels for 2010. Pediatr Res 2013;74:S35–49.

105. O'Connor A, Fielder A. Long term ophthalmic sequelae of prematurity. Early Hum Dev 2008;84:101–6.

106. Molnar AEC, Andréasson SO, Larsson EKB, et al. Reduction of rod and cone function in 6.5-year-old children born extremely preterm. JAMA Ophthal 2017; 135(8):854–61.

107. Fierson W. American Academy of Pediatrics Section on Ophthalmology. Screening examination of premature infants for retinopathy of prematurity. Pediatrics 2013;131:189–95.

108. Farooqi A, Hagglof B, Sedin G, et al. Growth in 10 to 12 year old children born at 23 to 25 weeks' gestation in the 1990's: a Swedish national prospective follow-up study. Pediatrics 2006;118(5):e1452–65.

109. Tinnion R, Gillone J, Cheetham T, et al. Preterm birth and subsequent insulin sensitivity: a systematic review. Arch Dis Child 2014;99:362–8.

110. Hintz S, Kendrick D, Stoll B. Neurodevelopment and growth outcomes of extremely low birth weight infants after necrotizing enterocolitis. Pediatrics 2005;15:696–703.

111. Figueras-Aloy J, Alvarez-Dominguez E, Perez-Fernandez JM, et al. Metabolic bone disease and bone mineral density in very preterm infants. J Pediatr 2014;164:499–504.

112. Rigo J, De Curtis M, Pieltain C, et al. Bone mineral metabolism in the micropremie. Clin Perinatol 2000;27:147–70.

113. Grover TR, Brozanski BS, Barry J, et al. High surgical burden for infants with severe chronic lung disease (sCLD). J Pediatr Surg 2014;49:1202–5.

114. Malkar M, Gardner W, Welty S, et al. Antecedent predictors of feedings outcomes in premature infants with protracted mechanical ventilation. J Pediatr Gastroenterol Nutr 2015;61:591–5.

115. Jadcherla S, Khot T, Moore R, et al. Feeding methods at discharge predict long-term feeding and neurodevelopmental outcomes in preterm infants referred for gastrostomy evaluation. J Pediatr 2017;181:125–30.

116. Ottenbacher K, Msall M, Lyon N, et al. The WeeFIM instrument: its utility in detecting change in children with developmental disabilities. Arch Phys Med Rehabil 2000;81:1317–26.

117. Sparrow S, Chicchetti D, Saulnier C. Vineland-32016. Bloomington (MN): PsychCorp; 2016.
118. Haley S, Coster W, Ludlow L, et al. Pediatric evaluation of disability inventory: development, standardization and administration manual. Boston: Trustees of Boston University; 1992.
119. Spittle A, Orton J, Anderson P, et al. Early developmental intervention programs provided post hospital discharge to prevent motor and cognitive impairment in preterm infants. Cochrane Database Syst Rev 2015;(24):CD005495.
120. WHOQOL Group. Development of the WHOQOL: rationale and current status. Int J Ment Healt 1994;23:24–56.
121. Saigal S, Tyson J. Measurement of quality of life of survivors of neonatal intensive care: critique and implications. Semin Perinatol 2008;32:59–66.
122. Saigal S, Stoskopf B, Pinelli J, et al. Self-perceived health-related quality of life of former extremely low birth weight infants at young adulthood. Pediatrics 2006; 118:1140–8.

Biological and Social Influences on the Neurodevelopmental Outcomes of Preterm Infants

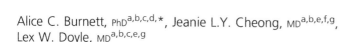

Alice C. Burnett, PhD[a,b,c,d,*], Jeanie L.Y. Cheong, MD[a,b,e,f,g], Lex W. Doyle, MD[a,b,c,e,g]

KEYWORDS

- Preterm infant • Neurodevelopment • Neurosensory • Cognition • Behavior
- Biomarkers • Environment

KEY POINTS

- Early biological factors (eg, brain injury and retinopathy of prematurity) and treatments (eg, postnatal corticosteroids and early surgery) are markers of later sensory and motor impairments.
- Cognitive and academic difficulties seem to be susceptible to some biological and social variables, but these influences vary across development.
- Behavior and mental health outcomes are not consistently associated with perinatal variables, but greater relationships exist with earlier behavioral difficulties and parental well-being.

INTRODUCTION

Preterm birth (birth at <37 weeks of gestation) is a substantial risk factor for poor neurodevelopmental outcomes in areas such as neurosensory, cognitive, and behavioral functioning. A gestational age gradient exists such that increasing immaturity at birth

Disclosure Statement: The authors have no conflicts of interests to disclose.
[a] Premature Infant Follow-Up Program, The Royal Women's Hospital, 20 Flemington Road, Parkville, Victoria 3052, Australia; [b] Victorian Infant Brain Studies, Murdoch Childrens Research Institute, Flemington Road, Parkville, Melbourne, Victoria 3052, Australia; [c] Department of Pediatrics, University of Melbourne, Parkville, Victoria 3010, Australia; [d] Department of Neonatal Medicine, The Royal Children's Hospital, 50 Flemington Road, Parkville, Victoria 3052, Australia; [e] Department of Obstetrics and Gynaecology, University of Melbourne, Parkville, Victoria 3010, Australia; [f] Neonatal Services, The Royal Women's Hospital, 20 Flemington Road, Parkville, Victoria 3052, Australia; [g] Newborn Research, The Royal Women's Hospital, Level 7, 20 Flemington Road, Parkville, Melbourne, Victoria 3052, Australia
* Corresponding author. Victorian Infant Brain Studies, Murdoch Childrens Research Institute, The Royal Children's Hospital, Flemington Road, Parkville, Melbourne, Victoria 3052, Australia.
E-mail address: alice.burnett@mcri.edu.au

is associated with greater risks of neurodevelopmental difficulties,[1,2] with those born extremely preterm or extremely low birthweight (EP/ELBW; <28 weeks/<1000 g) comprising a small proportion of births[3,4] but facing the greatest risk of adverse outcomes. Other categorizations of maturity at birth include very preterm (VP) and very low birthweight (<32 weeks/<1500 g), and moderate and late preterm (32–36 weeks). Traditionally, prematurity research has involved cohorts defined by birthweight rather than gestational age, which may have included more mature but growth-restricted infants than cohorts selected according to gestational age alone. In addition, survival of the most immature infants has improved dramatically since the 1970s, changing the profile of survivorship. It is, therefore, imperative to understand the biological and social–environmental influences that shape long-term outcomes in contemporary cohorts of preterm children. These biological and social–environmental effects may be direct or interactive and there may be critical windows of development within which such variables have amplified effects. Although moderate and late preterm infants are increasingly recognized as being at developmental risk,[5] they enter the ex utero environment later in gestational development than EP or VP infants, who are likely to have different biological vulnerabilities and environmental susceptibilities. Thus, this review examines the biological and social influences on neurosensory outcomes, cognitive and academic functioning, and behavior and mental health in contemporary VP and very low birthweight and EP/ELBW survivors, across key periods of development. We focus mainly on data from large longitudinal studies of prospective cohorts born since 1990 (the era of modern neonatal intensive care).

NEUROSENSORY OUTCOMES

Perhaps the most commonly reported outcome in studies of prematurity is a composite outcome of neurosensory impairment, also called neurodevelopmental impairment. Neurosensory impairments generally include cerebral palsy (CP), impaired vision, impaired hearing, and developmental delay in younger children or intellectual impairment in older children. Neurosensory impairments are generally categorized according to the degree of impairment observed (eg, mild/moderate/severe). Permanent motor and sensory impairments are generally identified early in life and have important implications for other aspects of children's functioning, including in cognitive, academic, and social domains.

Biological Influences on Neurosensory Outcomes

Biological influences are strong markers of later vision, hearing, and motor impairments in preterm children. Vulnerabilities of various organ systems as well as medical treatments have been linked with later sensorimotor impairments.

Cerebral palsy

CP is a family of nonprogressive movement disorders[6] that reportedly affects from 6%[7] to 14%[8] of children born EP. Brain injury identified in the perinatal period is a key predictor of later CP diagnosis. Major abnormalities on cranial ultrasound studies are associated with later CP (adjusted odds ratio, 8.8; 95% confidence interval, 2.6–30.1),[9] with risks greatest for those with cystic periventricular leukomalacia (PVL) or intraparenchymal involvement of an intraventricular hemorrhage (IVH; adjusted odds ratio, 28.4; 95% confidence interval, 15.7–51.6).[10] However, not all infants who later develop CP have a lesion identifiable on neonatal cranial ultrasound examination with evidence that 1 in 3 infants[10] to 1 in 2 infants[11] who later develop CP have normal cranial ultrasound findings as neonates. Compared with cranial ultrasound examination, abnormalities on neonatal brain MRI are more sensitive indicators of later CP.[12,13] Beyond early brain injury, inflammatory responses to infection have been highlighted as a potential contributor, including proven sepsis (adjusted odds ratio, 3.2; 95% confidence interval, 1.2–8.5).[9] However, whereas 16% of VP infants with necrotizing enterocolitis (NEC) had a diagnosis of CP at 5 years of age in 1 study, this was not a significant predictor after accounting for brain injury and other perinatal variables.[10] In terms of treatment exposures, antenatal corticosteroid administration to mothers at risk of preterm delivery enhances fetal lung maturation and, indeed, seems to be protective for a range of organ systems.[14,15] Consistent with these findings, infants whose mothers received a complete course of antenatal corticosteroid are reported to be at one-half the risk of those with no antenatal corticosteroid for later diagnosis of any CP.[16,17] Postnatally, systemic corticosteroids are used to prevent or treat bronchopulmonary dysplasia, but the risks of short- and long-term adverse outcomes, including CP,[18,19] have led to suggestions to restrict their use to those at greatest risk of developing bronchopulmonary dysplasia.[20] Finally, the sex of the infant is also relevant to the risk of CP. Males born EP are at increased risk of CP relative to females (11% vs 7%),[21] and this pattern has been reported in some studies, irrespective of the presence of major brain injury.[10,22]

Vision and hearing

Severe hearing and vision deficits are infrequent in contemporary cohorts of EP children, with rates in toddlers of less than 2% and 3%, respectively.[7,23] Vision impairments can arise from retinopathy of prematurity (ROP), a condition that involves abnormal development of the retinal vasculature and is more common in the most immature babies (ie, EP infants) and those with other medical conditions, including respiratory distress, inadequate oxygen control (both hypoxia and hyperoxia), infections, and hyperglycaemia.[24] Although ROP generally resolves without causing blindness, its prevalence and severity are greater in lower resource settings than in higher resource settings.[24] ROP treatments include laser therapy and anti-vascular endothelial growth factor treatments, including ranibizumab and bevacizumab.[25] Both focal and diffuse brain injury associated with preterm birth can damage visual cortex and pathways, resulting in impaired visual function across development.[26,27] However, ROP and focal brain injury (eg, IVH and cystic PVL) account for only some of the variance in visual outcomes, suggesting that other variables are also at play.[27] Other medical morbidities, including cardiac anomalies such as patent ductus arteriosus and its treatments, have been variably associated with ROP, although confounding by indication has been raised as a concern in the literature.[28,29]

Etiologic factors for hearing difficulties in preterm infants are also not fully understood. Antibiotics such as gentamicin, commonly used to treat infections in preterm infants, have ototoxic side effects such as causing death of hair cells in the cochlea.[30] VP infants with patent ductus arteriosus receiving treatment (either medical or surgical) are at increased risk of hearing impairment in toddlerhood (5%–6% vs 2% in infants with no or mild patent ductus arteriosus).[31] Genetic factors may be relevant, but greater investigation in human studies is required.[30,32] The majority of preterm infants with severe hearing loss can be detected by early newborn hearing screening; however, some VP infants with normal neonatal hearing screens may nevertheless experience sensorineural hearing loss in the toddler period.[33] Moreover, other hearing deficits, such as figure-ground perceptual loss and poor short-term auditory memory, which can interfere with classroom learning, are more common in children born preterm,[34] but cannot be detected by newborn hearing screening.

Social Influences on Neurosensory Outcomes

Less evidence exists regarding how social or environmental influences may shape neurosensory outcomes, compared with biological influences, in preterm children. However, early diagnosis and intervention of permanent sensory or motor problems can assist in minimizing the functional consequences of neurosensory impairments; social variables may play a role in determining access to and delivery of early intervention. With respect to hearing, exposure to high noise levels in the neonatal intensive care unit (NICU) may interact with biological exposures, such as gentamicin, to accelerate damage to the hearing system.[30] Exposure to high-frequency sounds seems to be particularly problematic for cochlear development.[30] In the general population, earlier identification of hearing impairment, participation in early intervention programs, and highly engaged parents are all beneficial in reducing the impact of hearing impairment on later language functioning.[32,35] Early therapeutic interventions can also improve motor outcomes for preterm infants more generally, although these effects are not large and long-term effects are not widely found, partly because they are infrequently reported.[36]

Summary

Biological influences are important markers of later motor, vision, and hearing impairments, although the mechanisms behind these outcomes remain incompletely understood. Environmental influences including exposures and interventions have the potential to improve the broader outcomes of children with permanent sensory and motor impairments.

COGNITIVE AND ACADEMIC OUTCOMES

Cognitive deficits are the most commonly identified difficulties after preterm birth. In toddlerhood, early cognitive and language abilities are now primarily assessed using the Bayley Scales of Infant and Toddler Development–Third Edition.[37] For older samples assessed with the second edition of this test, cognitive and language abilities at this age were measured with a single index (Mental Developmental Index) and, thus, could not be distinguished from each other. In older children, many studies focus on full-scale IQ, whereas some delve more deeply into different cognitive domains. Importantly, different cognitive skills emerge and mature at different points in development, and thus may have different windows of susceptibility to external influences. Further, cognitive and academic deficits can emerge in children whose earlier development seemed to be normal.

Biological Influences on Cognitive and Academic Outcomes

Medical conditions and exposures, including brain injury, treatments, and systemic illness, as well as sex, have been investigated for links with later cognitive outcomes, although precise causal pathways remain unknown in some cases. Major focal brain injury (generally comprising severe IVH or cystic PVL) and more diffuse PVL in early life both have the potential for direct and secondary disruption of brain development, and hence cognitive function.[38] Although major brain injuries are now less common compared with earlier eras, they are nonetheless associated with decreased general intellectual ability in childhood and adolescence,[39] and with school-age literacy and numeracy for EP children.[40] Examination of the relationships of other brain abnormalities with later outcome is beyond the scope of this review, and interested readers are directed to recent reviews on advanced neuroimaging correlates of cognitive function.[41]

Metaanalytic evidence suggests that perinatal infections and inflammatory conditions, predominantly NEC and meningitis, have moderate effects on Bayley-II Mental Developmental Index and Psychomotor Development Index scores for VP and very low birthweight toddlers.[42] A small effect size has been reported for chorioamnionitis as a predictor of later cognitive function, particularly evident with respect to chorioamnionitis with clinical manifestations.[43] However, this finding has not been supported in a metaanalysis.[42] Similarly, sepsis does not seem to be linked strongly with cognitive development in toddlerhood, despite its relationships with physical development and CP.[9,42] In some data from older children, NEC has a strong independent relationship with later reading and mathematics abilities.[40]

Although many studies have reported correlates and precursors of later cognitive functioning, very little longitudinal evidence exists regarding change in the relative importance of biological and social predictors of cognitive and academic function. In a prospective longitudinal cohort of EP/ELBW children, Doyle and colleagues[39] examined multivariable associations of biological and environmental influences with cognitive function at ages 2, 5, 6, and 18 years of age (**Fig. 1**) and academic skills at 8 and 18 years of age (**Fig. 2**). They found that gestational age at birth did not independently predict cognitive functioning after accounting for other medical and social variables, although in a larger EP cohort those born at 23 to 24 weeks of gestation were most at risk of poor cognitive and academic functioning at 10 years of age compared with children born more maturely.[2] Doyle and colleagues found that

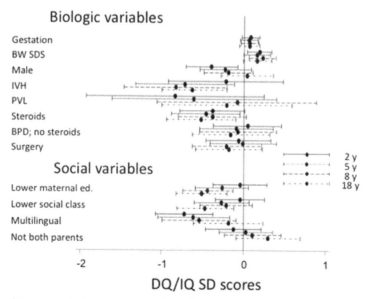

Fig. 1. Relationship of biological and social variables with cognitive test scores at each age standardized relative to the control group. Results are regression coefficients (and 95% confidence intervals) from a single multivariable model for each outcome and represent the mean difference in cognitive scores (SD [Standard Deviation] units) between those with and without the exposure of interest or per-unit increase in continuous variables. The results for each variable are adjusted for the presence of all other variables. Steroids refer to postnatal corticosteroids. BPD, bronchopulmonary dysplasia; BW SDS, birth weight SD score; DQ, developmental quotient; IVH, intraventricular hemorrhage; PVL, periventricular leukomalacia. (*From* Doyle LW, Cheong JLY, Burnett AC, et al. Biological and social influences on outcomes of extreme-preterm/low-birth-weight adolescents. Pediatrics 2015;136(6):e1517; with permission.)

biological influences other than gestational age were more variably associated with cognitive function at different time points, although the direction of effects was generally consistent over time: severe IVH predicted poorer intellectual function at ages 5, 8, and 18 years of age, as did postnatal corticosteroid exposure for function at ages 8 and 18 years of age. Postnatal corticosteroid exposure was also associated with poorer reading, spelling, and mathematical skills at 18 years of age, although not at 8 years of age; bronchopulmonary dysplasia without corticosteroid treatment was not related to academic outcomes at either time point (see **Fig. 2**).[39] Higher birthweight z-scores were associated with better cognitive function at 2 and 8 years, whereas cystic PVL, bronchopulmonary dysplasia without corticosteroid treatment, and neonatal surgery had negligible effects.[39]

Sex differences have also been reported in the literature, with around 42% of EP boys having an Mental Developmental Index of less than 70 compared with 27% of EP girls in toddlerhood.[21] A small male disadvantage has also been reported in Swedish 6-year-olds born at less than 27 weeks of gestation for intellectual functioning, although this was not adjusted for other medical or social influences.[44] However, as shown in **Fig. 1**, sex may also differ in its relationships with cognition across development, with male sex being associated with poorer cognitive function only in the toddler period and not at school age (ages 5, 8, or 18 years).[39] Conflicting evidence exists for

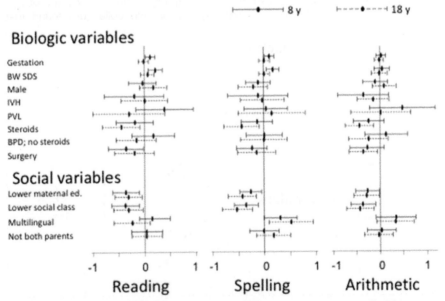

Fig. 2. Relationships of biological and social variables with academic achievement test scores at 8 and 18 years of age standardized relative to the control group. Results are regression coefficients (and 95% confidence intervals) from a single multivariable model for each outcome, and they represent the mean difference in academic scores (SD units) between those with and without the variable of interest or per-unit increase in continuous variables. The results for each variable are adjusted for the presence of all other variables. Arithmetical refers to arithmetical skills at 8 years of age and math computation skills at 18 years of age; steroids refer to postnatal corticosteroids. BPD, bronchopulmonary dysplasia; BW SDS, birth weight SD score; IVH, intraventricular hemorrhage; PVL, periventricular leukomalacia. (*From* Doyle LW, Cheong JLY, Burnett AC, et al. Biological and social influences on outcomes of extreme-preterm/low-birth-weight adolescents. Pediatrics 2015;136(6):e1518; with permission.)

associations between sex and academic functioning, with some evidence for a male disadvantage for reading in the middle school years in 1 study[40] and little evidence for an effect of sex at both 8 and 18 years in another study (see **Fig. 2**).[39]

Associations of earlier developmental status with later cognitive functioning and the contribution of child-specific cognitive influences to academic achievement have also been explored. The size of the difference between preterm and term-born children in general intellectual ability and academic achievement seems to be stable through childhood until late adolescence.[39] Adverse findings in early development, including lower performance on cognitive testing in toddlerhood, are also associated with later reading and mathematics difficulties for EP children.[40] Vulnerability for preterm children may be even more pronounced for mathematical skills than literacy skills,[40] although there are conflicting reports.[45] Mathematical difficulties have been linked with concurrent neuropsychological deficits including attention, executive functioning, and visuospatial processing.[40,46]

Social Influences on Cognitive and Academic Outcomes

Various social–environmental influences have been linked with cognitive functioning, or at least performance on cognitive testing, in preterm samples, including features of the NICU environment, access to early developmental intervention, parental education and socioeconomic status, and the main language spoken in the home. Preterm infants are admitted to the NICU at a time of rapid brain development and the level of sensory stimulation experienced during this period is relevant to children's later functioning. Although it is recognized that excessive auditory exposures are harmful for infants in the NICU, data from randomized, controlled trials of sound reduction interventions to improve long-term outcomes are limited.[47] However, VP infants in single NICU rooms may have poorer language and motor outcomes at 2 years than those cared for in an open ward, suggesting the need to optimize rather than solely minimize sound exposure for preterm infants.[48,49] Greater exposure to painful procedures may also have implications for cognitive development; however, the evidence base is currently small.[50] Early developmental intervention after hospital discharge has the capacity to improve cognitive development into at least the preschool years, although wide variation in the nature and content of early intervention programs makes interpretation difficult.[36]

Although studies to date have measured parental education and socioeconomic status heterogeneously, these influences seem to associate with cognitive functioning.[51] In their longitudinal analysis, Doyle and colleagues[39] found that lower maternal education and lower social class had increasing negative associations with children's cognitive functioning from 2 to 18 years of age, with maternal education of less than a high school completion level ultimately accounting for a decrement of around one-half of a standard deviation in general intellectual ability (see **Fig. 1**).[39] This finding was consistent with evidence from a recent systematic review[52] and these influences also predicted poorer reading, spelling, and mathematical abilities consistently at ages 8 and 18 years (see **Fig. 2**).[39]

The language spoken in the home is also likely to contribute to performance on developmental or cognitive testing, at least in the early years. For instance, tests of language development that are presented in English are biased against children from non–English-speaking households, with the latter performing around 0.3 standard deviation below their English-speaking peers after accounting for medical and socioeconomic variables.[53] Importantly, this relationship may only be evident at particular points in development; Doyle and colleagues[39] found that living in a multilingual household was associated with lower IQ performances from toddlerhood to school age, but this effect dissipated by adolescence (see **Fig. 1**).

Summary

Cognitive difficulties and reduced academic achievement remain high-prevalence sequelae of preterm birth in the current era, and both biological and social influences are associated with these outcomes. Major brain injury is associated with substantial cognitive difficulties, but occurs infrequently. Perinatal infections and inflammatory conditions such as NEC and meningitis carry risks for later cognitive development. Developmental difficulties identified in early life also signal risk for later cognitive and academic outcomes. Male sex and having a language other than English spoken in the home are associated with lower cognitive performance earlier in life, but these effects may dissipate as children grow up. However, parental education and other socioeconomic influences have strong relationships with cognitive and academic outcomes that may be more pronounced as children grow older.

BEHAVIOR AND MENTAL HEALTH

Difficulties in behavior and mental health are widely reported among preterm cohorts, with anxiety, attention problems, and peer/social difficulties, as well as clinical diagnoses of attention deficit and hyperactivity disorder (ADHD; predominantly the inattentive subtype) and autism spectrum disorder (ASD) highlighted.[54] A range of methodologic issues is relevant to this area of literature. Most studies examining behavior and mental health have used questionnaires, targeting either overall behavior problems or measuring specific domains of behavior continuously. Although questionnaires have many strengths, a limitation particularly noted in regard to ASD screening is the potential for confounding by other sequelae of prematurity, such as difficulties in movement, vision, hearing, and language.[55] Few studies have used diagnostic tools, with reported outcomes focusing similarly on any mental health disorder or on specific conditions. Assessments in childhood necessarily rely on parental or teacher reports of emotions and behavior, whereas assessments in adolescence also permit self-report, which may yield divergent information from parental perspectives.[56] Age at follow-up is also an important factor, because disorders differ in their timing of peak onset, with ASD and ADHD generally recognized earlier in childhood, and disorders such as anxiety and depression having a later onset for the majority of cases. The balance of symptoms or disorders that predominate in composite outcomes, such as overall behavior problems or any diagnosis, therefore, may change across development, which has implications for the prediction of these outcomes.

Biological Influences on Behavior and Mental Health

Neonatal biological influences have not been associated consistently with behavior and mental health outcomes for preterm children and adolescents. Of these influences, brain injury and/or altered brain development present as likely candidates for adverse outcomes in this domain, but evidence remains equivocal. Major abnormalities on cranial ultrasound examination (such as severe IVH or cystic PVL) have been associated with a doubling of the odds of overall behavior problems in toddlerhood,[57] but this finding was not observed in the same sample at 5 years of age.[58] Such abnormalities have also not yielded strong relationships with ADHD, ASD, or anxiety symptoms at 8 years of age,[59] clinical diagnosis of overall psychiatric disorder at 11 years of age,[60] or with ADHD or mood/anxiety disorder diagnosis at 18 years of age[61] in EP and ELBW samples. Although cranial ultrasound abnormalities were related to continuously measured ADHD symptoms at 11 years in models of only neonatal variables, behavior and development later in childhood were much stronger correlates.[62] Taken together, these findings may reflect differences in the nature and severity of symptoms assessed (screening questionnaire vs clinical diagnosis), or perhaps an adaptation across the course of development. Studies using brain MRI are more limited, but MRI abnormalities at term-equivalent age have been linked with later behavior and mental health. For instance, white matter abnormalities on MRI have been associated with poorer self-regulation in VP toddlers.[63] VP children with severe abnormalities on MRI had more than 5 times the odds of a mental health disorder diagnosis at 7 years of age compared with those without brain abnormalities,[64] although such a relationship was not observed between questionnaire-based ratings of overall behavior difficulties and MRI abnormalities in the same cohort.[65] In addition to qualitative assessment of brain injury or abnormality, MRI studies have linked more localized structural alterations of the neonatal brain with later outcome. For instance, reduced hippocampal volumes at term-equivalent age were associated with increased hyperactivity and inattentiveness, and peer problems in VP girls at age 5 years.[66]

Other perinatal medical influences do not seem to be strong indicators of later difficulties in this domain. Regarding the degree of prematurity, some data have not shown gradient effects in EP/ELBW children for overall behavior difficulties,[67] whereas an ASD diagnosis was more common with decreasing gestation in a large sample of EP 10-year-old children.[68] In other, smaller EP studies, little evidence has been found for univariable associations of gestational age or birthweight with overall risk of psychiatric disorder at 11 years of age[60] or with ADHD or mood/anxiety disorder diagnosis at 18 years of age.[61] Indeed, in the latter study, EP/ELBW group membership was not associated with increased lifetime mood and anxiety disorders or current mood and anxiety symptoms compared with controls.[61] Further, there is minimal evidence for features such as multiple birth,[60,63,64,69] birthweight relative to gestational age/small for gestational age status,[60,61] postnatal corticosteroid use and/or bronchopulmonary dysplasia[60,63,64,69](cf.[59]), neonatal surgery,[61] or duration of hospitalization[60] relating to mental health symptoms or disorders. Exposure to antenatal corticosteroid may be protective for self-regulation[63] and emotional–behavioral problems[70] in toddlerhood, although this effect has not been found at the level of clinical diagnosis later in childhood.[60,64]

In the broader population, sex differences are observed in some aspects of behavioral functioning and mental health diagnoses. For instance, female sex is a risk factor for depression and anxiety from adolescence onward,[71] whereas ADHD diagnoses are more common in males.[72] Sex differences are also observed in preterm samples, with higher rates of ASD symptoms and diagnosis as well as symptoms of hyperactivity and impulsivity in males than females[62,73] A male bias in ADHD diagnosis is not reported universally,[60] however, this finding may reflect the predominance of inattentive-type ADHD symptoms in preterm populations. Although sex differences are observed to some extent, sex does not seem to interact with extreme prematurity to further elevate risk of poor behavioral functioning or mental health problems in childhood and adolescence.[61,69,74] An exception to this may exist for ASD, where the male:female ratio is lower in EP 10-year-olds than expected from the general population (2.1:1 vs 4:1, respectively).[68]

As noted, cognitive impairment is common in preterm children, and it may also co-occur with behavioral symptoms and psychiatric disorders. In early school age, lower cognitive ability is associated with greater overall behavior difficulties for VP[58] and EP[75] children, although this factor does not account entirely for the excess of morbidity in behavior compared with controls. Associations with cognitive ability seem to be particularly notable for ADHD and ASD, but less so for emotional disorders.[60,75] Major cognitive impairment seems to be associated with ASD to a similar extent in EP children as in the general population, with IQ scores in the intellectual disability range (<70) occurring in around 40% of EP children with an ASD diagnosis.[68] The presence of a chronic medical condition (including neurosensory impairment and nonpsychiatric medical illnesses) has been associated with mood and anxiety symptoms in EP 11-year-olds.[74] Similarly, major neurosensory disability (including cognitive impairment) in childhood predicted the presence of ADHD in older adolescence, although not mood or anxiety disorder.[61] Behavioral difficulties earlier in childhood are also strongly associated with later difficulties in this domain.[60,64]

Social Influences on Behavior and Mental Health

Relationships between social–environmental influences and children's behavior and mental health have been reported more widely. The home environment plays a critical role in any child's development of appropriate coping strategies and emotional regulation. In preterm samples, families' level of social advantage or socioeconomic status is variably linked with behavioral outcomes, although methodologic differences in the measurement of this broad construct hamper direct comparisons. For instance, higher social risk (including family structure, caregiver education and occupation, language spoken in the home, and maternal age at birth) is associated with externalizing behaviors in VP toddlers,[76] and an increased risk of concurrent psychiatric diagnosis in the same sample at 7 years of age.[64] In the more immature EPICure cohort, however, socioeconomic status defined by parental occupation was not related to psychiatric disorders.[60] Young maternal age at birth may also be a relevant factor, and these families often face a variety of adverse social influences. For instance, EP infants born to adolescent mothers have around 1.6 times the odds of emotional–behavioral problems than those born to mothers aged 20 years or older after accounting for other maternal and infant influences.[70]

Reciprocal relationships exist between parenting behaviors and parental well-being and children's behavior and well-being. Parents of preterm infants are at increased risk of anxiety and depression symptoms,[77] although this risk does seem to diminish over time at the group level.[78] Supportive maternal behaviors[63] and low levels of parental mental health symptoms[79] are related to better self-regulation in VP toddlers. There is some suggestion that VP toddlers may have disproportionately poorer self-regulation in the context of parental mental health problems than term-born toddlers,[79] which may have longer term implications for their own behavioral and emotional well-being.

Summary

Methodologic differences abound in studies of behavior and mental health after preterm birth. Overall, perinatal medical influences do not seem to be strong predictors of later behavior and mental health, with conflicting evidence for the value of neonatal cranial ultrasound abnormalities and term-equivalent age MRI. Cognitive and neurosensory impairments may co-present with behavioral and emotional difficulties in preterm children, but are generally not sufficient to explain the increased frequency of these problems. Earlier behavioral difficulties are related to later functioning; monitoring is needed in the early years to promote positive behavioral outcomes. Family influences, including parental mental health and well-being, are also likely to be amenable to intervention.

FUTURE DIRECTIONS

Biological and social influences are associated with outcomes after preterm birth, but more work is needed to characterize the relative importance of and interplay between these influences for different outcomes throughout development. For instance, although it is beyond the scope of this review, prenatal exposures to maternal stress or other biological challenges may program long-term responses to the environment. Gene–environment interaction studies are also a potentially fruitful avenue for future research. This review has focused on preterm birth as the index event. However, it is possible that, for some outcomes, preterm birth is in fact an intermediate event on a broader risk pathway beginning before conception. This does not preclude preterm birth from having its own substantial consequences for later functioning, but highlights the value of life-span perspectives in understanding the mechanisms of outcome.

Recommendations for Future Studies

The evidence summarized herein suggests a number of opportunities for future research to improve knowledge in this area. High-quality longitudinal cohort studies and intervention studies are ideally placed to identify early indicators and predictors of outcomes as opposed to their cross-sectional counterparts. Future studies should report the quantitative contribution of biological and social–environmental predictors to outcome in addition to the primary predictors of interest, and focus on longitudinal relationships between biological and social events that precede outcomes. Ultimately, this will permit the construction of risk models to predict longer term outcomes and facilitate investigations into potential mechanisms behind these outcomes. In addition, individual patient data metaanalyses could use the large extant literature to better interrogate relative contributions of biological and social–environmental influences to long-term outcome, particularly for outcomes that are clinically important but occur relatively infrequently. It is also important to note that some variables associate with outcomes to a similar extent in preterm as in term-born children, although they may occur more frequently in preterm children. In contrast, some variables seem to have disproportionate relationships with adverse outcomes in those born preterm than in controls. This pattern emphasizes the importance of well-matched term-born control groups and the need for comprehensive data about biological and social features of study participants. Finally, this review focused on those with the greatest immaturity at birth, and investigation of the common and unique influences on outcomes in more mature preterm infants is an important area for future research.

SUMMARY

Ultimately, greater knowledge of the contributions of biological and social influences to outcomes for preterm children will enhance our capacity to identify and intervene to support children at high developmental risk.

Best Practices

What is the current practice?

Children born very preterm and very low birthweight are at high risk of sensory, cognitive, academic, and behavioral difficulties, but these risks are shaped by biological and social influences.

What changes in current practice are likely to improve outcomes?

Major Recommendations
- Increased reporting of relationships of biological and social influences with outcomes.
- Individual patient metaanalyses of predictors of outcomes.
- Randomized, controlled trials of influences that are amenable to such studies, particularly medications or other medical procedures, or early intervention programs.

Summary Statement

More research is needed to understand biological and social influences on outcomes for preterm children and to develop effective interventions.

REFERENCES

1. Johnson S. Cognitive and behavioural outcomes following very preterm birth. Semin Fetal Neonatal Med 2007;12(5):363–73.
2. Joseph RM, O'Shea TM, Allred EN, et al. Neurocognitive and academic outcomes at age 10 years of extremely preterm newborns. Pediatrics 2016;137(4) [pii:e20154343].
3. Australian Institute of Health and Welfare. Australia's mothers and babies 2014-in brief. Canberra (Australia): AIHW; 2016.
4. Hamilton BE, Martin JA, Osterman MJ, et al. Births: final data for 2014. Natl Vital Stat Rep 2015;64(12):1–64.
5. Cheong JL, Doyle LW, Burnett AC, et al. Association between moderate and late preterm birth and neurodevelopment and social-emotional development at age 2 years. JAMA Pediatr 2017;171(4):e164805.
6. Bax M, Goldstein M, Rosenbaum P, et al. Proposed definition and classification of cerebral palsy, April 2005. Dev Med Child Neurol 2005;47(8):571–6.
7. Synnes A, Luu TM, Moddemann D, et al. Determinants of developmental outcomes in a very preterm Canadian cohort. Arch Dis Child Fetal Neonatal Ed 2017;102(3):F234–5.
8. Cheong JLY, Anderson PJ, Burnett AC, et al. Changing neurodevelopment at 8 years in children born extremely preterm since the 1990s. Pediatrics 2017; 139(6):e20164086.
9. Schlapbach LJ, Aebischer M, Adams M, et al. Impact of sepsis on neurodevelopmental outcome in a Swiss National Cohort of extremely premature infants. Pediatrics 2011;128(2):e348–57.
10. Beaino G, Khoshnood B, Kaminski M, et al. Predictors of cerebral palsy in very preterm infants: the EPIPAGE prospective population-based cohort study. Dev Med Child Neurol 2010;52(6):e119–25.
11. Kuban KCK, Allred EN, O'Shea TM, et al. Cranial ultrasound lesions in the NICU predict cerebral palsy at age 2 years in children born at extremely low gestational age. J Child Neurol 2009;24(1):63.
12. Mirmiran M, Barnes PD, Keller K, et al. Neonatal brain magnetic resonance imaging before discharge is better than serial cranial ultrasound in predicting cerebral palsy in very low birth weight preterm infants. Pediatrics 2004;114(4):992–8.
13. de Vries LS, van Haastert IC, Benders MJ, et al. Myth: cerebral palsy cannot be predicted by neonatal brain imaging. Semin Fetal Neonatal Med 2011;16(5): 279–87.
14. Wapner RJ, Gyamfi-Bannerman C, Thom EA. What we have learned about antenatal corticosteroid regimens. Semin Perinatol 2016;40(5):291–7.
15. Roberts D, Brown J, Medley N, et al. Antenatal corticosteroids for accelerating fetal lung maturation for women at risk of preterm birth. Cochrane Database Syst Rev 2017;(3):CD004454.
16. Chawla S, Natarajan G, Shankaran S, et al. Association of neurodevelopmental outcomes and neonatal morbidities of extremely premature infants with differential exposure to antenatal steroids. JAMA Pediatr 2016;170(12):1164–72.
17. Sotiriadis A, Tsiami A, Papatheodorou S, et al. Neurodevelopmental outcome after a single course of antenatal steroids in children born preterm: a systematic review and meta-analysis. Obstet Gynecol 2015;125(6):1385–96.
18. Doyle LW, Ehrenkranz RA, Halliday HL. Early (< 8 days) postnatal corticosteroids for preventing chronic lung disease in preterm infants. Cochrane Database Syst Rev 2014;(5):CD001146.

19. Doyle LW, Ehrenkranz RA, Halliday HL. Late (> 7 days) postnatal corticosteroids for chronic lung disease in preterm infants. Cochrane Database Syst Rev 2014;(5):CD001145.
20. Doyle LW, Halliday HL, Ehrenkranz RA, et al. An update on the impact of postnatal systemic corticosteroids on mortality and cerebral palsy in preterm infants: effect modification by risk of bronchopulmonary dysplasia. J Pediatr 2014;165(6):1258–60.
21. Hintz SR, Kendrick DE, Vohr BR, et al. Gender differences in neurodevelopmental outcomes among extremely preterm, extremely-low-birthweight infants. Acta Paediatr 2006;95(10):1239–48.
22. Wood NS, Costeloe K, Gibson AT, et al. The EPICure study: associations and antecedents of neurological and developmental disability at 30 months of age following extremely preterm birth. Arch Dis Child Fetal Neonatal Ed 2005;90(2): F134–40.
23. Doyle LW, Roberts G, Anderson PJ, Victorian Infant Collaborative Study Group. Outcomes at age 2 years of infants <28 weeks' gestational age born in Victoria in 2005. J Pediatr 2010;156(1):49–53.
24. Blencowe H, Lawn JE, Vazquez T, et al. Preterm-associated visual impairment and estimates of retinopathy of prematurity at regional and global levels for 2010. Pediatr Res 2013;74(Suppl 1):35–49.
25. Fielder A, Blencowe H, O'Connor A, et al. Impact of retinopathy of prematurity on ocular structures and visual functions. Arch Dis Child Fetal Neonatal Ed 2015; 100(2):F179–84.
26. Glass HC, Fujimoto S, Ceppi-Cozzio C, et al. White matter injury is associated with impaired gaze in premature infants. Pediatr Neurol 2008;38(1):10–5.
27. Molloy CS, Wilson-Ching M, Anderson VA, et al. Visual processing in adolescents born extremely low birth weight and/or extremely preterm. Pediatrics 2013; 132(3):e704–12.
28. Weisz DE, More K, McNamara PJ, et al. PDA ligation and health outcomes: a meta-analysis. Pediatrics 2014;133(4):e1024–46.
29. Weisz DE, Mirea L, Rosenberg E, et al. Association of patent ductus arteriosus ligation with death or neurodevelopmental impairment among extremely preterm infants. JAMA Pediatr 2017;171(5):443–9.
30. Zimmerman E, Lahav A. Ototoxicity in preterm infants: effects of genetics, aminoglycosides, and loud environmental noise. J Perinatol 2013;33(1):3–8.
31. Janz-Robinson EM, Badawi N, Walker K, et al. Neurodevelopmental outcomes of premature infants treated for patent ductus arteriosus: a population-based cohort study. J Pediatr 2015;167(5):1025–32.e3.
32. Vohr BR. Language and hearing outcomes of preterm infants. Semin Perinatol 2016;40(8):510–9.
33. van Noort-van der Spek IL, Goedegebure A, Hartwig NG, et al. Normal neonatal hearing screening did not preclude sensorineural hearing loss in two-year-old very preterm infants. Acta Paediatr 2017;106(10):1569–75.
34. Davis NM, Doyle LW, Ford GW, et al. Auditory function at 14 years of age of very-low-birthweight. Dev Med Child Neurol 2001;43(3):191–6.
35. Moeller MP. Early intervention and language development in children who are deaf and hard of hearing. Pediatrics 2000;106(3):E43.
36. Spittle A, Orton J, Anderson PJ, et al. Early developmental intervention programmes provided post hospital discharge to prevent motor and cognitive impairment in preterm infants. Cochrane Database Syst Rev 2015;(11):CD005495.
37. Bayley N. Bayley scales of infant and toddler development, third edition. San Antonio (TX): Pearson PsychCorp; 2006.

38. Volpe JJ. Brain injury in premature infants: a complex amalgam of destructive and developmental disturbances. Lancet Neurol 2009;8(1):110–24.
39. Doyle LW, Cheong JLY, Burnett AC, et al. Biological and social influences on outcomes of extreme-preterm/low-birth-weight adolescents. Pediatrics 2015;136(6): 1513–20.
40. Johnson S, Wolke D, Hennessy E, et al. Educational outcomes in extremely preterm children: neuropsychological correlates and predictors of attainment. Dev Neuropsychol 2011;36(1):74–95.
41. Anderson PJ, Cheong JL, Thompson DK. The predictive validity of neonatal MRI for neurodevelopmental outcome in very preterm children. Semin Perinatol 2015; 39(2):147–58.
42. van Vliet EO, de Kieviet JF, Oosterlaan J, et al. Perinatal infections and neurodevelopmental outcome in very preterm and very low-birth-weight infants: a meta-analysis. JAMA Pediatr 2013;167(7):662–8.
43. Pappas A, Kendrick DE, Shankaran S, et al. Chorioamnionitis and early childhood outcomes among extremely low-gestational-age neonates. JAMA Pediatr 2014; 168(2):137–47.
44. Serenius F, Ewald U, Farooqi A, et al. Neurodevelopmental outcomes among extremely preterm infants 6.5 years after active perinatal care in Sweden. JAMA Pediatr 2016;170(10):954–63.
45. Aarnoudse-Moens CSH, Weisglas-Kuperus N, van Goudoever JB, et al. Meta-analysis of neurobehavioral outcomes in very preterm and/or very low birth weight children. Pediatrics 2009;124(2):717–28.
46. Aarnoudse-Moens CSH, Weisglas-Kuperus N, Duivenvoorden HJ, et al. Executive function and IQ predict mathematical and attention problems in very preterm children. PLoS One 2013;8(2):e55994.
47. Almadhoob A, Ohlsson A. Sound reduction management in the neonatal intensive care unit for preterm or very low birth weight infants. Cochrane Database Syst Rev 2015;1:Cd010333.
48. Pineda RG, Neil J, Dierker D, et al. Alterations in brain structure and neurodevelopmental outcome in preterm infants hospitalized in different neonatal intensive care unit environments. J Pediatr 2014;164(1):52–60.
49. Pineda R, Durant P, Mathur A, et al. Auditory exposure in the neonatal intensive care unit: room type and other predictors. J Pediatr 2017;183:56–66.e3.
50. Vinall J, Grunau RE. Impact of repeated procedural pain-related stress in infants born very preterm. Pediatr Res 2014;75(5):584–7.
51. Wong HS, Edwards P. Nature or nurture: a systematic review of the effect of socio-economic status on the developmental and cognitive outcomes of children born preterm. Matern Child Health J 2013;17(9):1689–700.
52. Linsell L, Malouf R, Morris J, et al. Prognostic factors for poor cognitive development in children born very preterm or with very low birth weight: a systematic review. JAMA Pediatr 2015;169(12):1162–72.
53. Lowe JR, Nolen TL, Vohr B, et al. Effect of primary language on developmental testing in children born extremely preterm. Acta Paediatr 2013;102(9):896–900.
54. Johnson S, Marlow N. Growing up after extremely preterm birth: lifespan mental health outcomes. Semin Fetal Neonatal Med 2014;19(2):97–104.
55. Pritchard MA, de Dassel T, Beller E, et al. Autism in toddlers born very preterm. Pediatrics 2016;137(2):e20151949.
56. De Los Reyes A, Kazdin AE. Informant discrepancies in the assessment of childhood psychopathology: a critical review, theoretical framework, and recommendations for further study. Psychol Bull 2005;131(4):483–509.

57. Delobel-Ayoub M, Kaminski M, Marret S, et al. Behavioral outcome at 3 years of age in very preterm infants: the EPIPAGE study. Pediatrics 2006;117(6): 1996–2005.
58. Delobel-Ayoub M, Arnaud C, White-Koning M, et al. Behavioral problems and cognitive performance at 5 years of age after very preterm birth: the EPIPAGE Study. Pediatrics 2009;123(6):1485–92.
59. Hack M, Taylor GH, Schluchter M, et al. Behavioral outcomes of extremely low birth weight children at age 8 years. J Dev Behav Pediatr 2009;30(2):122–30.
60. Johnson S, Hollis C, Kochhar P, et al. Psychiatric disorders in extremely preterm children: longitudinal finding at age 11 years in the EPICure study. J Am Acad Child Adolesc Psychiatry 2010;49(5):453–63.
61. Burnett A, Davey CG, Wood SJ, et al. Extremely preterm birth and adolescent mental health in a geographical cohort born in the 1990s. Psychol Med 2014; 44(7):1533–44.
62. Johnson S, Kochhar P, Hennessy E, et al. Antecedents of attention-deficit/hyperactivity disorder symptoms in children born extremely preterm. J Dev Behav Pediatr 2016;37(4):285–97.
63. Clark CAC, Woodward LJ, Horwood LJ, et al. Development of emotional and behavioral regulation in children born extremely preterm and very preterm: biological and social influences. Child Dev 2008;79(5):1444–62.
64. Treyvaud K, Ure A, Doyle LW, et al. Psychiatric outcomes at age seven for very preterm children: rates and predictors. J Child Psychol Psychiatry 2013;54(7): 772–9.
65. Anderson PJ, Treyvaud K, Neil JJ, et al. Associations of newborn brain magnetic resonance imaging with long-term neurodevelopmental impairments in very preterm children. J Pediatr 2017;187:58–65.e1.
66. Rogers CE, Anderson PJ, Thompson DK, et al. Regional cerebral development at term relates to school-age social-emotional development in very preterm children. J Am Acad Child Adolesc Psychiatry 2012;51(2):181–91.
67. Anderson PJ, Doyle LW. Neurobehavioural outcomes of school-age children born extremely low birth weight or very preterm in the 1990s. JAMA 2003;289(24): 3264–72.
68. Joseph RM, O'Shea TM, Allred EN, et al. Prevalence and associated features of autism spectrum disorder in extremely low gestational age newborns at age 10 years. Autism Res 2017;10(2):224–32.
69. Fevang SK, Hysing M, Markestad T, et al. Mental health in children born extremely preterm without severe neurodevelopmental disabilities. Pediatrics 2016;137(4) [pii:e20153002].
70. Hoffman L, Bann C, Higgins R, et al. Developmental outcomes of extremely preterm infants born to adolescent mothers. Pediatrics 2015;135(6):1082–92.
71. Mendelson T, Kubzansky LD, Datta GD, et al. Relation of female gender and low socioeconomic status to internalizing symptoms among adolescents: a case of double jeopardy? Soc Sci Med 2008;66(6):1284–96.
72. Rucklidge JJ. Gender differences in attention-deficit/hyperactivity disorder. Psychiatr Clin North Am 2010;33(2):357–73.
73. Johnson S, Hollis C, Kochhar P, et al. Autism spectrum disorders in extremely preterm children. J Pediatr 2010;156(4):525–31.e2.
74. Farooqi A, Hägglöf B, Sedin G, et al. Mental health and social competencies of 10- to 12-year-old children born at 23 to 25 weeks of gestation in the 1990s: a Swedish national prospective follow-up study. Pediatrics 2007;120(1):118–33.

75. Samara M, Marlow N, Wolke D. Pervasive behavior problems at 6 years of age in a total-population sample of children born at ≤25 weeks of gestation. Pediatrics 2008;122(3):562–73.
76. Spittle AJ, Treyvaud K, Doyle LW, et al. Early emergence of behavior and social-emotional problems in very preterm infants. J Am Acad Child Adolesc Psychiatry 2009;48(9):909–18.
77. Pace CC, Spittle AJ, Molesworth CM, et al. Evolution of depression and anxiety symptoms in parents of very preterm infants during the newborn period. JAMA Pediatr 2016;170(9):863–70.
78. Treyvaud K. Parent and family outcomes following very preterm or very low birth weight birth: a review. Semin Fetal Neonatal Med 2014;19(2):131–5.
79. Treyvaud K, Anderson VA, Lee KJ, et al. Parental mental health and early social-emotional development of children born very preterm. J Pediatr Psychol 2010; 35(7):768–77.

Long-Term Functioning and Participation Across the Life Course for Preterm Neonatal Intensive Care Unit Graduates

Frances A. Carter, BA[a], Michael E. Msall, MD[b],*

KEYWORDS

- NICU graduates • Academic performance • Learning disorders • Survival rates
- Neurodevelopmental disorders • Functional outcomes
- Lifecourse health development

KEY POINTS

- There is increased recognition that the major functional sequelae of preterm birth is a spectrum of cognitive, executive function, coordination, learning, social and adaptive behavior disorders.
- Key outcomes include literacy, numeracy, and social skills.
- Proactively providing support to families and developmental and educational supports to children can optimize academic functioning and participation in adult learning, physical and behavioral health activities, community living, relationships, and employment.

Two frameworks inform assessing the complexity of children's risk and resilience after prematurity. The first is the *International Classification of Functioning, Disability and Health for Children and Youth* (ICF-CY).[1] The ICF-CY is derived from, and compatible with, the *International Classification of Functioning, Disability and Health* (ICF).[2] The

Dr M.E. Msall was supported in part by T73 MC11047 Health Resources and Services Administration/Department of Health and Human Services Leadership Education in Neurodevelopmental and Related Disorders Training Program (LEND), UG3 OD023348-01 National Institutes of Health/National Institute of Child Health and Human Development (NIH/NICHD) ELGAN-III: Environment, Epigenetics, Neurodevelopment & Health of Extremely Preterm Children, and UG3 OD023281-01 NIH/NICHD The Microbiome as a Potential Mediator of Socio-economic Disparities in Preterm Infant Neurodevelopmental Trajectories from NICU Discharge to School Age. Both of these NIH grants are part of the NICHD Environmental Influences on Child Health Outcomes (ECHO) Consortium. There were no conflicts of interest.
[a] Department of Psychology, The Center for Early Childhood Research, University of Chicago, 5848 S. University Avenue, Chicago, IL 60637, USA; [b] Department of Pediatrics, Section of Developmental and Behavioral Pediatrics, Kennedy Research Center on Intellectual and Neurodevelopmental Disabilities, University of Chicago Comer Children's Hospital, Woodlawn Social Services Center, 950 East 61st Street, Chicago, IL 60637, USA
* Corresponding author.
E-mail address: mmsall@peds.bsd.uchicago.edu

Clin Perinatol 45 (2018) 501–527
https://doi.org/10.1016/j.clp.2018.05.009
0095-5108/18/© 2018 Elsevier Inc. All rights reserved.

components of the ICF in the context of health include *body function and body structure impairments; activity and activity limitations; participation and participation restrictions;* and *environmental factors.* Environmental factors make up the physical, social and attitudinal contextual settings in which children and adolescents live and conduct their lives. This framework goes behind dichotomous classification of impairments (eg, cerebral palsy (CP), yes or no; intellectual disability, yes or no) and instead describes a spectrum of functioning at body structure and body function levels; for example, activities in whole-person tasks like running, reading, and dancing, and participation in roles with peers like being on a team, participating in church, temple, or mosque, or meeting friends for a movie. This ICF model is illustrated in **Fig. 1** for a child who was born late preterm.

Historically, functional measures in childhood included basic daily skills of feeding, dressing, toileting, and bathing; however, adaptive behaviors in daily living also include conceptual skills (literacy, numeracy, keyboarding, and written language), social skills (self-direction, maintaining relationships), and community-living skills (household chores, cooking, shopping, using transportation, and employment). These composite adaptive outcome skills impact on both becoming an independent adult and participation in community life and are illustrated in **Fig. 2** for a child who survived extreme prematurity.

The second framework, the *Life Course Health Development Model (LCHD),* holds that the trajectories of children are influenced by the dynamic interactions of multiple risks, protective factors, and promoting factors, especially during sensitive periods of health development.[3] From the standpoint of premature infants, due to critical human brain development in the second and third trimesters, this must consider complex maternal, placental, and fetal dynamic interactions. Likewise, infant, toddler, and childhood periods of development are indelibly influenced by multilevel, multidirectional, transactional, and long-lasting interactions, and critically emphasize the

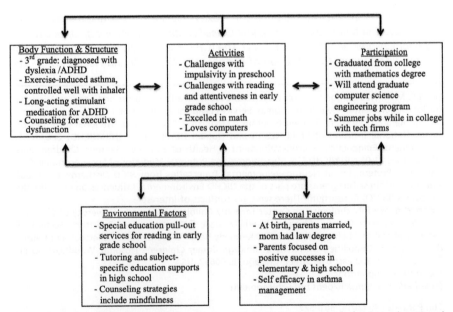

Fig. 1. ICF Case 1: 34 weeks' gestational age, maternal preeclampsia, behavior, educational, and stressors: resilience at age 22 years.

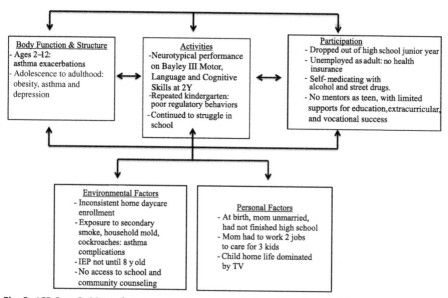

Fig. 2. ICF Case 2: 28 weeks' gestational age, cumulative adversity, adult jeopardy at 25 years. IEP, individualized education program.

importance of timing. Using an LCHD framework to analyze the origins and impact of prematurity and the opportunity to optimize health development outcomes suggests the following considerations for assessing outcomes across the life course[4]:

- Children who are born prematurely are assumed to be more developmentally vulnerable and are potentially more sensitive to a wide range and nested array of dynamic interacting influences.
- Because alterations in evolutionarily presumed, developmentally determined adaptive mechanisms are well documented, lags in developmental processes as well as catch-up and feed-forward processes that are specific to premature infants may influence the nature and dynamics of their health and developmental trajectories.
- Understanding how the caregiving environments of premature infants interact with emerging developmental capacities, and how different types of exposures, levels of supports, and adversity influence these emergent developmental trajectories is important if specific and targeted interventions are to be designed to modify developmental pathways based on specific risk profiles. The goal is to shift the health and developmental curves for the entire population of premature infants toward thriving and enablement.
- To implement a broader approach to improve the health and developmental outcomes of diverse preterm populations, it is important to determine what is known about the special developmental vulnerabilities of premature infants; how these vulnerabilities manifest (timing, context, specific risks); and whether the mechanisms involved are phase or period specific, modifiable, or of cumulative risk.

We illustrate our models with several tables, 2 cases using the ICF, and 2 figures.

Case 1 (Fig. 1): James was born late preterm at 34 weeks of gestation due to preeclampsia. His parents were married and his mother completed law school. She reported significant job-related stressors during pregnancy. The immediate newborn period was complicated by immature lungs leading to respiratory distress syndrome; however, ultimately James was discharged at 38 weeks' gestational age without a need for oxygen in the home. He was enrolled in full-day day care and preschool since the age of 2 years. James was found to have some challenges with impulsivity in preschool, which parents addressed with occupational and behavioral therapies. He entered kindergarten without an Individualized Education Program, and in early grade school was found to struggle with reading and inattentiveness. He received a formal diagnosis of a specific language learning disability (dyslexia) and attention-deficit/hyperactivity disorder (ADHD) in third grade. James received special education pull-out services for reading and language arts and started on a long-acting stimulant medication for ADHD with the guidance of a developmental and behavioral pediatrician. James received tutoring and subject-specific special education supports throughout high school. His parents focused on his positive successes, such as his strong performance in mathematics. James went to college and pursued a math and engineering program. His adult health is complicated by exercise-induced asthma well controlled on an inhaler, long-acting stimulant medications, and periodic counseling with a psychologist for management strategies for executive dysfunction and implementing mindfulness practices.

Case 2 (Fig. 2): Michael was born at 28 weeks of gestation due to preterm labor after premature rupture of membranes. His mother was unmarried and did not finish high school. His neonatal intensive care unit (NICU) course was complicated by intubation for the first 4 weeks of life, but he did not experience additional medical complications and was able to be slowly transitioned to room air and oral feedings. At 2 years of age he tested within the age-appropriate range on the Bayley Scales of Infant and Toddler Development, 3rd Edition. Between ages 2 and 4, he experienced asthma exacerbations complicated by environmental exposures to secondary tobacco smoke, household mold, and cockroach infestations, and was hospitalized on average 2 to 3 times per year. Until the age of 5 years, Michael was enrolled in inconsistent home day care programs and did not receive early intervention services because he was considered less than 30% delayed and thereby was deemed not eligible for services. He enrolled in kindergarten at age 5 years; however, he had to repeat kindergarten due to poor regulatory behaviors, impulsivity, and lack of familiarity with letters and numbers, which interfered with learning. Throughout his early elementary years, he continued to struggle in school. His home life was largely dominated by television watching while his mom worked 2 jobs to help care for him and his 2 siblings. In school he received an Individual Education Plan at age 8 years, but did not access pharmacotherapies for ADHD. He dropped out of high school in his junior year. His adult health is complicated by obesity, asthma, and depression. Because of unemployment, he does not have health insurance. His state has not expanded Medicaid access.

CHANGING SURVIVAL RATES, MORBIDITIES, AND EARLY NEURODEVELOPMENTAL DISORDERS AMONG EXTREMELY PRETERM INFANTS

Tables 1 and **2** explore the overall outcomes by gestational age stratum and early neurodevelopmental disabilities of children who survive extremely preterm (EPT) birth. These tables highlight both the increased survival rates of extreme prematurity as well as the spectrum of early and life course challenges impacting on health, education, behavior. Ancel and colleagues[16] examined survival and neonatal morbidities of infants born at 22 to 34 weeks' gestation using 2 waves of the EPIPAGE cohorts born in 1997 and 2011, respectively. The major outcomes included survival to discharge and survival without neonatal morbidities associated with high risk for

Table 1
Life course impact of prematurity

Weeks of Gestation	Children with Special Health Care Needs, %	Major Neurodevelopmental Disability, %	Educational Supports, %	Behavioral Disorders, %
22	80	70 (52–100)	75	NK
23–24	80	50–60	60–70	NK
25–26	60	56	50–67	NK
27–28	50	20	50	20
29–31	40	15	40	15
32–36	30	10	25	10
37+	20	5	15	5

Abbreviation: NK, not known.
Data from Refs.[5–15]

adverse developmental outcomes. The latter included grade 3 or 4 intraventricular hemorrhage, cystic periventricular leukomalacia, severe bronchopulmonary dysplasia, stage 3 or higher retinopathy of prematurity (ROP), or stage 2 or stage 3 necrotizing enterocolitis. In the 2011 cohort, 0.7% of infants born before 24 weeks, 31% at 24 weeks, 59% at 25 weeks, 75% at 26 weeks, 94% at 27 to 31 weeks, and 99% at 32 to 34 weeks survived to discharge. Between the 1997 and 2011 samples, the portion of infants surviving without severe morbidity increased by 14.4% at 25 to 29 weeks of gestation and by 6% at 30 to 31 weeks. The proportion did not significantly change for infants born at less than 25 weeks of gestation. Furthermore, rates of antenatal corticosteroid use, induced preterm deliveries, cesarean deliveries, and surfactant use significantly increased, except at gestational age 22 to 23 weeks. Overall, the significant improvement in survival to discharge for infants born at 25 to 31 weeks of gestation was associated with a decrease in severe morbidities.

Washburn and colleagues[5] examined infants born between 23 and 27 weeks of gestation with no congenital malformations enrolled from a 13-county region in North Carolina.[5] Outcomes at age 1 year between the 2 birth periods of 1990 to 1995 and 1995 to 2000 were compared. The percentage of live births was 67% in the first epoch and 71% in the second. Major neurodevelopmental impairment, defined as CP, Bayley II Scales Mental Development Index more than 2 SDs below the mean, or severe hearing loss or blindness, was present in 20% of survivors in the first period and 14% of survivors in the second period.

Amer and colleagues[25] compared the mortality and neurodevelopmental outcomes of infants born at less than 29 weeks of gestation who were outborn versus those who were inborn in the Canadian Neonatal Network and Canadian Neonatal Follow-up Network databases. Canada has a centralized perinatal care system whose purpose is to improve care of both mothers and neonates during the perinatal period by providing access to regional tertiary care centers for mothers with threatened labor before 30 to 32 weeks of gestation. However, 15% to 20% of these children are still not born in these specialized perinatal centers. Outborn infants had higher mean birth weight (940 ± 278 g vs 897 ± 237 g), lower rates of antenatal steroid treatment (54% vs 93%), lower rates of small for gestational age (SGA) status (5.3% vs 9.4%), and lower rates of maternal college education (44% vs 54%) than inborn infants. The median 5-minute Apgar score and Score for Neonatal Acute Physiology-II were higher for inborn infants. Furthermore, outborn infants had higher odds of death or severe

Table 2
Major neurodevelopmental disabilities at age 2 years among extremely low birth weight survivors in the 1990s and extremely preterm survivors in 2005 to 2015

Study	Sample	Cerebral Palsy, %	Developmental Disability, %	Hearing Impairment, %	Vision Impairment, %
Adams-Chapanis et al,[23] United States	Epoch 4 22–26 wk GA N = 2013				
	22 wk, n = 17	41	59	0	0
	23 wk, n = 161	22	42	6	2
	24 wk, n = 486	14	32	4	1
	25 wk, n = 657	8	25	3	2
	26 wk, n = 792	5	24	2	0
Younge et al, 2017,[18] United States	22–24 wk GA				
	Epoch 1 (2000–2003): N = 424	15	47	4	2
	Epoch 2 (2004–2007): N = 459	11	45	4	2
	Epoch 3 (2008–2011): N = 487	11	41	3	0.4
Synees 2009–2011,[21] Canada	N = 2340	6.4	21.8	2.6	1.6
Schmidt et al, 1996–1998,[45] Canada and United States	N = 944 500–999 g	12	27	2	2
Vohr et al, 1993–1998,[15] United States	N = 2291 22–26 wk	19	30	2	2
	N = 1494 27–32 wk GA	11.6	26	1	0.7

Study	N				
Moore et al,[17] 2006–2012, United Kingdom	N = 325	23	38	7	3
Wood et al,[62] 1995, United Kingdom	N = 235, 22–25 wk GA	25	31	4	6
Doyle et al,[74] 2005, Australia	N = 172, 22–27 wk GA (EP)	9.8	47.9	4	0
	N = 220, FT	0	20.3	0.5	0
Doyle et al,[75] 1997, Australia	N = 170, 500–999 g	11	22	1.8	2.4
Pierrat et al,[19] 2017, France	EPIPAGE-2 N = 5170				
24–26 wk GA		6.9	34 (V), 13–25 (NV)	1.4	0.7
27–31 wk GA		4.3	24 (V), 11–16 (NV)	0.6	0.3
32–34 wk GA		1	18 (V), 11–13 (NV)	0.5	0.2
Ishii et al,[61] 2013, Japan					
22 wk GA		22	52	0	8.7
23 wk GA		18	57	3.4	10.2
24 wk GA		8	37	1.2	3.4
25 wk GA		15	34	1.3	2.2
Serenius 2004–2007,[22] Sweden	N = 456; 22–26 6/7 wk GA	7	35.3	0.9	3.7

Developmental disability as defined as Bayley II Mental Developmental Index less than 70 or Bayley-III Cog SS <85.

Abbreviations: EP, extremely preterm; FT, full term; GA, gestational age; NV, nonverbal (problem solving and personal social); V, verbal.

Data from Refs. [15–24,45,61,62]

neurodevelopmental impairments attributed to higher rates of sonographic parenchymal brain injury.

Berry and colleagues[6] compared short-term mortality and major morbidities of infants born at 23 or 24 weeks of gestation in New Zealand. At the time of discharge, there was parenchymal brain injury in 13% of surviving 23-week infants and in 3% of surviving 24-week infants. The survival rate at 2-year follow-up was 58% for infants born at 23 weeks and 60% for infants born at 24 weeks. There was no difference in rates of disability at 2 years corrected age. The investigators argue that, with maximal perinatal care in a tertiary setting, it is possible to have comparable 2-year rates of survival with no significant brain structural injury or severe disability in infants born at 23 or 24 weeks' gestation.

Thus, these series of international studies highlight a changing picture of survival at the extremes of viability. Survival and outcomes after survival are strongly influenced by gestational age at birth, inborn versus outborn status, and era in which the child is born.

ACADEMIC PERFORMANCE AND LEARNING DISORDERS

It has been known for 2 decades that children born very preterm (VPT; <32 weeks of gestation) or with very low birth weight (VLBW; <1500 g) have higher rates of neurosensory abnormalities as well as behavioral and socialization difficulties, and lower performance on cognitive, language, and motor skill assessments than their normal birth weight term (NBWT) peers.[4] Furthermore, over the past decade there is evidence that these problems tend to be more severe and more common in children born EPT (<28 weeks of gestation) or with extremely low birth weight (ELBW; <1000 g) and that executive function, attention, and specific learning disorders are part of these difficulties. Past studies of educational outcomes in high-risk neonates predominantly focused on VLBW/VPT in the surfactant era. However, investigators in Australia, the United Kingdom, and Scandinavia have followed regional cohorts of EPT cohorts in the past decade. These cohorts have benefited from full-term controls and a commitment to collaborate with educational, disability, and community systems of care. The following portion of this review explores several important studies that have provided insight into the cognitive, academic, and behavioral outcomes of children, adolescents, and adults who were born EPT or with ELBW.

Academic achievement and school performance problems tend to become clear very soon after starting school. They often manifest as grade repetition, a need for special education assistance, parent and teacher reports of poor school performance, and low scoring on tests of reading, spelling, writing, and mathematics skills. There is evidence that difficulties related to academic performance are more common among preterm or low birth weight survivors than health disorders like asthma or epilepsy or more global development problems, such as significant intellectual disability (defined as intelligence quotient [IQ] <55 with concurrent adaptive behavior challenges). This is possibly due to a large number of children with mild cognitive impairments (standard scores 1–2 SDs below the mean) and specific neuropsychological weaknesses. These early childhood school performance difficulties are significant because they are often predictive of later adverse educational outcomes, including decreased long-term learning skills, difficulty competing with peers academically, and decreased rates of pursuing higher education after high school completion. Behavioral problems including impulsivity, inattention, anxiety, and depression too often compromise extracurricular, social, vocational, and community success.

When compared with NBWT children, VLBW/VPT children are more likely to repeat grades, to require special education assistance, and to be rated by their teachers as having school performance weaknesses. One multinational review based on cohorts from New Jersey, Ontario, Bavaria, and Holland found that these suboptimal educational outcomes were consistent for ELBW children across sites despite differences in education policy.[26] Another study found that rates of qualification for special education programs were 38% and 11% for ELBW and NBWT children, respectively, and another found that their rates of grade retention differed as well (20% vs 7%).[27,28] These and similar studies have revealed a "gradient" between degree of low birth weight/preterm status and educational outcomes. Klebanov and colleagues[29] examined the rates of grade failure and/or special education placements among 9-year-olds distributed across birth weights. There was a clear graded relationship with birth weight status categorized as less than 1000 g, 1001 to 1500 g, 1501 to 2500 g, and greater than 2500 g (normal birth weight). Rates of grade failure were 37%, 26%, 27%, and 14%, and rates of special education enrollment were 12%, 6%, 6%, and 4% across these birth weight categories. A Cleveland study found rates of grade retention were 30% for a group with birth weight less than 750 g, 13% for 750 to 1499 g, and 8% for term controls, and that rates of special education were 50%, 27%, and 8% for the same groups, respectively.[30] One study also found that VLBW children had higher rates of placement in nearly all special education programs than children with birth weight 3000 to 4749 g, with the exception of programs for the "emotionally handicapped," and that this difference was most pronounced in programming for more severe and multiple disabling conditions and less pronounced in programming for conditions that allowed for academic competitiveness.[31]

Many studies have found that VLBW/VPT and ELBW/EPT children perform worse than NBWT children on reading, spelling, writing, mathematics, and handwriting tests. In addition, ELBW/EPT children perform less well than VLBW/VPT children, and the sizes of these group differences range from moderate to large across studies. This pattern of results also holds when excluding children with global intellectual or neurosensory disability.

Among VLBW/VPT-born young adults, educational outcomes vary, with some studies reporting that there are no differences between groups on attained education levels, and other studies reporting that high school graduation rates, college enrollment rates, and performance on word recognition and mathematics tests are higher among NBWT individuals than among VLBW/VPT individuals. This wide variability in educational outcomes, both within and between samples, can be attributed to biological risks (eg, neonatal medical complications, postnatal neurosensory impairments, and subnormal head circumference) and to social risk factors (eg, low socioeconomic status, disadvantaged family environments, low parental educational achievement). Modifying factors that can impact the effect of these risks include quality early developmental interventions, family and teacher supports, prenatal drugs or alcohol exposure, and family history of learning difficulties.

Garfield and colleagues[32] used state academic testing from 1.3 million Florida children to examine how gestational age and kindergarten readiness impact on academic achievement trajectories. Children were born between 23 and 41 weeks of gestation and attended public school. Overall, kindergarten readiness performance, standardized academic achievement test scores, and gifted status were positively related to higher gestational ages, whereas low kindergarten and academic performance was inversely related to gestational age. It should be noted that standardized test data were unavailable for 16% of the sample, and the kindergarten readiness measure was unavailable in 56% of the sample. Among children surviving 23 to 24 weeks' gestation, 2 in 3 were kindergarten ready, compared with 85% of children born at term. Children born at 23 to 24 weeks of gestation scored 0.66 SD lower than those born at full-term. Although 9.5% of all students were considered gifted, this included only 1.8% of those born at 23 to 24 weeks of gestation; 5.8% of students were low performing, and 33.5% of these children had been born at 23 to 24 weeks of gestation. The Florida population data indicate that a large majority of children (65%) born near the limits of viability performed within expected school norms and that further investigation is needed to examine how and why some children are able to demonstrate resiliency after preterm birth.

Serenius and colleagues[7] examined the neurodevelopmental outcomes of a national cohort of Swedish children born EPT (<27 weeks of gestation) and compared them with matched term-born controls. Neurodevelopmental outcomes at age 6.5 years included intellectual disability measured by Weschler intelligence batteries, the diagnoses of CP, hearing impairment requiring amplification, and visual disability. Overall, 441 EPT children and 371 controls were assessed. The EPT children's adjusted mean IQ was 14.2 points lower than that of the term controls; 18.8% and 11.1% of EPT children had moderate and severe cognitive disability, respectively, compared with only 2.2% and 0.3% of controls. CP, blindness, and hearing impairment were observed in 9.5%, 2.0%, and 2.1% of EPT children, respectively, and in 0.0%, 0.0%, and 0.5% of controls. Overall, for EPT children, 30% experience mild, 20% moderate, and 13% severe disability. Among EPT children, moderate or severe disability decreased with increasing gestational age. Importantly, among children assessed at both 2.5 and 6.5 years, rates of disability increased from 1 in 4 to 1 in 3.

Heeren and colleagues[33] examined the nature and prevalence of cognitive functional limitations in US children born EPT using latent profile analysis. This statistical technique allows for the identification of subgroups of EPT children with similar IQ and executive functioning profiles. Four different neurocognitive profiles emerged in these Extremely Low Gestational Age Newborns (ELGAN) survivors: normal (34%), low-normal (41%), moderately impaired (17%), and severely impaired (8%). Children in the "low-normal" group showed impaired inhibition compared with their reasoning and working memory functional abilities, whereas children in "impaired" groups demonstrated global limitations across cognitive and executive function domains. The most preterm (23–24 weeks of gestation) survivors were the least likely to have a normal profile and the most likely to have a severely impaired profile; children in the moderately or severely impaired groups tended to perform worse on academic achievement measures of math and literacy; and children who had poorer cognitive function scores (based on IQ and executive functioning) tended to require more special education resources. Importantly, after categorizing the EPT children by IQ, there were still significant variations in executive functioning within each category. These results highlight that among EPT survivors in the modern era of neonatology, both IQ and executive functioning assessments are necessary for describing outcomes at school age. It is for this reason that we highlight middle childhood behavioral health impairments that impact on academic and social outcomes in **Table 3** and cognitive, executive function, and academic achievement outcomes in adolescence and adulthood in **Table 4**.

Hirschberger and colleagues[34] examined the prevalence of neurodevelopmental impairments in the US ELGAN cohort at age 10 years to create a categorization framework for neurologic limitations. A total of 889 10-year-old children(<28 weeks' gestation) were recruited, and cognitive impairment prevalence was assessed using multidomain cognitive assessments as well as observations of executive function, CP, autism spectrum disorder (ASD), and epilepsy. Three categories of neurodevelopmental impairment severity were assessed: I, no major neurodevelopmental impairment; II, normal cognitive ability with CP, ASD, and/or epilepsy; III, cognitive impairment (IQ and executive functioning). Category I included 68% of children,

Table 3
Middle childhood behavioral health outcomes after extreme prematurity

Study	Years of Inception of Birth Cohort	ELBW/EP NBW, n Tested	Age at Assessment, y	Mental Health Outcomes Eligible for Meta-Analysis	Estimates of Effect SMD, g, and SE (g)
Szatmari et al,[39] 1990, Canada	1980–1982	82 ELBW 208 NBW	5.0 5.0	P: Attention problems P: Emotion problems P: Conduct disorder T: Attention problems T: Emotion problems T: Conduct disorder	0.94 (0.73) 0.01 (0.60) 0.87 (1.22) 0.41 (0.52) 0.06 (0.60) −0.39 (1.07)
Szatmari et al,[40] 1993, Canada	1977–1981	129 ELBW 145 NBW	7.8 (0.4) 8.1 (0.5)	P: Attention problems P: Emotion problems P: Conduct disorder T: Attention problems T: Emotion problems T: Conduct disorder	1.50 (1.07) 0.69 (0.66) 0.69 (1.19) 0.37 (0.48) −0.36 (0.61) −0.78 (0.83)
Taylor et al,[41] 2000, United States	1982–1986	60 ELBW 49 NBW	6.7 (0.9) 7.0 (1.0)	C: Self-esteem P: Attention problems P: Behavior competence P: Hyperactivity T: Attention problems T: Social skills rating T: Hyperactivity	−0.19 (0.13) 0.76 (0.20) −0.47 (0.20) 0.58 (0.20) 0.48 (0.20) −0.14 (0.28) 0.25 (0.20)

(continued on next page)

Table 3
(continued)

Study	Years of Inception of Birth Cohort	ELBW/EP NBW, n Tested	Age at Assessment, y	Mental Health Outcomes Eligible for Meta-Analysis	Mean (SD)
Akshoomoff et al,[35] 2017, United States	2002–2004	668 <28 wk GA	10	Working memory	RD: 91.4 (10.2)
					MD: 88.2 (8.9)
					MD/RD:84.5 (11.5)
					No LD: 98.1 (12.3)
				Attention	RD: 8.4 (3.0)
					MD: 8.0 (2.7)
					MD/RD: 7.4 (2.8)
					No LD: 9.3 (2.5)
				Inhibition	RD: 6.6 (2.8)
					MD: 6.8 (2.7)
					MD/RD:5.7 (2.5)
					No LD: 8.3 (2.9)
				Visual perception	RD: 8.0 (2.4)
					MD: 7.1 (2.3)
					MD/RD:7.0 (2.5)
					No LD: 9.1 (2.5)
				Visuomotor precision	RD: 7.5 (3.3)
					MD: 7.6 (3.1)
					MD/RD:6.8 (3.7)
					No LD: 8.5 (3.4)

Hirschberger et al,[34] 2018, United States	2002–2004	873 <28 wk GA	10	Cognitive/Executive Function Class (CFC 1-4) CP; ASD; epilepsy	No. impairments (CFC 3–4,CP, ASD, epilepsy)
					23–24 wk GA:
					0: 48%
					1: 26%
					2: 21%
					3: 5%
					4: 0%
					25–26 wk GA:
					0: 68%
					1: 21%
					2: 10%
					3: 2%
					4: 0.25%
					27 wk GA:
					0: 79%
					1: 13%
					2: 4%
					3: 3%
					4: 0.3%

(continued on next page)

Table 3
(continued)

Study	Years of Inception of Birth Cohort	ELBW/EP NBW, n Tested	Age at Assessment, y	Mental Health Outcomes Eligible for Meta-Analysis	% Elevated Scores
Burnett et al,[36] 2017, Australia	1991–1992, 1997, 2005	613 EP/ELBW 564 controls	7–8	P: Disability status (blindness, deafness, CP, delayed development) at 2 and 8 y; BRI (inhibit, shift, emotional control); MI (initiate, working memory, plan/organize, organization of materials, monitor); GEC (BRI and MI); WM (working memory)	1991–1992 EP/ELBW vs FT GEC: 13 vs 8 BRI: 13 vs 8 MI: 15 vs 7 WM: 20 vs 7 1997 EP/ELBW vs C GEC: 9 vs 6 BRI: 13 vs 7 MI: 10 vs 5 WM: 15 vs 7 2005 EP/ELBW vs C GEC: 27 vs 11 BRI: 22 vs 9 MI: 29 vs 8 WM: 37 vs 9
Leviton et al,[37] 2018, United States	2002–2004	716 <28 wk GA	10	Cog: IQ (verbal, nonverbal); Working memory; Inhibition; Inhibition in switching; Executive dysfunction (ED)	% Z-scores ≤-1 WM: 24% Inhibition: 49% Switching: 50% All 3: 15% ED Risk Profiles 1. Low SES = 2. Prematurity = 3. inflammatory biomarkers Cog Limitation risks: FGR

Abbreviations: ASD, autism spectrum disorder; BRI, behavioral regulation index; C, child; Cog, cognitive; CP, cerebral palsy; ELBW, extremely low birthweight; EP, extremely preterm; FGR, fetal growth restriction; FT: full term; GA, gestational age; GEC, global executive composite; LD, learning disability (score <16th percentile); MD, mathematics-only LD; MD/RD, combined mathematics/reading LD; MI, metacognition index; NBW: normal birth weight; P, parent; RD, reading-only LD; SES, socioeconomic status; SE, standard error; SMD, standard mean difference. T, teacher.
Data from Refs.[34–41]

Table 4
Cognitive, executive function, and academic achievement outcomes in adolescence and adulthood

Authors	Cohort	Assessment Age	Developmental Outcome
Botting et al,[64] 1998	1980–1983 Liverpool, England 138 VLBW and 108 matched controls	12 y	1. Any psychiatric disorder: 28% VLBW vs 9% controls had any psychiatric disorder 2. ADHD: 23% VLBW vs 6% controls 3. VLBW lower IQ
Saigal et al,[67] 2000	1977–1982 Ontario, Canada 141 ELBW 124 matched controls	12–16 y	1. 28% reported neurosensory impairments 2. 25% of ELBW vs 6% repeated a grade 3. 49% of ELBW vs 10% required special education services 4. 22% ELBW required full-time educational assistance (vs 0%) 5. Lower mean IQ 6. Lower mean math, reading, and spelling 7. At age 22–25, 1.3% ELBW had ASD
Levy-Shiff et al,[69] 1994	Israel 90 VLBW and 90 NBW	13–14 y	Significantly increased hyperactive behavior among VLBW; however, paternal involvement was as predictive as birth weight for hyperactivity in childhood
Dahl et al,[63] 2006	1978–1989 Norway 99 VLBW	13–18 y	1. VLBW adolescents report less externalizing behaviors than NBW adolescents 2. Parents of VLBW adolescents report more externalizing behaviors and emotional problems than NBW adolescents

(continued on next page)

Table 4
(continued)

Authors	Cohort	Assessment Age	Developmental Outcome
Rushe et al,[66] 2001	1979–1980 London, England <33 wk; 75 premature and 53 FT	14–15 y	1. No differences for tests of executive function, verbal memory, attention 2. Preterm group had impaired verbal fluency
Grunau et al,[65] 2004	1981–1986 British Columbia 79 <800 g vs 31 term	17 y	1. No differences focus and attention 2. Significantly more parental re-ported internalizing, externalizing, and problem behaviors
Lefebvre et al,[68] 2005	1976–1981 Montreal, Canada 57 ELBW and 44 NBW	18 y	1. 56.1% ELBW vs 84.6% controls completed HS 2. 33% vs 9% required special education 3. Significant differences in low IQ (<85)
Linsell et al,[52] 2018	UK and Ireland Prospective, population-based cohort study 315 <26 wk GA, 160 term controls	19 y	1. EP IQ: 85.7, term IQ: 103.9 2. If moderate/severe brain injury, IQ: 78.4 3. If GA <25 wk, IQ: 83.1
Hack et al,[54] 2007	1977–1979 Cleveland, Ohio 242 VLBW and 233 controls	20 y	1. 74% VLBW graduated HS vs 83% NBW 2. 30% pursued secondary education vs 53% NBW 3. 40% repeated grade vs 27% NBW 4. Scored 1/3 SD lower on WAIS-R
Lindstrom et al,[70] 2007	1973–1979 Sweden 24–28 wk (EP) vs FT	1987–2002 national registry	71% EP vs 78.6% FT completed 12 or more years of school
Moster et al,[56] 2008	1976–1983 Norway 325 preterm (23–27 wk) vs 828,227 FT	20–36 y	1. 67.7% preterm vs 75.4% completed HS 2. 4.4% preterm vs 0.1% full-term with ID

Study	Sample	Age	Findings
Nomura et al,[71] 2011 Johns Hopkins Collaborative Perinatal Study	1960–1965 Baltimore 226 near-term and 1393 FT	27–33 y	1. Near-term birth associated with lower adult educational attainment only for those living below poverty line 2. SGA had no association with educational attainment
Saigal et al,[57] 2006	1977–1982 Ontario, Canada 166 ELBW and 145 controls	22–25 y	No significant difference in: 1. % graduation from high school 2. Pursuit of post-secondary education 1.3% ELBW had ASD
Breeman et al,[59] 2015	Bavarian Longitudinal study 260 VP/VLBW	26 y	1. VP IQ: 86.2, term IQ: 102.6 2. IQ <70: VP 27%, term 3.9%
Laerum et al,[72] 2017	44 VLBW, 63 SGA, and 81 controls	26 y	1. Mood disorders: 18% VLBW, 14% SGA, 0% controls 2. Anxiety disorders: 27% VLBW, 20% SGA, 9% controls 3. Employed: 66% VLBW, 64% SGA, 67% controls 4. Receiving disability benefits: 14% VLBW, 3% SGA, 0% controls 5. Completed Bachelor's degree or higher: 25% VLBW, 40% SGA, 55% controls
Sullivan et al,[73] 2012	Providence Prospective NICU and FT cohort, stratified by SES	17 y	

	HPT	MPT	NPT	SGAPT	FT
COG	99	100	97	99	101
AA	96	101	96	99	101
EF	98	104	92	99	103

Abbreviations: AA, academic achievement; ADHD, attention-deficit/hyperactivity disorder; ASD, autism spectrum disorder; COG, cognitive; EF, executive function; ELBW, extremely low birth weight (<1000 g); EP, extremely preterm; FT, full-term; GA, gestational age; HPT, healthy preterm; HS, high school; ID, intellectual disability; IQ, intelligence quotient; MPT, medical preterm; NBW, normal birth; NPT, neurological preterm; SGA, small for gestational age; SGAPT, small for gestation age preterm; VLBW, very low birth weight (<1500 g); VP, very preterm; WAIS-R, Wechsler Adult Intelligence Scale-Revised.

Data from Refs. 52–59,63–73

category II included 8%, and category III included 24%. One in 4 children had cognitive disability, 11% had CP, 7% had ASD, and 6% had epilepsy. Nineteen percent of participants had 1 neurodevelopmental disability, 10% had 2, and 3% had 3. Furthermore, gestational age was inversely associated with number of neurodevelopmental disabilities. Approximately half of children with cognitive disability and one-third of children with either CP, ASD, or epilepsy had only 1 impairment. In terms of resilience, approximately 75% of children were considered to have normal intellect at 10 years of age, and nearly 70% had no neurodevelopmental disability.

According to the existing literature, there are certain neuropsychological functions that seem to be especially influenced by preterm birth. There is evidence that very preterm children who have learning difficulties tend to have both decreased IQ and selective cognitive impairments. There is also evidence that, among VPT children, academic achievement is associated with a variety of factors, including low socioeconomic status. Akshoomoff and colleagues[35] examined academic achievement, rates of learning disability (LD), and neuropsychological outcomes at 10 years of age of children born between 23 and 27 weeks of gestation from the US ELGAN study cohort. Both grade-based and age-based academic achievement measures were used. Children with IQ ≥ 2 SD below the mean were excluded. The investigators examined the rates of LD in reading and math (defined as standard scores <16th percentile) as well as the neuropsychological test correlates of reading and math LD. Socioeconomic status (as indicated by maternal education) was correlated with academic achievement, IQ, and neuropsychological measures. However, after controlling for socioeconomic status, the sample still had higher than expected rates of LD, especially in mathematics. The risk of low math scores was 27%, 1.5 times greater than the risk of low reading scores (17%); 6.4% of the sample was classified as having low reading achievement only, 16.2% was classified as having low math achievement only, and 8.3% was classified as having low math and reading achievement. All 3 of these groups exhibited multiple neuropsychological weaknesses when compared with the 69% of the sample with neither low math nor low reading scores. However, the low math group and low reading group differed in their neuropsychological profiles. These data suggest that there are specific cognitive weaknesses that differ between preterm children with low math achievement and low reading achievement.

Joseph and colleagues[42] examined whether or not maternal education, which is widely regarded to be an important marker of socioeconomic status, is associated with neurocognitive and academic outcomes for EPT children. Using 873 preterm children from the ELGAN cohort with gestational ages between 23 and 27 weeks, researchers compared the outcomes for children whose mothers had fewer years of education at time of delivery and children whose mothers advanced in education during the 10 years after birth. Adjustments were made for gestational age and potential confounding variables. It was found that children whose mothers were in the lowest educational bracket at their birth were significantly more likely to score at least 2 SDs worse than expected on 17 of the 18 neurocognitive and academic achievement tests given at age 10 years. Children whose mothers advanced in education were at a reduced risk of scoring at least 2 SDs worse than expectation on 15 of the 18 tests. However, this reduced risk was statistically significant for only 2 tests (inhibitory control and processing speed).

Leviton and colleagues[43] examined the antecedents of learning functional limitations at 10 years in 874 EPT children using multinomial logistic regression analyses in the US ELGAN cohort. Variables were entered in a chronologic, temporal order with earlier predictors and covariates entered first but not displaced by later covariates. Reading and math functional limitations were defined as scores of 1 or more

SD below the expected average on a reading or math examination. Of the 874 subjects, 56 were classified as reading limited, 132 as math limited, and 89 as having both. The risk profiles included indicators of socioeconomic status (maternal racial identity or eligibility for government-provided health insurance), medical vulnerability (such as a high illness severity score or receiving hydrocortisone for severe bronchopulmonary dysplasia), fetal growth restriction and inflammation (such as urinary tract infection during pregnancy), or late ventilator dependence. Overall fetal growth restriction and inflammation were antecedents of reading functional limitations and limitations in both reading and math functioning. Socioeconomic disadvantage and medical vulnerability were antecedents of educational underachievement in math, as well as in both reading and math.

Kuban and colleagues[44] reported on 889 children in the ELGAN cohort who underwent a comprehensive neuropsychological and autism assessment battery at age 10 years. Parents reported on health, behavior, development, and seizures. Twenty-eight percent of the boys and 21% of the girls had moderate/severe cognitive impairment. Furthermore, boys had a higher prevalence of impairment in nearly all measures of cognition, were more likely to have microcephaly (15% vs 8%), and more frequently required assistive devices to walk (6% vs 4%). However, boys and girls were at similar risk for current epilepsy (7% of cohort overall, although 10% had had seizures in the past). The prevalence of ASD was 9% in boys and 5% in girls, reflecting substantially higher risks in ELGAN than the 2% risk in term control boys and 1% risk in term control girls.

Caffeine citrate therapy for apnea of prematurity has been known to reduce rates of bronchopulmonary dysplasia, severe retinopathy, and neurodevelopmental disability at 18 months and improve motor function at 5 years. Schmidt and colleagues[45] investigated if neonatal caffeine therapy is associated with improved functional outcomes at 11 years. A total of 920 children from the multicenter international randomized, placebo-controlled Caffeine for Apnea of Prematurity trial were assessed in follow-up: 457 VPT/EPT (birth weight 500–1249 g) had received caffeine, and 463 placebo. The functional outcome was a composite of academic performance (at least 1 score of <2 SD below the mean on the Wide Range Achievement Test-4), motor impairment (percentile rank ≤5 on the Movement Assessment Battery for Children-Second Edition), and behavior problems (Total Problem T score ≥2 SD above the mean on the Child Behavior Checklist). The composite rate of functional limitations was not significantly different between the treatment (32%) and placebo (38%) groups. However, the treatment group did have a lower risk of motor impairment (20%) compared with the placebo group (28%). This study demonstrated that neonatal caffeine improved motor functioning, did not adversely impact long-term cognitive and behavioral performance, and was safe.

Luu and colleagues[46] examined 275 children born between 1989 and 1992 with birthweight 600 to 1250 g who were enrolled in the New England Indomethacin Intraventricular Hemorrhage (IVH) Prevention Trial. Concurrently at 12 years there were an additional 111 term controls. All participants were assessed with neuropsychometric testing and received a neurologic examination. Parents provided information about educational needs. The preterm group's scores were 6 to 14 points lower than those of the term group on all psychometric tests, after adjustment for socio-demographic factors. On a test of basic language skills, 22% to 24% of preterm children scored in the abnormal range (<70), compared with 2% to 4% of term children. Furthermore, preterm children both with and without sonographic brain injury required more school services than full-term children (76% and 44% vs 16%) and supports in reading (44% and 28% vs 9%), writing (44% and 20% vs 4%), and mathematics (47% and 30% vs 6%). The preterm group also had more internalizing and externalizing behavioral challenges. The strongest predictors of lower cognitive scores were severe neonatal brain injury, and minority status also was associated with worse cognition. Predictors of higher cognitive performance scores included antenatal steroids as well as the social capital of higher maternal education, and 2-parent family status.

Roze and colleagues[47] conducted a prospective cohort study of preterm infants less than 37 weeks of gestation with periventricular hemorrhagic infarction (PVHI) to examine motor, cognitive, and behavioral outcomes at school age. Motor outcomes at 4 and 12 years of age were classified using the Gross Motor Function Classification System (GMFCS) and the Manual Ability Classification System (MACS). Participants were assessed for cognition, visual-motor integration, visual perception, and verbal memory, and behavior was assessed using the Child Behavior Checklist and the Behavior Rating Inventory of Executive Function. Fifteen of the original 38 infants died, and 21 of the survivors were included in the follow-up. In this small study, characteristics of the PVHI were not related to functional motor outcomes or intelligence. Post-hemorrhagic ventricular dilatation was a risk factor for lower full-scale IQ, performance IQ, and fine motor dysfunction. Most of the surviving participants with PVHI had mild CP with the ability to walk (GMFCS <3) or perform manipulative tasks (MACS <3) across home and school activities. Importantly, intelligence was within 1 SD of the norm of preterm children without lesions in 60% to 80% of the children. However, verbal memory was often impaired, and behavioral and executive functional challenges occurred with high frequencies in those preterm infants with and without lesions.

Yu and Garcy[48] investigated cognitive and educational outcomes of adults born SGA, including the potential impact of family attitudes toward education on the effects of SGA birth on educational outcomes. A total of 9598 subjects of the Stockholm Birth Cohort were followed from infancy through age 50 years, with educational measures at age 13 years and 48 years. The verbal, spatial, and numerical test scores were lower for individuals born SGA (n = 798) than for individuals born appropriate for gestational age (AGA, n = 7364) or large for gestational age (n = 1436). The differences between the SGA and AGA groups were statistically significant, although small, and the effects of being born SGA were mediated by family attitudes toward education. Importantly, attainment of higher education after high school was largely (although not entirely) explained by family attitudes toward education.

Vohr and colleagues[49] assessed neurocognitive functioning at age 16 years in 338 preterm infants (birthweight 600–1250 g) born in New England. The cohort consisted of 11 preterm participants with grades 3 to 4 IVH, 44 with grade 2 IVH, 31 with grade 1 IVH, and 251 without IVH. Regression models were used to identify associations between low-grade hemorrhage and cognitive, executive function, and memory deficits. Preterm adolescents with grade 2 hemorrhage were at increased risk for learning challenges, including cognitive and executive function limitations, as well as higher rates of functional challenges on activities of verbal intelligence, receptive vocabulary, phonemic fluency, cognitive flexibility, and phonological fluency. The comparison groups included preterm adolescents with grade 1 hemorrhage or no hemorrhage, or term controls (n = 102). Preterm adolescents with grade 2 hemorrhage and no cystic periventricular leukomalacia were at an increased risk of cognitive and executive functional limitations when compared with term controls, and at a higher risk of cognitive challenges than preterm adolescents with no hemorrhage.

Brydges and colleagues[50] performed a systematic review to evaluate the association between VPT birth (<32 weeks of gestation) and intelligence, executive function, and processing speed through childhood and adolescence. Inclusion criteria were English-speaking subjects who had an age-matched control group born at term, and were tested with standardized measures between ages 4 and 16 years. A total of 6163 VPT children and 5471 term-born controls from 60 different studies were included. The investigators found that VPT children tended to score 0.82 SD lower on intelligence measures, 0.51 SD lower on executive functioning measures, and 0.49 SD lower on processing speed measures compared with their age-matched term-born controls. The investigators concluded that there may be a cascade effect: preterm birth predicts processing speed, which predicts executive functioning (including working memory), and working memory predicts math and reading abilities.

Doyle and colleagues[51] examined the relative importance of biological versus social factors on long-term outcomes of EPT using cognitive ability and academic achievement assessments in a regional Australian cohort. A total of 298 EPT survivors (gestational age <28 weeks or birthweight <1000 g) and 262 FTNB (full term normal birthweight) controls were evaluated at ages 2, 5, 8, and 18 years. IVH and postnatal corticosteroid therapy were the biological variables most associated with cognitive and educational functioning. Among social variables, being reared in a multilingual household was disadvantageous early on, whereas social class and maternal education became important for later outcomes. Although the strengths of the biological associations equaled or exceeded the strengths of the social associations throughout all age points, both factors contributed to long-term cognitive and educational outcomes. It is important to note that settings of social disadvantage, access to health services, and quality of education in public schools may be more adverse in the United States.

Linsell and colleagues[52] followed until age 19 years the UK EPICure cohort of surviving individuals born less than 26 weeks of gestation. The investigators compared cognitive development trajectories between EPT and term children using the Bayley Scales of Infant Development-Second Edition (2.5 years), the Kaufman Assessment Battery for Children (6 and 11 years), and the Wechsler Abbreviated Scale of Intelligence-Second Edition (19 years). At 19 years, researchers were able to assess 129 of the original 315 EPT subjects (41%) and 65 term-born matched controls. They found significantly lower cognitive performance in EPT survivors with an IQ of 85.7 compared with 103.9 in term-born controls (mean difference 18.2, effect size 1.2 Z). Importantly, the cognitive test scores of EPT participants with moderate or severe neonatal brain injury were 10.9 points below participants with no or mild brain injury. On average, male individuals and those who experienced brain injury early in life were at highest risk. These data suggest that among preterm children there are ongoing vulnerabilities that limit brain function and plasticity and that these cumulative challenges impact on long-term physical, cognitive, and social health. **Table 5** highlights several studies of adult outcomes focusing on employment, educational attainment, and health-related quality of life.

Severe ROP is associated with increased risk for visual disability, but the long-term impact on other neurodevelopmental domains is not as well understood. Molloy and colleagues[58] examined the relationship between severe ROP and cognitive, educational, and visual outcomes in 180 EPT individuals between the ages of 17 and 18 years. Rates of CP were 11%, intellectual disability 7%, and severe ROP (grade 3–5) 15%. The participants were sequentially assessed at ages 2, 5, 8, and 17 to 18 years using a wide range of neurodevelopmental measures, including academic achievement, cognition, visual processing, and visual-motor integration. Severe ROP was associated with an almost 9.8 IQ point difference (effect size 0.67 Z) and 6 to 7 standard score achievement point differences for reading, spelling, and mathematics (effect size 0.4–0.47 Z). In multiple logistic regression, severe ROP significantly increased the odds for IQ <85 (odds ratio 2.85). Thus, even without sequelae of blindness, EPT children with severe ROP are at an increased risk for difficulties with higher cortical visual processing, cognition, and educational achievement. This study demonstrates the critical role that ROP has on both visual and neurodevelopmental functioning.

Table 5
Adult outcomes after very and extremely preterm birth

Authors	Cohort	Age at Assessment	Developmental Outcome
Baumgardt et al,[53] 2012	1983–1985 Zurich, Switzerland 52 VLBW (<1250 g) 75 controls	23 y	No difference in overall self-reported quality of life
Hack et al,[54] 2007	1977–1979 Cleveland, Ohio 241 VLBW 232 NBW	20 y	1. No difference on self-reported health satisfaction 2. No difference on self-reported comfort (physical or emotional) 3. Decreased self-reported resiliency 4. Increased self-reported risk avoidance
Hille et al,[55] 2008	1983 Netherlands 959 adult survivors of prematurity (<32 wk or VLBW)	19 y	1. 50% had moderate/severe problem with profession 2. of individuals with moderate/severe problems in education had full-time employment
Moster et al,[56] 2008	1976–1983; Norway 325: 23–27 wk 1608: 28–30 wk 6363: 31–33 wk 31,169: 34–36 wk 828,227: full-term	20–36 y	1. 10.6% for 23–27 wk preterm vs 1.7% term receiving disability pension 2. Lower gestation less likely to have found life partner 3. Lower gestation less likely to have children
Saigal et al,[57] 2006	1977–1982 Ontario, Canada 166 ELBW and 145 controls	22–25 y	No significant difference in rates of: • Employment • Independent living • Married/cohabitation • Parenthood

Abbreviations: ELBW, extremely low birth weight (<1000 g); NBW, normal birth weight (>2500 g); VLBW, very low birth weight (<1500 g).
  Data from Refs.[53–57]

Breeman and colleagues[59] sought to determine the stability of cognitive functions from childhood to adulthood for preterm (less than 32 weeks' gestational age) and VLBW individuals when compared with individuals born at term, as well as how early adult cognitive functioning can be predicted. They used the cohort of the Bavarian Longitudinal Study, which is a prospective cohort study following 260 VPT/VLBW individuals and 229 controls born at term from birth through adulthood. Developmental and IQ tests were administered at 5 and 20 months, as well as at 4, 6, 8, and 26 years of age. For all assessments, VPT/VLBW individuals had significantly lower IQs than the controls born at term. This finding held even when individuals with severe cognitive impairment were excluded. IQ scores tended to be more stable over time for VPT/VLBW individuals compared with term-born individuals, although this effect went away when the subjects with cognitive impairment were excluded from analysis. Adult IQ scores could be predicted with a fair amount of certainty starting as early as 20 months of age for the VPT/VLBW sample, and as early as 6 years of age for the term-born control sample. These persistent deficits emphasize that proactive strategies are required for vulnerable preterm children to support their information, reading, and math vulnerabilities.

Mathewson and colleagues[60] performed a systematic review and meta-analysis to examine the risk for mental health problems in ELBW survivors compared with NBWT (>2.5 kg) term controls in childhood, adolescence, and adulthood. Previous evidence indicated that there may be gradient effects within preterm groups, with earlier gestational birth associated with higher rates of cognitive problems, attentional difficulties, hyperactivity, internalizing problems, and total psychological problems. In total, 41 studies with 2712 ELBW children, adolescents, and adults, and 11,127 NBWT peers were included. Researchers analyzed the impacts of birthplace, birth era, and neurosensory impairment on outcomes. In particular, they chose to examine the effects of birth era to compare outcomes in cohorts before and after the widespread availability of surfactant and steroid therapies. They also compared rates and types of mental health problems in participants with and without neurosensory impairment. The standardized mean difference from every study was used as the effect estimate, because difference measurement scales were used across studies. According to parent and teacher reports, ELBW children were at significantly greater risk for inattention and hyperactivity, internalizing symptoms, and externalizing symptoms when compared with NBWT controls. However, *self-reports* of inattention, hyperactivity, and oppositional behavior were lower for ELBW teens compared with NBWT controls. ELBW young adults had higher self-reported levels of internalizing problems and shyness than their NBWT peers. ELBW adults showed elevated levels of depression, anxiety, and social difficulties. Group differences were found to be robust for region of birth, birth era, and neurosensory impairments.

SUMMARY

If we are to understand the trajectories of risk and resilience in the vulnerable preterm and neonatal brain, we must go beyond survival and critically examine on a population basis the functional outcomes of children, adolescents, and adults across their life course. Our evaluations must go well beyond Bayley assessments and counts of neonatal morbidities, such as bronchopulmonary dysplasia, ROP, sonographic brain injury, sepsis, and necrotizing enterocolitis. We must proactively provide supports to families and developmental and educational supports to children to optimize academic functioning and participation in adult learning, physical and behavioral health activities, community living, relationships, and employment. We must better understand what underlies resiliency and how cumulative missed opportunities influence trajectories of physical, developmental, and social health. In this way, we can truly develop prenatal, perinatal, and postnatal neuroprotective interventions.

REFERENCES

1. World Health Organization(WHO). International classification of functioning, disability and health—children and youth version. Geneva (Switzerland): ICF-CY; 2009.
2. World Health Organization. International classification of functioning, disability and health (ICF). Geneva (Switzerland): 2001.
3. Halfon N, Hochstein M. Life course health development: an integrated framework for developing health, policy, and research. Milbank Q 2002;80(3):422–79.
4. Msall ME, Sobotka SA, Dmowska A, et al. Life-course health development outcomes after prematurity: developing a community, clinical and translational

research agenda to optimize health, behavior and functioning. In: Halfon N, Forrest C, Lerner R, et al, editors. Handbook of life course health development science. Cham (Switzerland): Springer Publishers; 2017. p. 321–48.

5. Washburn LK, Dillard RG, Goldstein DJ, et al. Survival and major neurodevelopmental impairment in extremely low gestational age newborns born 1990-2000: a retrospective cohort study. BMC Pediatr 2007;7:20–8.

6. Berry MJ, Saito-Benz M, Gray C, et al. Outcomes of 23- and 24-weeks gestation infants in Wellington, New Zealand: a single centre experience. Sci Rep 2017;7: 12769.

7. Serenius F, Ewald U, Farooqi A, et al. Neurodevelopmental outcomes among extremely preterm infants 6.5 years after active perinatal care in Sweden. JAMA Pediatr 2016;170:954–63.

8. Morse SB, Zheng H, Tang Y, et al. Early school-age outcomes of late preterm infants. Pediatrics 2009;123(4):e622–9.

9. Allen MC, Cristofalo EA, Kim C. Outcomes of preterm infants: morbidity replaces mortality. Clin Perinatol 2011;38(3):441–54.

10. Stephens BE, Vohr BR. Neurodevelopmental outcome of the premature infant. Pediatr Clin North Am 2009;56(3):631–46. Table of contents.

11. Vohr B. Long-term outcomes of moderately preterm, late preterm, and early term infants. Clin Perinatol 2013;40(4):739–51.

12. Saigal S, Doyle LW. An overview of mortality and sequelae of preterm birth from infancy to adulthood. Lancet 2008;371(9608):261–9.

13. Herber-Jonat S, Streiftau S, Knauss E, et al. Long-term outcome at age 7-10 years after extreme prematurity—a prospective, two centre cohort study of children born before 25 completed weeks of gestation (1999-2003). J Matern Fetal Neonatal Med 2014;27(16):1620–6.

14. Sharp M, French N, McMichael J, et al. Survival and neurodevelopmental outcomes in extremely preterm infants 22-24 weeks of gestation born in Western Australia. J Paediatr Child Health 2018;54(2):188–93.

15. Vohr BR. Neurodevelopmental outcomes of extremely preterm infants. Clin Perinatol 2014;14:241–55.

16. Ancel P-Y, Goffinet F, Group E-W. Survival and morbidity of preterm children born at 22 through 34 weeks' gestation in France in 2011: results of the EPIPAGE-2 cohort study. JAMA Pediatr 2015;169:230–8.

17. Moore T, Hennessy EM, Myles J, et al. Neurological and developmental outcome in extremely preterm children born in England in 1995 and 2006: the EPICure studies. BMJ 2012;345:e7961.

18. Younge N, Goldstein RF, Bann CM, et al. Survival and neurodevelopmental outcomes among periviable infants. N Engl J Med 2017;376(7):617–28.

19. Pierrat V. Neurodevelopmental outcome at 2 years for preterm children born at 22 to 34 weeks' gestation in France in 2011: EPIPAGE-2 cohort study. BMJ 2017; 358:j3448.

20. Doyle LW, Roberts G, Anderson PJ, Victorian Infant Collaborative Study Group. Outcomes at age 2 years of infants < 28 weeks' gestational age born in Victoria in 2005. J Pediatr 2010;156:49–53.e1.

21. Synnes A, Luu TM, Moddemann D, et al. Determinants of developmental outcomes in a very preterm Canadian cohort. Arch Dis Child Fetal Neonatal Ed 2017;102:235–43.

22. Serenius F, Källén K, Blennow M, et al. Neurodevelopmental outcome in extremely preterm infants at 2.5 years after active perinatal care in Sweden. JAMA 2013;309(17):1810–20.

23. Adams-Chapman I, Heyne RJ, DeMauro SB, et al. Neurodevelopmental impairment among extremely preterm infants in the neonatal research network. Pediatrics 2018;141(5) [pii:e20173091].
24. Msall ME. Neurodevelopmental surveillance in the first 2 years after extremely preterm birth: evidence, challenges, and guidelines. Early Hum Dev 2006;82: 157–66.
25. Amer R, Moddemann D, Seshia M, et al. Neurodevelopmental outcomes of infants born at <29 weeks of gestation admitted to Canadian Neonatal Intensive Care Units based on location of birth. J Pediatr 2018;196(5):31–7.e1.
26. Saigal S, den Ouden L, Wolke D, et al. School-age outcomes in children who were extremely low birth weight from four international population-based cohorts. Pediatrics 2003;111:943–50.
27. Taylor H, Klein N, Drotar D, et al. Consequences and risks of <1000-g birth weight for neuropsychological skills, achievement, and adaptive functioning. J Dev Behav Pediatr 2006;27(6):459–69.
28. Anderson P, Doyle L, Group VICS. Neurobehavioral outcomes of school-age children born extremely low birth weight or very preterm in the 1990s. JAMA 2003; 289(24):3264–72.
29. Klebanov P, Brooks-Gunn J, McCormick M. School achievement and failure in very low birth weight children. J Dev Behav Pediatr 1994;15(4):248–56.
30. Taylor H, Klein N, Minich N, et al. Middle-school-age outcomes in children with very low birthweight. Child Dev 2000;71(6):1495–511.
31. Resnick M, Gueorguieva R, Carter R, et al. The impact of low birth weight, perinatal conditions, and sociodemographic factors on educational outcome in kindergarten. Pediatrics 1999;104(6):e74.
32. Garfield CF, Karbownik K, Murthy K, et al. Educational performance of children born prematurely. JAMA Pediatr 2017;171:764–70.
33. Heeren T, Joseph RM, Allred EN, et al. Cognitive functioning at the age of 10 years among children born extremely preterm: a latent profile approach. Pediatr Res 2017;82(4):614–9.
34. Hirschberger RG, Kuban KCK, O'Shea TM, et al. Co-occurrence and severity of neurodevelopmental burden (cognitive impairment, cerebral palsy, autism spectrum disorder, and epilepsy) at age ten years in children born extremely preterm. Pediatr Neurol 2018;79:45–52.
35. Akshoomoff N, Joseph RM, Taylor HG, et al. Academic achievement deficits and their neuropsychological correlates in children born extremely preterm. J Dev Behav Pediatr 2017;38:627–37.
36. Burnett AC, Anderson PJ, Lee KJ, et al. Trends in executive functioning in extremely preterm children across 3 birth eras. Pediatrics 2018;141(1) [pii: e20171958].
37. Leviton A, Joseph RM, Allred EN, et al. Antenatal and neonatal antecedents of executive dysfunctions in extremely preterm children. J Child Neurol 2018; 33(3):198–208.
38. Saigal S. Functional outcomes of very premature infants into adulthood. Semin Fetal Neonatal Med 2014;19:125–30.
39. Szatmari P, Saigal S, Rosenbaum P, et al. Psychiatric disorders at five years among children with birthweights less than 1000g: a regional perspective. Dev Med Child Neurol 1990;32(11):954–62.
40. Saigal S, Rosenbaum P, Szatmari P, et al. Learning disabilities and school problems in a regional cohort of extremely low birth weight (less than 1000 g) children: a comparison with term controls. J Dev Behav Pediatr 1991;12(5):294–300.

41. Taylor HG, Klein N, Hack M. School-age consequences of birth weight less than 750 g: a review and update. Dev Neuropsychol 2000;17(3):289–321.

42. Joseph RM, O'Shea TM, Allred EN, et al. Maternal educational status at birth, maternal educational advancement, and neurocognitive outcomes at age 10 years among children born extremely preterm. Pediatr Res 2017. https://doi.org/10.1038/pr.2017.267.

43. Leviton A, Joseph RM, Allred EN, et al. Antenatal and neonatal antecedents of learning limitations in 10-year old children born extremely preterm. Early Hum Dev 2018;118(4):8–14.

44. Kuban KCK, Joseph RM, O'Shea TM, et al. Girls and boys born before 28 weeks gestation: risks of cognitive, behavioral, and neurologic outcomes at age 10 years. J Pediatr 2016;173(6):69–75.

45. Schmidt B, Roberts RS, Anderson PJ, et al. Academic performance, motor function, and behavior 11 years after neonatal caffeine citrate therapy for apnea of prematurity: an 11-year follow-up of the CAP randomized clinical trial. JAMA Pediatr 2017;171:564–72.

46. Luu TM, Ment LR, Schneider KC, et al. Lasting effects of preterm birth and neonatal brain hemorrhage at 12 years of age. Pediatrics 2009;12:1037–44.

47. Roze E, Van Braeckel KNJA, van der Veere CN, et al. Functional outcome at school age of preterm infants with periventricular hemorrhagic infarction. Pediatrics 2009;123:1493–500.

48. Yu B, Garcy AM. A longitudinal study of cognitive and educational outcomes of those born small for gestational age. Acta Paediatr 2017;107:86–94.

49. Vohr BR, Allan W, Katz KH, et al. Adolescents born prematurely with isolated grade 2 haemorrhage in the early 1990s face increased risks of learning challenges. Acta Paediatr 2014;103:1066–71.

50. Brydges CR, Landes JK, Reid CL, et al. Cognitive outcomes in children and adolescents born very preterm: a meta-analysis. Dev Med Child Neurol 2018;60(5):452–68.

51. Doyle LW, Cheong JLY, Burnett A, et al. Biological and social influences on outcomes of extreme-preterm/low-birth weight adolescents. Pediatrics 2015;136:e1513–20.

52. Linsell L, Johnson S, Wolke D, et al. Cognitive trajectories from infancy to early adulthood following birth before 26 weeks of gestation: a prospective, population-based cohort study. Arch Dis Child 2018;103(4):363–70.

53. Baumgardt M, Bucher HU, Mieth RA, et al. Health-related quality of life of former very preterm infants in adulthood. Acta Paediatr 2012;101(2):e59–63.

54. Hack M, Cartar L, Schluchter M, et al. Self-perceived health, functioning and well-being of very low birth weight infants at age 20 years. J Pediatr 2007;151(6):635–41, 641.e1–2.

55. Hille ET, Weisglas-Kuperus N, van Goudoever JB, et al, for Dutch Collaborative POPS 19 Study Group. Functional outcomes and participation in young adulthood for very preterm and very low birth weight infants: the Dutch Project on Preterm and Small for Gestational Age Infants at 19 years of age. Pediatrics 2007;120(3):e587–95.

56. Moster D, Lie RT, Markestad T. Long-term medical and social consequences of preterm birth. N Engl J Med 2008;359(3):262–73.

57. Saigal S, Stoskopf B, Streiner D, et al. Transition of extremely low-birth-weight infants from adolescence to young adulthood: comparison with normal birth-weight controls. JAMA 2006;295(6):667–75.

58. Molloy CS, Anderson PJ, Anderson VA, et al. The long-term outcome of extremely preterm (<28 weeks' gestational age) infants with and without severe retinopathy of prematurity. J Neuropsychol 2016;10:276–94.
59. Breeman LD, Jaekel J, Baumann N, et al. Preterm cognitive function into adulthood. Pediatrics 2015;136:415–23.
60. Mathewson KJ, Chow CHT, Dobson KG, et al. Mental health of extremely low birth weight survivors: a systematic review and meta-analysis. Psychol Bull 2017;143: 347–83.
61. Ishii N, Kono Y, Yonemoto N, et al. Outcomes of infants born at 22 and 23 weeks' gestation. Pediatrics 2013;132(1):62–71.
62. Wood NS, Costeloe K, Gibson AT, et al. The EPICure study: growth and associated problems in children born at 25 weeks of gestational age or less. Arch Dis Child Fetal Neonatal Ed 2003;88(6):F492–500.
63. Dahl LB, Kaaresen PI, Tunby J, et al. Emotional, behavioral, social, and academic outcomes in adolescents born with very low birth weight. Pediatrics 2006;118(2): e449–59.
64. Botting N, Powis A, Cooke RW, et al. Cognitive and educational outcome of very-low-birthweight children in early adolescence. Dev Med Child Neurol 1998; 40(10):652–60.
65. Grunau RE, Whitfield MF, Fay TB. Psychosocial and academic characteristics of extremely low birth weight (< or = 800g) adolescents who are free of major impairment compared with term-born control subjects. Pediatrics 2004;114(6): e725–32.
66. Rushe TM, Rifkin L, Stewart AL, et al. Neuropsychological outcome at adolescence of very preterm birth and its relation to brain structure. Dev Med Child Neurol 2001;43:226–33.
67. Saigal S. Follow-up of very low birthweight babies to adolescence. Semin Neonatol 2000;5(2):107–18.
68. Lefebvre F, Mazurier E, Tessier R. Cognitive and educational outcomes in early adulthood for infants weighing 1000 grams or less at birth. Acta Paediatr 2005; 94(6):733–40.
69. Levy-Shiff R, Einat G, Mogilner MB, et al. Biological and environmental correlates of developmental outcome of prematurely born infants in early adolescence. J Pediatr Psychol 1994;19(1):63–78.
70. Lindstrom K, Winbladh B, Haglund B, et al. Preterm infants as young adults: a Swedish national cohort study. Pediatrics 2007;120(4):936.
71. Nomura Y, Gilman SE, Buka SL. Maternal smoking during pregnancy and risk of alcohol use disorders among adult offspring. J Stud Alcohol Drugs 2011;72: 199–209.
72. Laerum A, Reitan S, Evensen K, et al. Psychiatric disorders and general functioning in low birth weight adults: a longitudinal study. Pediatrics 2017;139(2): e20162135.
73. Sullivan MC, Miller RJ, Msall ME. 17-year outcome of preterm infants with diverse neonatal morbidities: Part 2, impact on activities and participation. J Spec Pediatr Nurs 2012;17(4):275–87.
74. Doyle LW, Roberts G, Anderson PJ. Victorian Infant Collaborative Study Group. Outcomes at age 2 years of infants < 28 weeks' gestational age born in Victoria in 2005. J Pediatr 2010;156(1):49–53.
75. The Victorian Infant Collaborative Study Group. Outcome at 2 years of children 23–27 weeks' gestation born in Victoria in 1991–92. J Paediatr Child Health 1997;33(2):161–5.

Behavioral and Socioemotional Development in Preterm Children

Myriam Peralta-Carcelen, MD, MPH[a],*, Justin Schwartz, MD[a],
Andrea C. Carcelen, MPH[b]

KEYWORDS

- Socioemotional • Behavior • Prematurity • Autism • ADHD

KEY POINTS

- Development of socioemotional competence is crucial for optimal long-term neurodevelopmental outcomes in preterm children.
- Preterm children are at increased risk for behavior and socioemotional difficulties (including attention deficit disorder, attention deficit/hyperactivity disorder and autism spectrum disorder) given brain vulnerability, which is sensitive to environmental stressors during critical periods of brain development.
- Clinicians, researchers, and parents should recognize that a complete assessment of outcomes on prematurity should include behavioral and socioemotional functioning.
- Accessibility to early-intervention programs to improve socioemotional functioning and behavioral problems can potentially improve long-term neurodevelopmental outcomes on preterm children.

INTRODUCTION

Advances in technology and health care delivery have resulted in an increased number of preterm infants at lower gestational ages surviving, both with and without clinical complications.[1] However, these children develop significant morbidities at higher rates than their term counterparts. Preterm children are at risk for neurologic injury associated with immaturity, hypoxia, inflammation, painful procedures, and stressful treatments. These injuries can have long-lasting effects, including cognitive, behavioral, motor language, and neurosensory impairment. Given the increased survival

Disclosure Statement: The authors have no commercial or financial conflicts of interests and no funding sources for all authors.
[a] Division of Developmental and Behavioral Pediatrics, Department of Pediatrics, University of Alabama at Birmingham, Dearth Tower Suite 5602, McWane. 1600 7th Avenue South, Birmingham, AL 35233-1711, USA; [b] International Health Department, John Hopkins Bloomberg School of Public Health, 615 North Wolfe Street, Room 5517, Baltimore, MD, USA
* Corresponding author.
E-mail address: mperalta@peds.uab.edu

rate of preterm children, clinicians should be made aware of the behavioral and socio-emotional difficulties experienced by preterm children and their families in addition to other traditional outcomes.

Definitions

It has been reported that children born preterm have decreased socioemotional functioning.[2–5] Socioemotional functioning involves the ability to learn to successfully interact and communicate within a social context and to efficiently deal with emotions. It requires skillful coordination of multiple psychological processes.[6,7] Furthermore, the term "social competence" refers to a variety of mental mechanisms aimed at supporting successful social functioning, including emotional self-regulation, social cognitive processing, positive communication, and prosocial social relationships.[8] The term "social cognition" refers to the fundamental abilities to perceive, store, analyze, process, categorize, reason with, and behave toward others.[9]

To develop effective social interactions and social adjustments, it is important to recognize facial emotional expressions. Deficits in emotional understanding are associated with socioemotional and psychiatric disorders.[10] Preterm children have difficulties recognizing emotion.[11,12] A study in 8-year-old to 11-year-old very preterm children described problems interpreting each other's emotions using a complex test of social perceptual skills.[13]

Emotion regulation has increasingly been recognized as a potential crucial marker of later psychosocial risk.[14,15] Emotion regulation refers to a child's ability to modulate his or her emotions in response to people and situations, using a range of cognitive, physiologic, and behavioral processes and strategies, allowing for empathic and socially appropriate behavior. Emotional regulation was longitudinally tested in a group of very preterm children at 2 and 4 years. Higher mean levels of emotional dysregulation emerged at both time points in the very preterm group compared with controls.[8,16]

Social cognitive skills related to theory of mind are also impaired in preterm children.[17,18] Theory of mind is defined as the ability to understand that other people may have different motivations and emotions from one's own and that people's behavior is guided by their inner states.[19] Impaired theory of mind has been described as a core deficit in autism spectrum disorder (ASD) and has been linked to social anxiety and low popularity with peers.[7]

The developmental regulation process initially involves physiologic regulation during the neonatal period, emotional regulation during infancy, attention regulation during toddlerhood, and self-regulation during preschool years.[20] Specific brain networks have been found to subserve these processes and to form the so-called "social brain."[21] The cornerstone of successful social adjustment is social competence achieved in the context of its typically developing neural substrates.

The increased social vulnerability seen in preterm children occurs as a result of specific alterations in the social brain, part of the neurodevelopmental sequelae of very preterm birth.[22]

SOCIOEMOTIONAL DEVELOPMENT AND PREMATURITY
Perinatal Brain Injury Related to Behavioral Difficulties and Socioemotional Problems

The etiology of the behavioral abnormalities noted in preterm children is not clear but very likely to be multifactorial, and perinatal brain injury has been implicated as a contributing cause. Children born preterm are at high risk for brain injury, with the most common abnormality being white matter injury.[23,24] Inder and colleagues[25] showed that 20% of preterm children display moderate to severe white matter abnormalities, and another 51% have mild abnormalities. Additionally, gray matter abnormalities in certain brain regions have been reported to have a role in behavioral outcomes.[26] Early cerebellar injury noted on cranial ultrasound and confirmed with MRI of the brain was associated with behavioral, cognitive, language, and motor deficits in children born very preterm at 34 months of age.[27] The cerebellum has significant interconnectedness with cerebral hemispheres; therefore, the cerebellum is vital in cognitive and emotional functioning.[28]

Social adjustment and anxiety problems have been associated with smaller volume of left caudate nucleus[29] and right superior temporal lobe.[30] Caudate abnormalities have also been found in children with ASD,[31] suggesting the role of the caudate nucleus in reciprocal social and communicative behavior possibly due to its complex connections within cortical-basal ganglia.

The data of Limperopoulous and colleagues[26] suggest that the immature cerebellum may impact neurologic function through mechanisms that disrupt subsequent development of remote regions in the cerebral cortex.[26] Injury is not as "static" as previously thought, as the remote effects of primary cerebellar injury may continue to influence cerebral development for months and even years. Similar mechanisms are likely to operate following any premature related brain lesions, including periventricular leukomalacia or hemorrhage. It is important to understand how these secondary delayed effects on brain development are occurring to try to prevent further damage to the brain. Smith and colleagues[32] presented evidence that in 44 children born at less than 26 weeks' gestation who underwent a brain MRI, stressors to which the infant is exposed may be directly associated with decreased frontal and parietal width, altered diffusion measures, and functional connectivity in the temporal lobes. Additionally, increased abnormalities in motor behavior were observed during neurobehavioral examinations in this study.

These studies highlight the complex interplay among different brain structures and the role of their connectivity in maintaining unimpaired social cognition and social behaviors.

Environment and Behavioral and Socioemotional Difficulties

The biological immaturity of infants born preterm can cause deficits in their developmental regulatory processes.[33] Therefore, infants born preterm may be unable to manage environmental stimuli and may exhibit hyperactive responses and low tolerance to minimal stimulation.[34] However, when examining the processes of regulation in children born preterm from 0 to 5 years of age, the differences between preterm infants born with high and low medical risk changed during their development.[35] Over time, the effects of the environment on regulatory functions can improve the balance between biological and environmental regulation shifting toward the direction of environmental provisions, thus changing developmental outcomes.[36]

Psychosocial variables, such as positive parental interactions and low parental stress, can potentially protect children born preterm from behavioral problems.[37] These variables have an interactive effect with behavioral problems, specifically in children born very preterm. Individuals vary[38,39] in the degree to which they are affected by experiences and qualities of the environment to which they are exposed. By contrast, less susceptible individuals are less affected by parental rearing practices that either support or weaken well-being. Preterm children's social development is affected by parents' behavior and mental conditions, as well as interactions in the family.[40] Positive parenting during early childhood resulted in better cognitive as well as social-emotional outcomes when preterm children entered kindergarten.[41]

Early in life the hypothalamic-pituitary-adrenal axis (HPA) of very preterm infants is characterized by an inability to secret sufficient glucocorticoids for the degree of stress and illness. Emerging evidence suggests that the axis becomes overactive with age, which might offer an explanation for increased abdominal fat contents, insulin resistance, elevated blood pressure, shorter adult stature, and internalizing problems more often than found in preterm children.[42] In humans poor quality of parental care, such as neglect or emotional or physical maltreatment early in childhood was associated with greater HPA axis activity, mental illness, and cardiometabolic disease.[43] In an autopsy study, childhood abuse was associated with increased DNA methylation at the glucocorticoid receptor (GR) promotor and decreased expression of GR messenger RNA in the hippocampus.[44] Whether such findings could be extrapolated to very preterm infants, who receive less parental care and are exposed to stressors like invasive procedures, pain interruption of sleep states, and noise during their admission to the neonatal intensive care unit (NICU), remains to be explored.

There is a complex interplay between biological vulnerabilities and environmental influences, including functional and structural brain alterations, neonatal pain and stress, and nonoptimal parenting strategies.

Studies on Prevalence and Risk Factors Associated with Behavioral and Socioemotional Problems on Preterm Children

Studies examining preterm children's socioemotional development, including social competence and behaviors, are emerging more in the literature. Some researchers have suggested the "preterm behavioral phenotype" consists of inattention, anxiety, and social difficulties.[45] Behavioral problems, including poor self-regulation and social functioning, have been reported as early as 2 years of age in children born preterm.[5] There is also some evidence that deficits found at preschool age remain stable from early childhood through school age[46]; longitudinal studies, although infrequent, have also been reported[45]

A systematic review of studies on the relationship of prematurity, neonatal health status, and behavioral and emotional problems in school-age children confirmed that being preterm combined with neonatal risk factors increased the risk of behavioral and/or emotional problems in children.[35] A study from the Eunice Kennedy Shriver National Institute of Child Health and Development (NICHD) Neonatal Research Network (NRN) on 2205 extremely preterm children showed that lower birth weight was associated with both behavioral problems and socioemotional competence at 18 to 22 months of corrected age. Boys were more likely to have behavioral problems than girls. Other neonatal factors like intraventricular hemorrhage, bronchopulmonary dysplasia, and necrotizing enterocolitis were not found to be associated with behavioral or emotional problems after controlling for other variables. Social factors, such as having public medical insurance and lower maternal education, were also associated with behavioral or emotional problems. The effect of these risk factors on the presence of behavioral and competence problems were mediated by cognitive and language development measured by the Bayley Scales of Infant Development-third edition (Bayley-III) scores at 18 to 22 months old.[2]

Implications for Clinical Care Practice

The importance of recognizing socioemotional concerns and problem behaviors early is crucial, as several effective interventions currently exist. Unfortunately, parents and providers may not be aware of the implications on long-term outcomes in preterm children and are not screening for these difficulties. Furthermore, they may not be aware of the interventions available to address them.

The elucidation of mechanisms linking preterm birth, and socioemotional and psychiatric problems could provide an evidence-based rationale for developing and delivering new effective interventions meant to specifically reinforce protective factors (for example, interventions on parental stress) or to target specific risk factors found to be precursors of socioemotional and psychiatric difficulties in preterm-born individuals.

Interventions for optimal socioemotional development of children born preterm should be given prenatally, during NICU stay and after discharge. Children born preterm should be screened frequently for risk factors that may impact their socioemotional development. Prenatally, interventions may include providing optimal maternal care, including nutrition and social support for the pregnant mother. During the NICU stay, different approaches can be used. One of these is developmental care, which is a philosophy that embraces the concept of dynamic interaction among the infant, family, and surrounding environment. This provides a framework in which the environment and processes of delivering care are modified. Care of the infant focuses heavily on including parents in the care of the child; avoids overstimulation, stress, pain, and isolation; and supports self-regulation, social competence, and goal orientation. A specific program for developmental care, The Newborn Individualized Developmental Care and Assessment Program (NIDCAP) has published data supporting using the NIDCAP principles to improve brain development, functional competence, health, and quality of life.[47] Other interventions that have demonstrated efficacy in improving outcomes is Kangaroo care, which focuses on skin-to-skin contact between the parents and newborns.[48]

An increasing number of studies in the literature have been focusing on what to do after hospitalization. Spittle and Treyvaud[49] emphasized that interventions that focus on parent-infant relationship and infant development have the greatest impact on cognitive development in infancy. The importance of promoting optimal development by implementing screening for behavioral and emotional problems has been emphasized in a clinical report.[50] There is strong empirical support for family-focused interventions for young children with emotional, behavioral, and relationship problems.[51] For additional information on interventions refer to the American Academy of Pediatrics (AAP) technical report.[52]

There are a few studies that focused on therapies to enhance the overall functional development, including socioemotional development in preterm children.[49,52,53] However, it is agreed that to have an impact on long-term neurobehavioral outcomes, interventions should start early in life, and it is important to involve and support parents, given the high influence of the parent-infant relationship on developmental outcomes.[49]

ATTENTION DEFICIT/HYPERACTIVITY DISORDER IN PRETERM CHILDREN

Attention deficit/hyperactivity disorder (ADHD) is a pattern of behavioral features characterized by poor attention span, increased activity level, and impulsivity, which significantly limit one's functioning across multiple settings (eg, school, home, work). Prevalence rates in the general population have varied widely, in part due to inconsistencies in interpretation and application of diagnostic criteria and differences in behavior sampling across settings.[54] However, more rigorous population-based and community-based studies have found rates between 8.7% and 15.5% of school-aged children, above the 3.0% to 7.0% prevalence rate quoted by the *Diagnostic and Statistical Manual of Mental Disorders-4th Edition-Text Revision* (DSM-IV-TR).[54,55] Individuals with ADHD have been shown to have poorer outcomes, including increased rates of grade retention, poorer academic achievement, high school dropout, poorer occupational achievement, substance use, mental health conditions, and suicide.[56–58] Thus, ADHD is thought to be of significant public health importance.

Prematurity and low birth weight have been generally accepted as risk factors for the future development of ADHD. Numerous studies have documented the increased difficulties with attention span and activity level among this population. A meta-analysis from 2016 encompassing 64,061 children and including studies conducted between 1980 and 2016 found that those born preterm had higher odds of ADHD diagnosis compared with those born at term, with those born very and moderately preterm having a threefold higher odds of ADHD diagnosis.[59] Evidence supports the role of decreasing gestational age at birth in increasing the chances of developing ADHD later in life. One population-based study by Harris and colleagues[60] found no difference between rates of diagnosis of ADHD in late preterm children (34 to <37 weeks' gestation) versus term-born children. Another population-based study by Sucksdorff and colleagues[61] using Finnish nationwide registers found that risk for ADHD increased with each gestational week. In general, the association between prematurity and ADHD held even when controlling for sociodemographic factors and other risk conditions. Several studies have suggested an independent relationship between prematurity and ADHD risk[62]; however, an independent effect of low birth weight has also been documented. One longitudinal study by Heinonen and colleagues[63] found no association between prematurity and ADHD symptoms, but did find threefold higher likelihood of having clinically significant ADHD symptoms in infants born small for gestational age compared with children born appropriate for gestational age. In contrast, the Finnish population-based study by Sucksdorff, and colleagues[61] showed not only an association between prematurity and ADHD, but also a U-shaped relationship between birth weight and ADHD symptoms, with those infants born at greater than 2 SDs above and below the mean weight for gestational age having twice the odds or greater of receiving an ADHD diagnosis in childhood.

Despite the associations between prematurity, low birth weight, and ADHD, other perinatal conditions have also been shown to be associated with ADHD independent of prematurity. One study by Getahun and colleagues[64] reported an increased risk in ADHD related to ischemic-hypoxic conditions, such as preeclampsia, birth asphyxia, and prolapsed/nuchal cord; although these associations were strongest in the 28-week to 33-week gestation group, they were noted to be mildly to moderately associated in the term group as well. Other studies have demonstrated associations between ADHD and induction of labor, although this finding was not replicated in larger studies.[62] Maternal smoking, which is also associated with prematurity and low birth weight, has been found in several studies to be associated with ADHD.[62,65,66] However, genetic or hereditary factors may be an important confounder in this association, as its strength lessened when comparing exposed children with nonexposed siblings or cousins[67]; parents who smoke were also found to have a higher burden of mental health conditions than nonsmoker parents.[68] It has been suggested, however, that genetic factors play less of a role in the pathogenesis of ADHD among children born extremely preterm, given the contributions of common neonatal illnesses that occur in this population, such as necrotizing enterocolitis, intraventricular hemorrhage, neonatal infection, and chronic lung disease.[69]

Many of the changes observed in the brain among premature infants, which have been well connected to many adverse neurocognitive outcomes,[70] have been implicated in the development of attention problems. White matter volume differences have been well documented among individuals with ADHD who were not born prematurely.[71–74] Similarly, in individuals born premature, thinning of the corpus callosum and reduced white matter volume have been associated with increased attention difficulties but not hyperactivity.[75] Murray and colleagues[76] demonstrated that in very preterm/very low birth weight children, white matter abnormalities, including cystic degeneration, focal signal abnormalities, delayed myelination, thinning of corpus callosum, dilated lateral ventricles, and/or reduction of white matter volume, on MRI at term-equivalent age were predictive of attention and processing speed deficits at 7 years of age. This study also found that deep gray matter abnormalities also predicted difficulties in shifting attention, divided attention, and processing speed.[70] In contrast, a study by Bora and colleagues[77] showed that the severity of white matter abnormalities did not correlate with later risk of persistent attention or hyperactivity difficulties at 9 years of age; rather, persistence of ADHD symptoms was associated with volumetric reductions in the dorsal prefrontal, orbitofrontal, premotor, sensorimotor, and parieto-occipital subregions of the brain, with the dorsal prefrontal region showing the greatest volumetric reduction among those with persistent attention difficulties. These results are consistent with the most widely held model of ADHD neuropathology, which implicates abnormalities of the frontostriatal pathways in disorders of attention and self-regulation.[78] Striatal neurons are particularly susceptible to hypoxic-ischemic injury during the perinatal period,[79] lending support to the notion that the genesis of ADHD in preterm infants may rely more on perinatal factors than genetic factors, as noted previously.

As inflammation has been proposed as an important modulator of white matter injury, interventions to reduce inflammation theoretically have the potential to lessen the risk of ADHD symptoms. However, use of antenatal glucocorticoids, antibiotics, or magnesium sulfate have not yet been shown to reduce the risk of attention problems.[69] Scarce data are available to suggest that reductions in leading causes of postnatal inflammation (bacteremia, mechanical ventilation, and necrotizing enterocolitis) would be successful at reducing attention problems as well.[69] At the time of writing, no postnatal interventions to reduce inflammation have documented long-term effects on outcomes, including attention. However, many interventions, including hypothermia, magnesium sulfate, and erythropoietin, have shown promise as neuroprotective in the short term.[80–83]

The public health implications of increased attention problems among preterm infants have necessitated heightened surveillance and treatment in this population throughout the life span. Several studies have documented the continuing burden of ADHD symptoms on individuals born preterm.[45,84,85] Breeman and colleagues[86] observed that although attention regulation in very preterm/very low birth weight individuals improved from childhood to adulthood, there was moderate stability of ADHD diagnosis in this group as compared with term-born individuals. Krasner and colleagues[87] showed 3 different trajectories of ADHD symptoms among low birthweight/preterm children: most (44%) had no symptoms by 9 years of age, 39% had symptoms at 9 but that they slowly declined by age 16, and 17% showed a persistent inattentive symptom burden while hyperactivity declined. Those with persistent inattention had poorer outcomes, including increased experiences of bullying, depressive symptoms, and poorer adaptive functioning. Symptoms at school age were shown to increase likelihood of special education services and below-expected grade performance. Consistent with the results of this study, several prior studies had previously described the ADHD phenotype of children born preterm as a primarily inattentive presentation,[4,45,88] which may predispose these children's difficulties to be underappreciated. Mainstays of treatment of ADHD include both behavioral (parent training, classroom accommodations) and pharmacologic approaches.[89] However, data are scarce on the efficacy of these treatments in populations of individuals born preterm. Due to the theoretic differences in underlying neuropathology and documented differences in neuropsychological presentation, this remains an area ripe for further study.

AUTISM SPECTRUM DISORDER AND PRETERM CHILDREN

ASD is a heterogeneous neurodevelopmental disorder characterized by impairments in reciprocal social interactions, verbal and nonverbal communication, as well as the presence of restricted or repetitive atypical behavioral patterns. ASD is a clinical diagnosis based on criteria from the *Diagnostic and Statistical Manual of Mental Disorders, Fifth Edition* (DSM V).[90] The most recent prevalence of ASD has been reported as 1 in 59 (Centers for Disease Control and Prevention) in the general population.[91] The cardinal features of ASD manifest early in childhood. These early signs have a significant impact on long-term cognitive function and quality of life. Genetics and environmental factors are known to contribute to autism risk; however, the pathogenesis of ASD continues to be an area of active investigation.

Prevalence of Autism in Preterm Children

Several studies have evaluated the prevalence and associated risk factors of developing autism in children born preterm. Epidemiologic studies in Europe have identified preterm birth and low birth weight as significant risk factors for ASD. In a large case-control study in Denmark of infants born between 1973 and 2000, a birth gestational age less than 35 weeks was associated with a nearly 2.5-fold increased risk of autism.[92] In Norway, Moster and colleagues[93] used the compulsory National Medical Registry to study nearly 1 million children born more than 23 weeks' gestation between 1967 and 1983. The relative risk for autism increased nearly 10-fold in children born between 23 and 28 weeks' gestation as compared to term-born children; for children born between 28 and 31 weeks' gestation, the relative risk increased 7-fold. In a population-based case-control study conducted in Finland, birthweight less than 2500 g and small-for-gestational-age status were each independently associated with increased ASD risk.[94] Preterm infants weighing less than 1500 g at birth had threefold higher odds of being diagnosed with ASD than term-born controls. However, the association between preterm birth and autism risk has not been entirely consistent across studies, due in part to varying methodologies and heterogeneous populations.[95]

Autism screening instruments have been used in several studies and demonstrate an increased prevalence of abnormal autism screens among preterm children. Limperopoulos and colleagues[96,97] assessed 91 former preterm infants with birth weights less than 1500 g and found that 26% of children had a positive result on the Modified Checklist for Autism in Toddlers (M-CHAT), a questionnaire used in screening children with ASD. In a cohort of extremely low gestational age newborns (<28 weeks' gestation) Kuban and colleagues[98] found that major neurosensory impairments accounted for more than half of positive M-CHAT results. After excluding children with neurosensory impairments, 10% still had a positive M-CHAT screen at 2 years of age, twice the expected rate in the general population. Similarly, Moore and colleagues[99] found that 41% of former preterm infants less than 26 weeks' gestation had a positive M-CHAT screen at 2 years of age, and the prevalence of a positive M-CHAT screen decreased as gestational ages increased. Preterm children without comorbid disabilities had a 16.5% prevalence of a positive screen. More recently Fevang and colleagues[100] found that in extremely preterm children without severe neurodevelopmental disability, the odds of screening positive for symptoms of autism were increased fourfold compared with term controls. Clinicians who use the M-CHAT screening for very preterm children should be cautioned about possible misclassification and may need supplementation with other screening measures.[101] The M-CHAT has been revised to the M-CHAT-R/F and now includes a follow-up interview that should be used together with the M-CHAT screen to improve the predictive value of the screening. It has been recommended that both parts of the screening should be completed.[102] Stephens and colleagues[103] reported the use of 3 screening methods (Pervasive Developmental Disorders Screening Test, second edition, Stage 2 and the response to name and joint attention items from the Autism Diagnostic Observation Schedule), on 554 extremely preterm children who did not have severe neurodevelopmental impairment (severe cerebral palsy, deafness, and blindness) at 18 to 22 months of age. Twenty percent of children had at least 1 positive screen for ASD consistent with prevalence in the literature; however, only 1% had all 3 screens positive, which caution us against this increase in prevalence using different screening instruments.

A few studies have focused on accurate prevalence of clinically diagnosed ASD in the preterm population. Johnson and colleagues[104] screened 11-year-old former preterm children with the Social Communication Questionnaire (SCQ) and ASD was confirmed using a semistructured diagnostic interview: the Development and Well-Being Assessment. Eight percent of former extremely preterm infants born at less than 26 weeks' gestation were diagnosed with autism, whereas none of the children in the term gestation control group had autism. Pinto-Martin and colleagues[105] studied a regional birth cohort of children with birth weights less than 2000 g and followed them with periodic assessments until 21 years of age. A subset of the sample was assessed using the Autism Diagnostic Observation Schedule (ADOS) and/or the Autism Diagnostic Interview-Revised (ADI-R) and estimated diagnostic prevalence of autism was 5%.[106] In a retrospective cohort study of infants born in the Kaiser Permanente Healthcare system, the prevalence of clinically diagnosed ASD in children born at less than 27 weeks' gestation was 3 times more prevalent compared with children born at term. Each week of shorter gestation was associated with an increased risk of ASD.[106] In a study of 889 extremely low gestational age children (<28 weeks' gestation) the estimated prevalence of ASD was 7.1% using the SCQ for screening, followed by the ADI-R and the ADOS-2.[107]

Clinical Autism Spectrum Disorder Features in Preterm Children

ASD may present differently in preterm children when compared with term counterparts. Comparable to the "behavioral phenotype" on preterm children, an "autism phenotype" has been described in preterm children.[108] Preterm children with ASD are thought to have more impairment in social interaction and communication but fewer symptoms of repetitive and stereotypic behavior. Introversion and difficulties with social engagement may persist to adulthood.[109] A recent study of Bowers and colleagues[110] looked at 883 individuals with a diagnosis of autism and compared 115 individuals who were born preterm with those who were born at term. There were more male preterm individuals with ASD with sleep apnea, seizures, and ADHD compared with term male individuals. Female individuals and with ASD were more likely to be nonverbal.

Brain Differences in Preterm Children with Autism Spectrum Disorder

Although neuropathology of ASD varies across cases, the most consistent pathology includes curtailment of normal development of the limbic system and abnormal development of the cerebellum and associated nuclei.[111,112] The pathways underlying brain connectivity and higher cortical function after extreme prematurity are not clearly understood.[113,114] Neuroimaging studies of preterm children with ASD have reported disrupted cerebellar growth[115] and impaired connectivity. A study that looked at term-equivalent brain MRI in extremely preterm children subsequently diagnosed with ASD demonstrated reduced volumes in the temporal, occipital, insular, and limbic regions, as well as regions involved in social behaviors.[116] Adolescents who were born preterm and had high scores on the autism spectrum questionnaire were associated with lower fractional anisotropy in specific white matter tracts, including the external capsule and superior fascicle.[117]

Although the pathogenesis of ASD is not fully understood, evidence supports the hypothesis that ASD develops in children with genetic susceptibility that experience abnormal stressors during a critical period of brain development.[26] Preterm birth is associated with high rates of perinatal brain injury and interrupts a critical period for brain growth and structural differentiation.[24]

Risk Factors for Autism Spectrum Disorder in Preterm Children

Prematurity seems to be a rather nonspecific risk factor compared with the specific risk factors for autism that have been previously suggested. Low birth weight has been associated with an increased risk of developing ASD. Biological vulnerability factors in preterm children seem to be obvious. Additionally, there is developing evidence that psychological factors are also important.

Joint attention skills have been described as important precursors of social development[118] and have been extensively investigated in the context of autism spectrum research. Studies by Landry and Chapieski[119] reported difficulties in joint attention in 6-month-old infants born preterm. These infants showed more problems engaging in joint play and initiating joint attention interactions with their mothers and exhibited more gaze aversion compared with their term-born peers.[120] Lower birth weight, gestational age, male gender, chorioamnionitis, acute intrapartum hemorrhage, illness severity, and lower birth weight have been associated with an abnormal autism screening.[97]

In terms of maternal characteristics, maternal infection and prenatal inflammation may be associated with development of ASD.[121] Stress during the perinatal period has been associated with the development of ASD.[122] Maternal obesity has also been associated with increased risk of ASD in preterm studies.[123] However, much work remains to understand these associations.

Clinical Practices for Early Detection of Autism Spectrum Disorder in Preterm Children

Currently there are no clinical guidelines specific for ASD screening in preterm children. The AAP recommends specific autism screening for all children at 18 months and 24 months of age in addition to global developmental screening.[124] Screening instruments recommended for early diagnoses have been published.[125] The most common instrument used in general practices is the M-CHAT-R/F, which recommends using a follow-up interview.[102] At each surveillance visit, clinicians should evaluate risk factors that include having a sibling with ASD or suspicion of ASD by the caregiver or provider. The AAP is in agreement with the Academy of Neurology and the Child Neurology Society Statement on Autism.[126] There has been reported improved outcome for ASD with early-intervention programs aimed at specific targets. Although the evidence for improving ASD symptoms in preterm children is not available, effective therapies are available for children with ASD if detected early[127] and should be offered to preterm children in a timely manner.

Best Practices

What is the current practice?

Behavior and socioemotional difficulties are not routinely included in evaluation of outcomes of preterm children.

Objective: To increase awareness among clinicians who care for preterm children on the importance of recognizing behavioral and socioemotional difficulties, identifying risk factors and providing early screening and referral for early intervention for children at risk of developing these difficulties.

What changes in current practice are likely to improve outcomes?

Early recognition of risk factors in preterm children who will have difficulties in their behavior and socioemotional development will confer improved long-term behavioral and cognitive outcomes. Providers need to be aware of practices being researched to improve socioemotional functioning.

Is there a clinical algorithm? If so, please include.

Currently there are no clinical algorithms for evaluation of behavior and socioemotional difficulties in preterm children. The AAP has published guidelines for behavioral evaluation in primary care settings, but no algorithm was provided. A report from the AAP addresses ASD screening in the primary care setting and provides an algorithm. Some guidelines have been published regarding assessments in NICU follow-up clinics, but these are not comprehensive. There are several ongoing studies to address the effects of early intervention on socioemotional development and behavioral outcomes in preterm and low birth weight children.

Recommendations

Providers caring for preterm children during their newborn period and after discharge should be doing periodic assessments on social-emotional development and behavioral problems as well as psychosocial problems, as recommended in the clinical report of the AAP for optimizing emotional and behavioral outcomes. A separate report for ASD screening has also been published by the AAP. Providers should also arrange for access to services for children and their families.

Families would benefit from attending a high-risk follow-up clinic, where more comprehensive evaluations can be done. High-risk clinics should evaluate children for behavioral and socioemotional difficulties and provide social support to families, as well as communicate and work with primary care providers. The efficacy of follow-up programs has not yet been well documented.

Summary statement

Preterm children are at risk for behavioral and socioemotional difficulties, given brain immaturity and vulnerability during critical periods of development. It is important that clinicians are aware and monitor these difficulties to optimize the overall neurodevelopmental function of preterm children and their families.

REFERENCES

1. Saigal S, Doyle LW. An overview of mortality and sequelae of preterm birth from infancy to adulthood. Lancet 2008;371(9608):261–9.
2. Peralta-Carcelen M, Carlo WA, Pappas A, et al. Behavioral problems and socio-emotional competence at 18 to 22 months of extremely premature children. Pediatrics 2017;139(6):e20161043.
3. Peralta-Carcelen M, Bailey K, Rector R, et al. Behavioral and socioemotional competence problems of extremely low birth weight children. J Perinatol 2013;33(11):887–92.
4. Hack M, Taylor HG, Schluchter M, et al. Behavioral outcomes of extremely low birth weight children at age 8 years. J Dev Behav Pediatr 2009;30(2):122–30.

5. Spittle A, Treyvaud K, Doyle L, et al. Early emergence of behavior and social-emotional problems in very preterm infants. J Am Acad Child Adolesc Psychiatry 2009;48(9):909–18.

6. Iarocci G, Yager J, Elfers T. What gene-environment interactions can tell us about social competence in typical and atypical populations. Brain Cogn 2007;65(1):112–27.

7. Happé F, Frith U. Annual research review: towards a developmental neuroscience of atypical social cognition. J Child Psychol Psychiatry 2014;55(6):553–7.

8. Jones KM, Champion PR, Woodward LJ. Social competence of preschool children born very preterm. Early Hum Dev 2013;89(10):795–802.

9. Fenoglio A, Georgieff MK, Elison JT. Social brain circuitry and social cognition in infants born preterm. J Neurodev Disord 2017;9:27.

10. Denham SA, Blair KA, DeMulder E, et al. Preschool emotional competence: pathway to social competence? Child Dev 2003;74(1):238–56.

11. Witt A, Theurel A, Tolsa CB, et al. Emotional and effortful control abilities in 42-month-old very preterm and full-term children. Early Hum Dev 2014;90(10): 565–9.

12. Potharst ES, van Wassenaer-Leemhuis AG, Houtzager BA, et al. Perinatal risk factors for neurocognitive impairments in preschool children born very preterm. Dev Med Child Neurol 2013;55(2):178–84.

13. Williamson KE, Jakobson LS. Social perception in children born at very low birthweight and its relationship with social/behavioral outcomes. J Child Psychol Psychiatry 2014;55(9):990–8.

14. Cole PM, Michel MK, Teti LO. The development of emotion regulation and dysregulation: a clinical perspective. Monogr Soc Res Child Dev 1994;59(2–3): 73–100.

15. Lawson KR, Ruff HA. Early focused attention predicts outcome for children born prematurely. J Dev Behav Pediatr 2004;25(6):399–406.

16. Clark CA, Woodward LJ, Horwood LJ, et al. Development of emotional and behavioral regulation in children born extremely preterm and very preterm: biological and social influences. Child Dev 2008;79(5):1444–62.

17. Pavlova M, Sokolov AN, Birbaumer N, et al. Perception and understanding of others' actions and brain connectivity. J Cogn Neurosci 2008;20(3):494–504.

18. Williamson KE, Jakobson LS. Social attribution skills of children born preterm at very low birth weight. Dev Psychopathol 2014;26(4 Pt 1):889–900.

19. Carlson SM, Moses LJ. Individual differences in inhibitory control and children's theory of mind. Child Dev 2001;72(4):1032–53.

20. Sameroff AJ, Rosenblum KL. Psychosocial constraints on the development of resilience. Ann N Y Acad Sci 2006;1094:116–24.

21. Kennedy DP, Adolphs R. The social brain in psychiatric and neurological disorders. Trends Cogn Sci 2012;16(11):559–72.

22. Healy E, Reichenberg A, Nam KW, et al. Preterm birth and adolescent social functioning-alterations in emotion-processing brain areas. J Pediatr 2013; 163(6):1596–604.

23. Inder TE, Volpe JJ. Mechanism of perinatal brain injury. Semin Neonatol 2000;5: 3–16.

24. Volpe JJ. Perinatal brain injury: from pathogenesis to neuroprotection. Ment Retard Dev Disabil Res Rev 2001;7(1):56–64.

25. Inder TE, Wells SJ, Mogridge NB, et al. Defining the nature of the cerebral abnormalities in the premature infant: a qualitative magnetic resonance imaging study. J Pediatr 2003;143(2):171–9.

26. Limperopoulos C, Chilingaryan G, Sullivan N, et al. Injury to the premature cerebellum: outcome is related to remote cortical development. Cereb Cortex 2014; 24(3):728–36.
27. Van Braeckel KN, Taylor HG. Visuospatial and visuomotor deficits in preterm children: the involvement of cerebellar dysfunctioning. Dev Med Child Neurol 2013;55(Suppl 4):19–22.
28. Panigrahy A, Wisnowski JL, Furtado A, et al. Neuroimaging biomarkers of preterm brain injury: toward developing the preterm connectome. Pediatr Radiol 2012;42(Suppl 1):S33–61.
29. Nosarti C, Allin MP, Frangou S, et al. Hyperactivity in adolescents born very preterm is associated with decreased caudate volume. Biol Psychiatry 2005;57(6): 661–6.
30. Rogers CE, Barch DM, Sylvester CM, et al. Altered gray matter volume and school age anxiety in children born late preterm. J Pediatr 2014;165(5):928–35.
31. Qiu A, Adler M, Crocetti D, et al. Basal ganglia shapes predict social, communication, and motor dysfunctions in boys with autism spectrum disorder. J Am Acad Child Adolesc Psychiatry 2010;49(6):539–51, 551.e1–4.
32. Smith GC, Gutovich J, Smyser C, et al. Neonatal intensive care unit stress is associated with brain development in preterm infants. Ann Neurol 2011;70(4): 541–9.
33. Feldman R. On the origins of background emotions: from affect synchrony to symbolic expression. Emotion 2007;7(3):601–11.
34. Als H, Duffy FH, McAnulty GB, et al. Early experience alters brain function and structure. Pediatrics 2004;113(4):846–57.
35. Cassiano RG, Gaspardo CM, Linhares MB. Prematurity, neonatal health status, and later child behavioral/emotional problems: a systematic review. Infant Ment Health J 2016;37(3):274–88.
36. Feldman R. The development of regulatory functions from birth to 5 years: insights from premature infants. Child Dev 2009;80(2):544–61.
37. Vinall J, Miller SP, Synnes AR, et al. Parent behaviors moderate the relationship between neonatal pain and internalizing behaviors at 18 months corrected age in children born very prematurely. Pain 2013;154(9):1831–9.
38. Belsky J. Theory testing, effect-size evaluation, and differential susceptibility to rearing influence: the case of mothering and attachment. Child Dev 1997;68(4): 598–600.
39. Belsky J, Pasco Fearon RM, Bell B. Parenting, attention and externalizing problems: testing mediation longitudinally, repeatedly and reciprocally. J Child Psychol Psychiatry 2007;48(12):1233–42.
40. Zmyj N, Witt S, Weitkämper A, et al. Social cognition in children born preterm: a perspective on future research directions. Front Psychol 2017;8:455.
41. Maupin AN, Fine JG. Differential effects of parenting in preterm and full-term children on developmental outcomes. Early Hum Dev 2014;90(12):869–76.
42. Finken MJJ, van der Voorn B, Hollanders JJ, et al. Programming of the hypothalamus-pituitary-adrenal axis by very preterm birth. Ann Nutr Metab 2017;70(3):170–4.
43. Francis DD, Champagne FA, Liu D, et al. Maternal care, gene expression, and the development of individual differences in stress reactivity. Ann N Y Acad Sci 1999;896:66–84.
44. McGowan PO, Sasaki A, D'Alessio AC, et al. Epigenetic regulation of the glucocorticoid receptor in human brain associates with childhood abuse. Nat Neurosci 2009;12(3):342–8.

45. Johnson S, Marlow N. Preterm birth and childhood psychiatric disorders. Pediatr Res 2011;69(5 Pt 2):11R–8R.

46. Gray RF, Indurkhya A, McCormick MC. Prevalence, stability, and predictors of clinically significant behavior problems in low birth weight children at 3, 5, and 8 years of age. Pediatrics 2004;114(3):736–43.

47. Als H, Duffy FH, McAnulty GB, et al. Is the Newborn Individualized Developmental Care and Assessment Program (NIDCAP) effective for preterm infants with intrauterine growth restriction? J Perinatol 2011;31(2):130–6.

48. Conde-Agudelo A, Díaz-Rossello JL. Kangaroo mother care to reduce morbidity and mortality in low birthweight infants. Cochrane Database Syst Rev 2016;(8):CD002771.

49. Spittle A, Treyvaud K. The role of early developmental intervention to influence neurobehavioral outcomes of children born preterm. Semin Perinatol 2016; 40(8):542–8.

50. Weitzman C, Wegner L, Section on Developmental and Behavioral Pediatrics, Committee on Psychosocial Aspects of Child and Family Health, Council on Early Childhood, Society for Developmental and Behavioral Pediatrics, American Academy of Pediatrics. Promoting optimal development: screening for behavioral and emotional problems. Pediatrics 2015;135(2):384–95.

51. Gleason MM, Goldson E, Yogman MW, AAP council on early childhood. Addressing early childhood emotional and behavioral problems. Pediatrics 2016; 138(6):e20163025.

52. Barlow J, Bergman H, Kornør H, et al. Group-based parent training programmes for improving emotional and behavioural adjustment in young children. Cochrane Database Syst Rev 2016;(8):CD003680.

53. Spittle A, Orton J, Anderson PJ, et al. Early developmental intervention programmes provided post hospital discharge to prevent motor and cognitive impairment in preterm infants. Cochrane Database Syst Rev 2015;(11):CD005495.

54. Rowland AS, Skipper BJ, Umbach DM, et al. The prevalence of ADHD in a population-based sample. J Atten Disord 2015;19(9):741–54.

55. Wolraich ML, McKeown RE, Visser SN, et al. The prevalence of ADHD: its diagnosis and treatment in four school districts across two states. J Atten Disord 2014;18(7):563–75.

56. Barbaresi WJ, Colligan RC, Weaver AL, et al. Mortality, ADHD, and psychosocial adversity in adults with childhood ADHD: a prospective study. Pediatrics 2013; 131(4):637–44.

57. Barbaresi WJ, Katusic SK, Colligan RC, et al. Long-term school outcomes for children with attention-deficit/hyperactivity disorder: a population-based perspective. J Dev Behav Pediatr 2007;28(4):265–73.

58. Klein RG, Mannuzza S, Olazagasti MA, et al. Clinical and functional outcome of childhood attention-deficit/hyperactivity disorder 33 years later. Arch Gen Psychiatry 2012;69(12):1295–303.

59. Allotey J, Zamora J, Cheong-See F, et al. Cognitive, motor, behavioural and academic performances of children born preterm: a meta-analysis and systematic review involving 64 061 children. BJOG 2018;125(1):16–25.

60. Harris MN, Voigt RG, Barbaresi WJ, et al. ADHD and learning disabilities in former late preterm infants: a population-based birth cohort. Pediatrics 2013; 132(3):e630–6.

61. Sucksdorff M, Lehtonen L, Chudal R, et al. Preterm birth and poor fetal growth as risk factors of attention-deficit/hyperactivity disorder. Pediatrics 2015;136(3): e599–608.

62. Sciberras E, Mulraney M, Silva D, et al. Prenatal risk factors and the etiology of ADHD-review of existing evidence. Curr Psychiatry Rep 2017;19(1):1.
63. Heinonen K, Raikkonen K, Pesonen AK, et al. Behavioural symptoms of attention deficit/hyperactivity disorder in preterm and term children born small and appropriate for gestational age: a longitudinal study. BMC Pediatr 2010;10:91.
64. Getahun D, Rhoads GG, Demissie K, et al. In utero exposure to ischemic-hypoxic conditions and attention-deficit/hyperactivity disorder. Pediatrics 2013;131(1):e53–61.
65. Silva D, Colvin L, Hagemann E, et al. Environmental risk factors by gender associated with attention-deficit/hyperactivity disorder. Pediatrics 2014;133(1): e14–22.
66. Langley K, Heron J, Smith GD, et al. Maternal and paternal smoking during pregnancy and risk of ADHD symptoms in offspring: testing for intrauterine effects. Am J Epidemiol 2012;176(3):261–8.
67. Skoglund C, Chen Q, D'Onofrio BM, et al. Familial confounding of the association between maternal smoking during pregnancy and ADHD in offspring. J Child Psychol Psychiatry 2014;55(1):61–8.
68. Thakur GA, Sengupta SM, Grizenko N, et al. Maternal smoking during pregnancy and ADHD: a comprehensive clinical and neurocognitive characterization. Nicotine Tob Res 2013;15(1):149–57.
69. O'Shea TM, Downey LC, Kuban KK. Extreme prematurity and attention deficit: epidemiology and prevention. Front Hum Neurosci 2013;7:578.
70. Kidokoro H, Neil JJ, Inder TE. New MR imaging assessment tool to define brain abnormalities in very preterm infants at term. AJNR Am J Neuroradiol 2013; 34(11):2208–14.
71. Valera EM, Faraone SV, Murray KE, et al. Meta-analysis of structural imaging findings in attention-deficit/hyperactivity disorder. Biol Psychiatry 2007;61(12): 1361–9.
72. Konrad K, Eickhoff SB. Is the ADHD brain wired differently? A review on structural and functional connectivity in attention deficit hyperactivity disorder. Hum Brain Mapp 2010;31(6):904–16.
73. Makris N, Buka SL, Biederman J, et al. Attention and executive systems abnormalities in adults with childhood ADHD: a DT-MRI study of connections. Cereb Cortex 2008;18(5):1210–20.
74. Cao Q, Sun L, Gong G, et al. The macrostructural and microstructural abnormalities of corpus callosum in children with attention deficit/hyperactivity disorder: a combined morphometric and diffusion tensor MRI study. Brain Res 2010;1310: 172–80.
75. Indredavik MS, Vik T, Heyerdahl S, et al. Psychiatric symptoms and disorders in adolescents with low birth weight. Arch Dis Child Fetal Neonatal Ed 2004;89(5): F445–50.
76. Murray AL, Scratch SE, Thompson DK, et al. Neonatal brain pathology predicts adverse attention and processing speed outcomes in very preterm and/or very low birth weight children. Neuropsychology 2014;28(4):552–62.
77. Bora S, Pritchard VE, Chen Z, et al. Neonatal cerebral morphometry and later risk of persistent inattention/hyperactivity in children born very preterm. J Child Psychol Psychiatry 2014;55(7):828–38.
78. Faraone SV, Biederman J. Neurobiology of attention-deficit hyperactivity disorder. Biol Psychiatry 1998;44(10):951–8.
79. Volpe JJ. Overview: normal and abnormal human brain development. Ment Retard Dev Disabil Res Rev 2000;6(1):1–5.

80. Juul SE, Pet GC. Erythropoietin and neonatal neuroprotection. Clin Perinatol 2015;42(3):469–81.
81. Chang E. Preterm birth and the role of neuroprotection. BMJ 2015;350:g6661.
82. Jacobs SE, Berg M, Hunt R, et al. Cooling for newborns with hypoxic ischaemic encephalopathy. Cochrane Database Syst Rev 2013;(1):CD003311.
83. Salmeen KE, Jelin AC, Thiet MP. Perinatal neuroprotection. F1000Prime Rep 2014;6:6.
84. Johnson S, Hollis C, Kochhar P, et al. Psychiatric disorders in extremely preterm children: longitudinal finding at age 11 years in the EPICure study. J Am Acad Child Adolesc Psychiatry 2010;49(5):453–63.e1.
85. Bhutta AT, Cleves MA, Casey PH, et al. Cognitive and behavioral outcomes of school-aged children who were born preterm: a meta-analysis. JAMA 2002; 288(6):728–37.
86. Breeman LD, Jaekel J, Baumann N, et al. Attention problems in very preterm children from childhood to adulthood: the Bavarian Longitudinal Study. J Child Psychol Psychiatry 2016;57(2):132–40.
87. Krasner AJ, Turner JB, Feldman JF, et al. ADHD symptoms in a non-referred low birthweight/preterm cohort: longitudinal profiles, outcomes, and associated features. J Atten Disord 2015 [pii:1087054715617532].
88. Jaekel J, Wolke D, Bartmann P. Poor attention rather than hyperactivity/impulsivity predicts academic achievement in very preterm and full-term adolescents. Psychol Med 2013;43(1):183–96.
89. Subcommittee on Attention-Deficit/Hyperactivity Disorder, Steering Committee on Quality Improvement and Management, Wolraich M, Brown L, Brown RT, et al. ADHD: clinical practice guideline for the diagnosis, evaluation, and treatment of attention-deficit/hyperactivity disorder in children and adolescents. Pediatrics 2011;128(5):1007–22.
90. American Psychiatry Association. Diagnostic and Statistical Manual of Mental Disorders 5th edition. Washington, DC; 2013.
91. Baio J, Wiggins L, Christensen DL, et al. Prevalence of autism spectrum disorder among children aged 8 years-autism and developmental disabilities monitoring Network, 11 sites, United States 2014. MMWR Surveillance Summaries 2018;67(5):1–15.
92. Larsson HJ, Eaton WW, Madsen KM, et al. Risk factors for autism: perinatal factors, parental psychiatric history, and socioeconomic status. Am J Epidemiol 2005;161(10):916–25 [discussion: 926–8].
93. Moster D, Lie RT, Markestad T. Long-term medical and social consequences of preterm birth. N Engl J Med 2008;359(3):262–73.
94. Lampi KM, Lehtonen L, Tran PL, et al. Risk of autism spectrum disorders in low birth weight and small for gestational age infants. J Pediatr 2012;161(5):830–6.
95. Kolevzon A, Gross R, Reichenberg A. Prenatal and perinatal risk factors for autism: a review and integration of findings. Arch Pediatr Adolesc Med 2007; 161(4):326–33.
96. Limperopoulos C, Bassan H, Gauvreau K, et al. Does cerebellar injury in premature infants contribute to the high prevalence of long-term cognitive, learning, and behavioral disability in survivors? Pediatrics 2007;120(3):584–93.
97. Limperopoulos C, Bassan H, Sullivan NR, et al. Positive screening for autism in ex-preterm infants: prevalence and risk factors. Pediatrics 2008;121(4):758–65.
98. Kuban KC, O'Shea TM, Allred EN, et al. Positive screening on the Modified Checklist for Autism in Toddlers (M-CHAT) in extremely low gestational age newborns. J Pediatr 2009;154(4):535–40.e1.

99. Moore T, Johnson S, Hennessy E, et al. Screening for autism in extremely preterm infants: problems in interpretation. Dev Med Child Neurol 2012;54(6): 514–20.

100. Fevang SK, Hysing M, Markestad T, et al. Mental health in children born extremely preterm without severe neurodevelopmental disabilities. Pediatrics 2016;137(4) [pii:e20153002].

101. Kim SH, Joseph RM, Frazier JA, et al. Predictive validity of the modified checklist for autism in toddlers (M-CHAT) born very preterm. J Pediatr 2016;178: 101–7.e2.

102. Robins DL, Casagrande K, Barton M, et al. Validation of the modified checklist for autism in toddlers, revised with follow-up (M-CHAT-R/F). Pediatrics 2014; 133(1):37–45.

103. Stephens BE, Bann CM, Watson VE, et al. Screening for autism spectrum disorders in extremely preterm infants. J Dev Behav Pediatr 2012;33(7):535–41.

104. Johnson S, Hollis C, Kochhar P, et al. Autism spectrum disorders in extremely preterm children. J Pediatr 2010;156(4):525–31.e2.

105. Pinto-Martin JA, Levy SE, Feldman JF, et al. Prevalence of autism spectrum disorder in adolescents born weighing <2000 grams. Pediatrics 2011;128(5): 883–91.

106. Kuzniewicz MW, Wi S, Qian Y, et al. Prevalence and neonatal factors associated with autism spectrum disorders in preterm infants. J Pediatr 2014;164(1):20–5.

107. Joseph RM, O'Shea TM, Allred EN, et al. Prevalence and associated features of autism spectrum disorder in extremely low gestational age newborns at age 10 years. Autism Res 2017;10(2):224–32.

108. Kalish BT, Angelidou A, Stewart J. Autism spectrum disorder in preterm children. Neoreviews 2017;18(7):e431–7.

109. Eryigit-Madzwamuse S, Strauss V, Baumann N, et al. Personality of adults who were born very preterm. Arch Dis Child Fetal Neonatal Ed 2015;100(6):F524–9.

110. Bowers K, Wink LK, Pottenger A, et al. Phenotypic differences in individuals with autism spectrum disorder born preterm and at term gestation. Autism 2015; 19(6):758–63.

111. Kemper TL, Bauman M. Neuropathology of infantile autism. J Neuropathol Exp Neurol 1998;57(7):645–52.

112. Sweeten TL, Posey DJ, Shekhar A, et al. The amygdala and related structures in the pathophysiology of autism. Pharmacol Biochem Behav 2002;71(3):449–55.

113. Msall ME. Central nervous system connectivity after extreme prematurity: understanding autistic spectrum disorder. J Pediatr 2010;156(4):519–21.

114. Msall ME. Optimizing early development and understanding trajectories of resiliency after extreme prematurity. Pediatrics 2009;124(1):387–90.

115. Limperopoulos C. Autism spectrum disorders in survivors of extreme prematurity. Clin Perinatol 2009;36(4):791–805, vi.

116. Padilla N, Eklöf E, Mårtensson GE, et al. Poor brain growth in extremely preterm neonates long before the onset of autism spectrum disorder symptoms. Cereb Cortex 2017;27(2):1245–52.

117. Skranes J, Vangberg TR, Kulseng S, et al. Clinical findings and white matter abnormalities seen on diffusion tensor imaging in adolescents with very low birth weight. Brain 2007;130(Pt 3):654–66.

118. Baron-Cohen S. Do people with autism understand what causes emotion? Child Dev 1991;62(2):385–95.

119. Landry SH, Chapieski ML. Joint attention and infant toy exploration: effects of Down syndrome and prematurity. Child Dev 1989;60(1):103–18.

120. Smith LEH. Pathogenesis of retinopathy of prematurity. Semin Neonatal 2003; 8(6):469–73.
121. Joseph RM, Korzeniewski SJ, Allred EN, et al. Extremely low gestational age and very low birthweight for gestational age are risk factors for autism spectrum disorder in a large cohort study of 10-year-old children born at 23-27 weeks' gestation. Am J Obstet Gynecol 2017;216(3):304.e1-16.
122. Beversdorf DQ, Manning SE, Hillier A, et al. Timing of prenatal stressors and autism. J Autism Dev Disord 2005;35(4):471–8.
123. Reynolds LC, Inder TE, Neil JJ, et al. Maternal obesity and increased risk for autism and developmental delay among very preterm infants. J Perinatol 2014;34(9):688–92.
124. Johnson CP, Myers SM, American Academy of Pediatrics Council on Children with Disabilities. Identification and evaluation of children with autism spectrum disorders. Pediatrics 2007;120(5):1183–215.
125. Zwaigenbaum L, Bauman ML, Fein D, et al. Early screening of autism spectrum disorder: recommendations for practice and research. Pediatrics 2015; 136(Suppl 1):S41–59.
126. Filipek PA, Accardo PJ, Ashwal S, et al. Practice parameter: screening and diagnosis of autism: report of the Quality Standards Subcommittee of the American Academy of Neurology and the Child Neurology Society. Neurology 2000; 55(4):468–79.
127. Zwaigenbaum L, Bauman ML, Choueiri R, et al. Early intervention for children with autism spectrum disorder under 3 years of age: recommendations for practice and research. Pediatrics 2015;136(Suppl 1):S60–81.

The Impact of Prematurity on Social and Emotional Development

Angela Leon Hernandez, MD

KEYWORDS

- Social and emotional development • Preterm birth • Screening and treatment

KEY POINTS

- High incidence of behavioral and emotional problems in children born prematurely have an impact on quality of life.
- Supporting social and emotional development in this high-risk population, with an emphasis on promoting protective factors and minimizing the factors that are known to be deleterious requires a multifaceted approach, and collaborative efforts among academic institutions, the private sector, and governmental programs.
- Lack of correlation between brain lesions and behavioral problems might indicate that premature birth affects social and emotional development through different mechanisms than brain injury, and that children affected by encephalopathy of prematurity may have impaired capabilities to adapt, respond, and overcome negative experiences, making them less resilient to the effects of psychosocial adversity.

INTRODUCTION

Advances in neonatal intensive care in the past 2 decades have led to an increase in survival rates of premature infants. Reports on long-term follow-up cohorts of children, adolescents, and young adults born prematurely, in particular very low birth weight infants (VLBW infants <1500 g), provide critical information about the prevalence of chronic conditions, functional outcomes, and quality of life in this population.[1,2] Among these chronic conditions, the high prevalence of behavioral and emotional problems, specifically deficits in attention, autism spectrum disorder (ASD), anxiety, and depression, have been a focus of concern due to their impact on family life, social interaction, and school performance.[3–6] In 2013, based on a study population of 96,677 children living in the United States aged 2 to 17 years old, Singh and colleagues[7] found 28.7% prevalence of parent-reported mental health problems among VLBW infants compared with 15% in children born full-term. Multiple studies have supported these findings, even after correcting for socioeconomic factors, severe developmental impairment, and other chronic

Neonatology Division, Emory University School of Medicine, 49 Jesse Hill Jr drive SE, Atlanta, GA 30030, USA
E-mail address: angela.leon-hernandez@emory.edu

Clin Perinatol 45 (2018) 547–555
https://doi.org/10.1016/j.clp.2018.05.010
0095-5108/18/© 2018 Elsevier Inc. All rights reserved.

conditions.[8–10] Johnson and colleagues[11] conducted an 11-year follow-up cohort study of 219 children born at less than 26 weeks' gestation compared with 153 term controls and found that premature infants were 3 times more likely to have a psychiatric disorder, had a significantly increased risk of attention-deficit/hyperactivity disorder (ADHD) (11.5% vs 2.9%; odds ratio [OR] 10.5; confidence interval [CI] 1.4–81.8); autism (8% vs 0%, $P = .000$), and other emotional disorders (9% vs 2.1%; OR 4.6; CI 1.3–15.9). Along with advances in neuroimaging and neurobiology have led to a better understanding of the extent of brain injury beyond intraventricular hemorrhage and periventricular leukomalacia (PVL) in premature infants. After the initial axonal injury hypomyelination or PVL, caused by the effects of hypoxemia, free radicals, and inflammatory mediators, a secondary insult to the developing brain, mediated by impaired cell-to-cell interactions, results in the arrest of neuronal and axonal proliferation in other areas of the brain and translates to the decreased volumes of cerebral cortex, thalamus, and basal ganglia seen in VLBW infants.[12] This widespread brain involvement or encephalopathy of prematurity has been postulated as an explanation for the high prevalence of sensory, cognitive, and behavioral deficits even in the absence of major motor impairment. However, unlike the patterns associated with motor outcomes and academic deficits, brain abnormalities on MRI are not predictors of behavioral outcomes.[13] Lack of correlation between brain lesions and behavioral problems might indicate that premature birth affects social and emotional development through different mechanisms than brain injury, and also that children affected by encephalopathy of prematurity may have impaired capabilities to adapt, respond, and overcome negative experiences, making them less resilient to the effects of psychosocial adversity.

EMOTIONAL-SOCIAL DEVELOPMENT AND PREMATURE BIRTH

To elucidate the different mechanisms by which premature birth affects behavior, it is important to start with the description of what it is known about normal early emotional and social development. According to the bio-behavioral synchrony model,[14] coordinated, predictable, and repetitive exchanges between mother-infant and father-infant establishes the framework for future stress reactions, emotional regulation, and socialization. These exchanges, mostly mediated by the epigenetic effects of oxytocin and cortisol on central nervous system (CNS) maturation and function, further enhances the ability of the infant and the parents to sense, process, and respond in a synchronous manner to each other.[15] Oxytocin not only plays a crucial role in reorganizing neuronal networks, but also affects stress, immune, and inflammatory responses.[16] According to this model, the potential for reorganization of neuronal networks, or neuronal plasticity, makes reparation possible during the first years of life.

In the event of premature birth, the need for intensive care support limits the opportunities for synchronous interactions. Following the bio-behavioral synchrony model, it is postulated that mother-infant separation and lack of synchronous interactions or "maternal deprivation" not only impairs an infant's ability to process information and to modulate responses, but also affects maternal responsiveness to the infant's ques. To support this theory, multiple studies of infant-maternal dyads, participating in kangaroo care programs in neonatal intensive care units (NICUs) have shown positive effects on infant and maternal responsiveness in addition to decreasing maternal anxiety when compared with the standard of care.[16–18] Long-term protective effects of kangaroo care have been reported, including a lower incidence of problems with in attention, impulsivity, and antisocial behavior.[18] Even though literature tends to focus on the negative effects of premature birth on bonding, there are reports of higher-quality mother-infant interactions among preterm dyads when compared with full-term counterparts, particularly in favorable social and supportive environments.[19] Furthermore, investigators have reported how premature infants are not only more sensitive to poor-quality mother-father-infant interactions, but more responsive to high-quality interactions than full-term infants,[20] which highlights the potential for long-term protective effects from these strategies. Breastfeeding is one of the most representative examples of synchronic interaction and it is affected by multiple factors associated with preterm birth, including infant-mother separation, delay in the attainment of mature feeding pattern, and need for fortification to promote growth. It is estimated that only 40% to 60% of VLBW infants are breastfed and are discharged from the NICU with a predominantly human milk diet.[21] The role of human milk in social and emotional development may be mediated by its direct effect on neurogenesis,[22] but also by the hormonal effect on CNS maturation and function, during infant-mother synchronic interactions. Some reports have shown a lower incidence of ADHD and other behavioral problems in children who received a human milk diet, suggesting the role of breastfeeding as a protective factor.[23,24] In addition to the limited opportunities for synchronic interactions, including breastfeeding, the exposure of the developing brain to noxious stimuli during NICU care has further potential to affect the infant's self-regulation and responsiveness (**Fig. 1**). In 2012, Montirosso and colleagues[25] reported a study of 178 VLBW infants from 25 NICUs and demonstrated how premature infants from NICUs with a commitment to developmental care defined by the frequency of use of kangaroo care, facilitation for parents to spent the night, and routine practices from nursing staff to support development, exhibited better attention and self-regulation, and less irritability than infants from NICUs with less structured commitment to developmental care. Furthermore, longer length of stay in the NICU has been associated with an increased risk for behavioral and emotional problems even after correcting for prematurity, chronic conditions such as bronchopulmonary dysplasia, and social factors.[26]

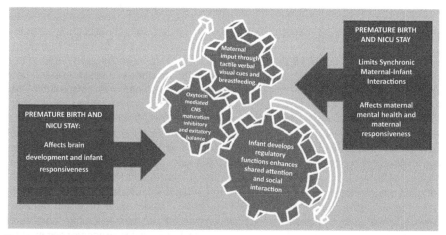

Fig. 1. Early stages of emotional-social development and premature birth. Repetitive and synchronic maternal-infant interactions establish the framework for emotional regulation and socialization mediated by oxytocin CNS maturation. Premature birth and NICU stay, affect both maternal and infant responsiveness resulting in dysregulation and impaired infant social interaction.

OTHER DETERMINANTS OF SOCIAL AND EMOTIONAL DEVELOPMENT AFTER PREMATURE BIRTH

The psychosocial environment, in particular maternal mental health and parental styles, are important determinants of behavioral outcomes of children born prematurely. Maternal mental health has been described as one of the most influential factors in on the emotional and social well-being of children.[27] Premature birth increases the risk for maternal depression, anxiety, and post-traumatic stress disorder (PTSD).[28] Maternal depression and anxiety have also been associated with attachment disorders and poor behavioral outcomes in children born prematurely.[27] In addition to the impact of maternal depression on children's mental health, the use of antidepressants during pregnancy, in particular selective serotonin reuptake inhibitors, has been a source of controversy due to reports that suggest an increased risk for ASD in children with prenatal exposure to these drugs.[29,30] Maternal substance abuse frequently coexists with other mental pathologies and has been associated with poor behavioral outcomes, most likely the result of a combination of in utero exposure, neurotoxicity, and adverse social environment.[31]

In addition to surveillance systems for maternal depression, anxiety, PTSD, and addiction, there is no question about the need for robust programs that support diagnosis and treatment of maternal mental health problems starting in pregnancy and continuing in the NICU and after discharge. Furthermore, there is a need for mental health professionals with experience in addressing issues related to attachment problems and with training in behavioral therapy. It is important to mention that high-quality developmental NICU practices, including family-centered approaches and home-visiting programs, have shown positive effects in decreasing parental symptoms of depression and anxiety.[17,24,32]

The role of parenting has been described as one of the most important determinants of social and emotional development. In particular, parental styles characterized by hostility, negativity, intrusiveness, and lack of structure have been associated with impaired child self-regulation and poor behavioral outcomes.[33] This highlights the importance of parent education regarding positive parenting practices starting from the NICU, as well as access to evidence-based behavioral interventions.[34,35]

CURRENT CHALLENGES IN THE SCREENING AND TREATMENT OF EMOTIONAL AND BEHAVIORAL PROBLEMS

Although there is a significant body of evidence that supports the importance of early detection and treatment of emotional and behavioral problems to improve functional outcomes, in the United States, it is estimated that primary care providers identify only half of children with serious behavioral and emotional problems, and when diagnosed only 1 of 8 children receive specialized treatment.[36,37] When analyzing obstacles that prevent pediatric patients from receiving mental health care services, the high cost, type of insurance, local governmental policies and limited availability of pediatric mental health providers are among the most critical factors. Medicaid covers only half of all costs of treatment for mental health conditions in children age 5 to 17 years, with an estimated per-child cost of $2000 per year.[38] Variation of coverage between states is affected by unfavorable local governmental policies, including the lack of adoption of Medicaid expansion, low rates for reimbursement of mental health care services, and no acceptance of developmentally specific diagnosis in children aged 0 to 5 years as reimbursable conditions in addition to the limited availability of pediatric mental health providers. The situation is maybe more critical for patients living in rural areas and for children younger than 5 years. Given the challenges of providing mental health services to children, models of collaborative efforts between mental health and primary care providers have been proposed to improve early detection and increase the probability of receiving treatment. Critical points to consider when developing these types of programs included identification of local mental health providers, the establishment of routine screening, tracking referrals, and obtaining psychiatric consultation.[36,37]

Similar models should be adopted at high-risk developmental follow-up clinics with an emphasis on early screening, in-house counseling when possible, and a surveillance system for referrals. Close contact with mental health providers in the community may help to improve the chances of getting adequate treatment. At the Developmental Progress Clinic at Emory University, as a result of the challenges in early diagnosis and treatment of behavioral and emotional problems in our population, a multidisciplinary focus group was created to evaluate the problem and to develop strategies to better support patients and families affected by these conditions. The adoption of a surveillance system for referrals, with follow-up calls and redirection of care, if needed, and the identification of reliable mental health resources that fit our population's needs and characteristics, increased the percentage of patients receiving treatment from 25% in 2015 to 60% and 65% in 2016 (Angela Leon Hernandez, 2016, unpublished data). Even though there is an improvement in the percentage of patients who are receiving therapies, insurance coverage and parental acceptance of need for behavioral intervention continues to be a challenge.

Developing models to support healthier behavioral and emotional development from NICU to school age in children born prematurely with an emphasis on the application of strategies that have proven to be protective, is a priority. High-risk follow-up clinics with the support of mental health providers can play a distinctive role in coordination and implementation of these strategies.

Given the complexity of the factors involved in social and emotional development, not a single strategy but a combination of actions starting from pregnancy and continuing in the NICU and after discharge at least for the first 5 years of life requires collaboration of academic institutions, the private sector, and governmental programs (**Fig. 2**).

Based on the current literature, implementation of various strategies is recommended:

- Promotion of early infant-mother, infant-father interactions and intervention when risks for attachment disorders are identified, systematic evaluation and treatment of maternal mental health problems during pregnancy, and continued evaluation at NICU and after discharge.
- Implementation of developmentally oriented strategies at NICU supporting human interaction through kangaroo care, and other positive experiences for premature infants, including family-centered care with involvement of both parents.
- Support and promote human milk–based diet and breastfeeding.
- Parental education about early social and emotional development, brain development, and positive parenting styles. Family support by social services for transportation, housing, and coordination of care and other social needs.
- After discharge, continue family education and support through home-visiting programs, parenting groups, and school readiness programs.
- Standardized screening for behavioral and emotional problems at specialized developmental clinics with surveillance systems for referrals with an option for consultation with mental health providers to guarantee early diagnosis and treatment.

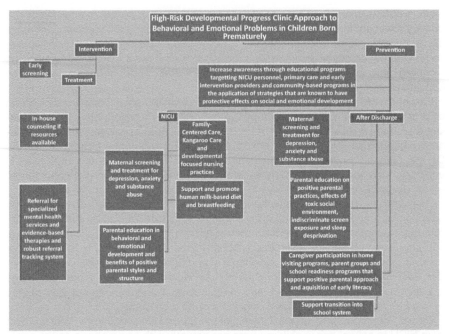

Fig. 2. Proposed model to support emotional and social development. High-risk follow-up developmental clinics have a critical role in the promotion and support of strategies that have been proven to have positive effects on social and emotional development in children born prematurely, providing continuous education and support to health care providers, early intervention programs, and community-based programs. Close contact with mental health providers and social services is essential.

- Establish collaborative efforts among academic institutions, the private sector, governmental programs, and community programs to guarantee access to high-quality and evidence-based preventive and therapeutic strategies, with special attention to children with history of prematurity and social adversity.

SUMMARY

Given the high incidence of behavioral and emotional problems in children born prematurely and their impact on quality of life, supporting social and emotional development in this high-risk population, with an emphasis on promoting protective factors and minimizing the factors that are known to be deleterious, requires a multifaceted approach and collaborative efforts among academic institutions, the private sector, and governmental programs.

REFERENCES

1. Doyle LW, Anderson PJ. Adult outcome of extremely preterm infants [review]. Pediatrics 2010;126(2):342–51.
2. Saigal S. Functional outcomes of very premature infants into adulthood [review]. Semin Fetal Neonatal Med 2014;19(2):125–30.
3. Aarnoudse-Moens CS, Weisglas-Kuperus N, van Goudoever JB, et al. Meta-analysis of neurobehavioral outcomes in very preterm and/or very low birth weight children. Pediatrics 2009;124(2):717–28.

4. Litt JS, McCormick MC. The impact of special health care needs on academic achievement in children born prematurely. Acad Pediatr 2016;16(4):350–7.
5. Scott MN, Hunter SJ, Joseph RM, et al. Neurocognitive correlates of attention-deficit hyperactivity disorder symptoms in children born at extremely low gestational age. J Dev Behav Pediatr 2017;38(4):249–59.
6. Lampi KM, Lehtonen L, Tran PL, et al. Risk of autism spectrum disorders in low birth weight and small for gestational age infants. J Pediatr 2012;161(5):830–6.
7. Singh GK, Kenney MK, Ghandour RM, et al. Mental health outcomes in US children and adolescents born prematurely or with low birthweight. Depress Res Treat 2013;2013:570743.
8. Richards JL, Chapple-McGruder T, Williams BL, et al. Does neighborhood deprivation modify the effect of preterm birth on children's first grade academic performance? Soc Sci Med 2015;132:122–31.
9. Gross SJ, Mettelman BB, Dye TD, et al. Impact of family structure and stability on academic outcome in preterm children at 10 years of age. J Pediatr 2001;138(2):169–75.
10. SKHysing M, Markestad T, Sommerfelt K. Mental health in children born extremely preterm without severe neurodevelopmental disabilities. Pediatrics 2016;137(4) [pii:e20153002].
11. Johnson S, Hollis C, Kochhar P, et al. Psychiatric disorders in extremely preterm children: longitudinal finding at age 11 years in the EPICure study. J Am Acad Child Adolesc Psychiatry 2010;49(5):453–63.e1.
12. Volpe JJ. The encephalopathy of prematurity–brain injury and impaired brain development inextricably intertwined [review]. Semin Pediatr Neurol 2009;16(4):167–78.
13. Anderson PJ, Treyvaud K, Neil JJ, et al. Associations of newborn brain magnetic resonance imaging with long-term neurodevelopmental impairments in very preterm children. J Pediatr 2017;187:58–65.e1.
14. Feldman R. Sensitive periods in human social development: new insights from research on oxytocin, synchrony, and high-risk parenting [review]. Dev Psychopathol 2015;27(2):369–95.
15. Carter CS. Oxytocin and human evolution. Curr Top Behav Neurosci 2017. https://doi.org/10.1007/7854_2017_18.
16. Cho ES, Kim SJ, Kwon MS, et al. The effects of kangaroo care in the neonatal intensive care unit on the physiological functions of preterm infants, maternal-infant attachment, and maternal stress. J Pediatr Nurs 2016;31(4):430–8.
17. Mendelson T, Cluxton-Keller F, Vullo GC, et al. NICU- based interventions to reduce maternal depressive and anxiety symptoms: a meta-analysis [review]. Pediatrics 2017;139(3) [pii:e20161870].
18. Charpak N, Tessier R, Ruiz JG, et al. Twenty-year follow-up of kangaroo mother care versus traditional care. Pediatrics 2017;139(1) [pii:e20162063].
19. Hoffenkamp HN, Tooten A, Hall RA, et al. The impact of premature childbirth on parental bonding. Evol Psychol 2012;10(3):542–61.
20. Gueron-Sela N, Atzaba-Poria N, Meiri G, et al. The caregiving environment and developmental outcomes of preterm infants: diathesis stress or differential susceptibility effects? Child Dev 2015. https://doi.org/10.1111/cdev.12359.
21. Kirchner L, Jeitler V, Waldhör T, et al. Long hospitalization is the most important risk factor for early weaning from breast milk in premature babies. Acta Paediatr 2009;98(6):981–4.

22. Belfort MB, Anderson PJ, Nowak VA, et al. Breast milk feeding, brain development, and neurocognitive outcomes: a 7-year longitudinal study in infants born at less than 30 weeks' gestation. J Pediatr 2016;177:133–9.e1.
23. Park S, Kim BN, Kim JW, et al. Protective effect of breastfeeding with regard to children's behavioral and cognitive problems. Nutr J 2014;13(1):111.
24. Oddy WH, Kendall GE, Li J, et al. The long-term effects of breastfeeding on child and adolescent mental health: a pregnancy cohort study followed for 14 years. J Pediatr 2010;156(4):568–74.
25. Montirosso R, Del Prete A, Bellù R, et al, Neonatal Adequate Care for Quality of Life (NEO-ACQUA) Study Group. Level of NICU quality of developmental care and neurobehavioral performance in very preterm infants. Pediatrics 2012; 129(5):e1129–37.
26. Cassiano RGM, Gaspardo CM, Faciroli RAD, et al. Temperament and behavior in toddlers born preterm with related clinical problems. Early Hum Dev 2017;112: 1–8.
27. Van den Bergh BRH, van den Heuvel MI, Lahti M, et al. Prenatal developmental origins of behavior and mental health: the influence of maternal stress in pregnancy [review]. Neurosci Biobehav Rev 2017. https://doi.org/10.1016/j.neubiorev.2017.07.003.
28. Yonkers KA, Smith MV, Forray A, et al. Pregnant women with posttraumatic stress disorder and risk of preterm birth. JAMA Psychiatry 2014;71(8):897–904.
29. Andalib S, Emamhadi MR, Yousefzadeh-Chabok S, et al. Maternal SSRI exposure increases the risk of autistic offspring: a meta-analysis and systematic review. Eur Psychiatry 2017;45:161–6.
30. Rai D, Lee BK, Dalman C, et al. Antidepressants during pregnancy and autism in offspring: population based cohort study. BMJ 2017;358:j2811.
31. Maguire DJ, Taylor S, Armstrong K, et al. Long-term outcomes of infants with neonatal abstinence syndrome [review]. Neonatal Netw 2016;35(5):277–86.
32. Melnyk BM, Feinstein NF, Alpert-Gillis L, et al. Reducing premature infants' length of stay and improving parents' mental health outcomes with the Creating Opportunities for Parent Empowerment (COPE) neonatal intensive care unit program: a randomized, controlled trial. Pediatrics 2006;118(5):e1414–27.
33. Treyvaud K, Doyle LW, Lee KJ, et al. Parenting behavior at 2 years predicts school-age performance at 7 years in very preterm children. J Child Psychol Psychiatry 2016;57(7):814–21.
34. Loe IM, Lee ES, Luna B, et al. Behavior problems of 9-16 year old preterm children: biological, sociodemographic, and intellectual contributions. Early Hum Dev 2011;87(4):247–52.
35. Landsem IP, Handegård BH, Ulvund SE, et al. Early intervention influences positively quality of life as reported by prematurely born children at age nine and their parents; a randomized clinical trial. Health Qual Life Outcomes 2015;13:25.
36. Council on Early Childhood, Committee on Psychosocial Aspects of Child and Family Health, Section on Developmental and Behavioral Pediatrics. Addressing early childhood emotional and behavioral problems. Pediatrics 2016;138(6) [pii: e20163023].
37. Weitzman C, Wegner L, Section on Developmental and Behavioral Pediatrics, Committee on Psychosocial Aspects of Child and Family Health, Council on Early Childhood, Society for Developmental and Behavioral Pediatrics, American Academy of Pediatrics. Promoting optimal development:

screening for behavioral and emotional problems. Pediatrics 2015;135(2): 384–95.

38. Davis K. Expenditures for treatment of mental health disorders among children, ages 5-17, 2009–2011: estimates for the U.S. Civilian Noninstitutionalized Population. The Agency for Healthcare Research and Quality. 2014. Available at: https://meps.ahrq.gov/data_files/publications/st440/stat440.shtml. Accessed June 13, 2018.

Burdens Beyond Biology for Sick Newborn Infants and Their Families

John A.F. Zupancic, MD, ScD[a,b,*]

KEYWORDS

- Infant • Newborn • Costs and cost analysis

KEY POINTS

- Outcomes in neonatology have focused mainly on the biological outcomes of the babies under our care, resulting in a "proband" and a "biological" bias in the literature.
- A "slower medicine" in the NICU would recognize the distinction between the remarkable technical capabilities of the modern medical world and how those intersect with our society, and its values, more broadly.
- Considering outcomes such as impact on families, as well as other financial and other stressors, would not require foregoing effective therapy or the improvements in mortality and morbidity it has brought.

The following is a modified transcript of the 2017 Kristine Sandberg Knisely Lectureship, which was delivered at the Children's Hospital of Philadelphia in May 2017. The Lectureship honors the memory of Kristine Sandberg Knisely, MD, a 1949 graduate of the University of Pennsylvania School of Medicine and The Children's Hospital of Philadelphia residency program, who became a neonatologist and Associate Professor of Pediatrics at the same institutions, and made significant contributions in public health initiatives and research involving newborns.

We are rightly proud of what we have accomplished in neonatology. According to traditional benchmarks, outcomes for sick newborn infants have never been better. Horbar and his colleagues[1] examined the outcomes of 408,000 very low birth weight infants at 756 centers in the Vermont Oxford Network, in 2005 and in 2014. They found that, in 2014, almost 100% of neonatal intensive care units (NICUs) reported mortality that was as good as the top 10% of units in 2005. There were similarly large

[a] Department of Neonatology, Beth Israel Deaconess Medical Center, 330 Brookline Avenue, Boston, MA 02215, USA; [b] Division of Newborn Medicine, Harvard Medical School, Boston, 300 Longwood Avenue, Boston, MA, 02115, USA
* Department of Neonatology, Beth Israel Deaconess Medical Center, 330 Brookline Avenue, Rose Building Room 318, Boston, MA 02215.
E-mail address: jzupanci@bidmc.harvard.edu

Clin Perinatol 45 (2018) 557–563
https://doi.org/10.1016/j.clp.2018.05.012
0095-5108/18/© 2018 Elsevier Inc. All rights reserved.

improvements in late-onset infection, necrotizing enterocolitis, severe intraventricular hemorrhage, and severe retinopathy of prematurity. Of course, absolute numbers of infants with these conditions remain high, but we can say unequivocally that, at the unit level, we are all being pulled up by a rising tide, and an infant is less likely to have these conditions now than a decade ago.

We have also long known that that is not the whole story. In part because the biological outcomes at borderline viability were poor, and in part because the cost, not just in financial terms but also human terms, such as time in the NICU, was high, neonatologists started examining outcomes that went beyond neurodevelopmental impairment rates, acute morbidity, and mortality. One of the earliest innovators in this arena was Saroj Saigal, who began to measure functional health outcomes, and to use these to quantify quality of life, using tools originally developed in economics.

Saigal assessed children in a geographically defined cohort of 141 extremely low birthweight (ELBW) adolescent survivors born between 1977 and 1982, and 124 term controls.[2] Instead of just cataloging rates of impairments, she collected measurements of functional health status, which included measures of the traditional sensory, mobility, and cognitive domains, but also emotion, self-care, and pain. Within each of those domains, there were 3 to 5 levels of increasing functional impairment. The domain of emotion, for example, might be anchored on 1, describing someone who is generally happy and free of worry, to 5, describing someone with extreme symptoms requiring high levels of psychiatric intervention. When comparing her ELBW patients with controls, functional health status differed between ELBW adolescents and controls in all domains. The really innovative contribution, though, was in measuring children's preferences for living in the state they were in. This involved assigning a value between 1 (for perfect health) and 0 (for death), using a process that is well-described in decision theory, called a standard gamble. Essentially, this was a subjective rating of how satisfied the children were with their overall health, including all the domains in the health status measure. It is a numerical estimate of quality of life, or conversely of "suffering." As expected, ELBW adolescents reported lower quality of life than the term adolescents, driven by a combination of the various domains. This finding continued into later life, as quality of life decreased steadily over time.[3] Importantly, while baseline rates were lowest among infants with neurosensory impairment (that is, cerebral palsy, blindness, deafness, or microcephaly at 3 years), they were still significantly different in adults without neurosensory impairment. There is thus a quality of life burden here that is not related to our traditional biological measures. What underlies these quality of life decrements?

A clue may lie in the fact that, in that same cohort, even those ex-preterm adults who did not meet the definition for neurosensory impairment had some indicators of underlying medical conditions, such as mental illness, learning disabilities, subtler motor problems such as self-reported clumsiness, or mild visual deficits. In other studies, these would typically not be enough to drive down numerical quality of life indicators to the levels observed. But importantly, the graduates also were less likely to work full-time, had substantially lower income, were more likely to receive social assistance, and were less likely to date or to be married. Whether these outcomes were secondary to biological deficits is not known.

These studies have really just started to tilt our perspective away from its traditional biological bias to a more holistic view of patient outcomes. Importantly, the work also applies to infants born in an era during which care in the NICU was very different. Just as is the case for neurodevelopmental impairment, though, that caveat is balanced by the fact that today's borderline viability is also much more biologically tenuous. The lesson is that measurement of pulmonary function tests, hypertension, even depression rates, in preterm adults will not be enough, that an infant exists as part of a society, and some of her suffering in the long run may be in how she interacts with the world.

So the literature has started at least to address some of the Biological Bias. But there is a second issue, that might be labeled the Proband Bias. Specifically, as neo-natologists, we understandably identify the infant as our patient, and follow her through her NICU course and into childhood and adulthood. But her condition obviously does not just affect her; every day, we see that it also affects families. It was not a foregone conclusion that it was relevant to measure this. The Proband Bias first came to light, for me, in studies of parental consent for resuscitative interventions at borderline viability and for research. In those questionnaire-based assessments, we noted that 77% of parents had anxiety above the median for the scale, and 30% had anxiety above the 90th percentile.[4,5]

Later, Lakshmanan and colleagues[6] surveyed 196 parents of preterm infants following discharge, and up to 24 months of age in a noncontrolled study that used 2 validated scales, the Impact on Family Scale and the Impact on Parent Scale. Lakshmanan and colleagues[6] made 2 important findings. First, 60% of parents of our patients reported financial worry, 50% unexpected costs, and 50% reported time off from work without pay. As seen in prior studies, large numbers also had ongoing medical issues, including prescriptions, technology dependence, and readmissions. Second, some of these, like bills, financial worry, unpaid time from work, and social isolation, had a higher impact on a family stress index, and others, like Early Intervention or Medicaid enrollment, tended to ameliorate that effect. There is thus a path forward to intervention.

Beyond the preschool period, the Victorian Infant Brain Study cohort examined 224 children born in Melbourne in the modern era of 2001 to 2003 and compared family outcomes with term controls at 2, 5, and 7 years.[7] They found that parents of ELBW infants, who were now 7 years of age, were more likely to report moderate to severe anxiety, depressive symptoms, poorer family functioning, and higher parenting stress. All of these persisted after adjusting for neurodevelopmental disability and for social risk (defined as a composite of family structure, education of primary caregiver, occupation and employment status of primary income earner, language spoken at home, and maternal age at birth). So, as for before, although degree of disability is important, it does not explain away all of the burden on the family.

Finally, in adolescence, parents of ELBW children in the Saigal cohort endorsed effects on their own emotional health or on family.[8] More than twice as many showed marital stress, 4% mentioned it as a significant contributing factor to divorce, there were impacts on decisions to have more children, to find employment, and 3 times as many stated that they had major financial worries.

That last point was illustrated less prosaically in the story of Andrew Stinson, as related by his parents.[9] Andrew Stinson was born at 24 and 1/2 weeks weighing 800 g in December 1976. He underwent several months of neonatal intensive care, and died on June 14, 1977, after a very difficult NICU course. His story was one of several that gave rise to the family-integrated care movement and highlighted the importance of autonomy and nonmaleficence. But there was also another message. In the final passage of the article, the Stinsons write, "At the end came a notice from the PHC business office, announcing in passionless figures that the hospital costs alone for Andrew Stinson's treatment came to $104,403.20…The bill reminds us… of the many times we tried to give attending physicians, residents, nurses, and business office clerks a sense of how financially destructive this experience was. Our marriage and family life came under substantial pressure…Hanging over our heads throughout the spring was the thought that …no matter how expensive our daily lives had become, we knew there would be hundreds and hundreds more to pay at the end. When this nightmare began, we had a small savings account, but this spring we saw it dwindle to nothing."

To be sure, the medical costs of neonatal intensive care are very high. Beam and colleagues[10] recently examined 700,000 infants in a paid claims database of 45 million patients, and confirmed that the bill for someone like Andrew in the first 6 months of life, in the current era, might be on the order of $200,000 to $300,000 on average. But those costs are typically not all borne by patients. In a questionnaire-based study of 1089 patients enrolled in 2 randomized trials of neonatal respiratory support (NIPPV and COT), we sought to determine what additional financial burdens families might experience.[11] The most frequently reported types of expenses for families were travel by car, and meals; these amounted to approximately 80 to 100 US dollars per week. These were far exceeded in dollar terms, however, by wage losses by parents and family members, which were some 5 to 10 times larger. In total, the median weekly out-of-pocket expenditure was approximately 424 US dollars. For many of us in the advantaged class, this might seem an expensive but doable option, but consider now that these represent median weekly costs in 2013 US dollars. The median US household income in 2013 was $51,939, or $1000 per week. The median weekly expenses borne by families of infants in the NICU in this study were thus 43% of the median US household income. The top 10% of families had expenses that were actually 30% HIGHER than the median household income. These findings were confirmed in the DOMINO trial, which randomized 363 infants below 1500 g to pasteurized human donor milk or formula when mother's milk was unavailable, and followed them through 18 to 24 months' postmenstrual age, including assessment of caregiver costs.[12] Over a median length of stay of about 10 weeks, caregiver costs were actually slightly higher than in the COT and NIPPV assessments, at almost $1000 per week.

These are potentially ruinous expenditures. In a survey and series of interviews of more than 1000 individuals affected by bankruptcy, Himmelstein and colleagues[13] determined that 62% had a medical cause, and that the majority were homeowners, college educated, and employed. Interestingly, they also specifically noted that "…a second common theme was sounded by parents of premature infants or chronically ill children; many took time from work or incurred large bills for home care."

I've argued that it is essential that we move beyond both a Biological Bias in which we as neonatologists concentrate only on the direct medical consequences of our treatment, and beyond a Proband Bias, in which we see only the patient in front of us, while ignoring the suffering in her family. One of the quirks of neonatology is that we have a Linnaeus-like predilection for description and classification. Almost all of the neonatal outcomes in literature for 2 decades was a listing of rates of bronchopulmonary dysplasia, patent ductus arteriosus, intraventricular hemorrhage, and sensory and neurodevelopmental impairment in various cohorts. This review has itself included a litany of nonbiological consequences of prematurity, stressors that I've argued are painful and unfair for families to bear. But what can we do about it? And must we?

An answer to that question might be found in the events in Rome on March 20, 1986. McDonald's was opening its doors at the Piazza di Spagna, and several thousand protesters were gathered together by Carlos Petrini, leader of the Save Rome committee. The organizers served pasta from large iron pots, there was Italian music playing, and they talked about how food had lost its way. It was the dawn of the Slow Food movement, which sought to preserve heritage plants, animals, and techniques, and to encourage regional food supply systems. Its principles were that food should be

Good (that is healthy, flavorful), Clean (meaning ecologically sound), and Fair (with respect to prices and conditions for both consumers and producers).

Just as Slow Food sought to address the rise of factory systems producing unhealthy and ecologically unsound calories, a Slow Medicine movement was suggested some 15 years ago to address similar problems in the medical world. In that first description, Alberto Dolara[14] wrote, "Such an approach would allow health professionals, and particularly doctors and nurses, to have a sufficiently long time to evaluate the personal, familial and social problems of patients extensively, to reduce anxiety whilst waiting for non-urgent diagnostic and therapeutic procedures, to evaluate new methods and technologies carefully, to prevent premature dismissals from hospital and finally to offer an adequate emotional support to the terminal patients and their families."

These ideas are not really new, but it does seem that we keep forgetting them. In the era of pre-modern medicine, there were relatively few effective therapies, and physicians consequently spent a great deal of time considering connections between patients and environment. With the dawn of effective treatment in the second half of the nineteenth century, the outcome was no longer the experience of the encounter, but the biological outcome itself. It was now possible to make the daily practice of medicine much more algorithmic, and to begin to deliver it at scale.

There were several inevitable results of such efficiency. First, because treatments were now effective in providing what to many of us is most important—return from illness for ourselves and our loved ones—the price of the service increased beyond its cost of production to the maximal cost that could be borne. That process was compounded by the simultaneous rise of insurance, which allowed some but not all patients and families to take advantage of new treatments for catastrophic illness at much higher cost. The pace of change and the new expectation that interventions would be effective meant that many treatments were introduced without being fully evaluated, leading to overdiagnosis, overtreatment, and waste. Finally, perverse incentives were created that ensured that the system concentrated on producing efficient therapies like medications and devices, often leaving time-intensive conditions, like mental illness or developmental delay, as therapeutic orphans, and ignoring the environmental and patient context in which illness occurs. No one gets paid for asking routinely about the patient's family.

I would argue that it is this fast medicine—costly, wasteful, poorly evidenced, algorithmic—that has allowed the Burdens Beyond Biology discussed previously to remain unaddressed. But what would the converse, Slow Medicine, look like in the NICU? Is it possible to undertake Slow Medicine in the very fast world in which we practice?

Let me offer some principles. The first of these principles might be to "Cultivate Curiosity." How many of us really know our patients? Have we asked about jobs, insurance, finances? I can personally say that I know about the outliers, but only infrequently do I have any idea who is taking time unpaid from work. A colleague does an exercise with his trainees in which he asks them to sit with a family and complete a version of the family costs questionnaire used alongside the trials noted earlier. The insights from such an exercise might lead to an understanding that, as clinicians, we need to sensitively make an offer to engage with our patients on these issues.

Second, we need to continue, more intensely, to commit to evidence-based medicine, to "Choose Wisely."[15,16] The costs that patients are exposed to are driven in part by the effectiveness of our therapies. Ineffective or unsafe therapies increase waste, and this is passed along to patients as premiums or as co-insurance. Unnecessarily long lengths of stay or fragmented follow-up recommendations may also directly increase parental out-of-pocket expenditures.

Finally, we as neonatologists have been too quiet during the health care financing debates over the past 2 decades. It is time to "Discard Discretion" and advocate more aggressively for universal pediatric health care coverage and paid parental leave. These will directly affect prenatal care, mental health and behavioral treatment, and school-based interventions for developmental delay, as well as ensuring that parental wage losses are at least partially mitigated. We have a powerful voice as pediatricians, and it should be put to use.

Implementing a Slower Medicine does not mean that we must forego effective therapy or the biological outcomes it has brought, but rather that we must move beyond the Proband and Biological Biases of our care. It requires us to understand the distinction between the remarkable technical capabilities of the modern medical world and how those intersect with our society, and its values, more broadly. It is a call for a more committed and compassionate view of medicine, and for us to lean in and engage outside the NICU to address the nonbiological suffering of the patients and families in front of us.

REFERENCES

1. Horbar JD, Edwards EM, Greenberg LT, et al. Variation in performance of neonatal intensive care units in the United States. JAMA Pediatr 2017;171(3): e164396.
2. Saigal S, Feeny D, Rosenbaum P, et al. Self-perceived health status and health-related quality of life of extremely low-birth-weight infants at adolescence. JAMA 1996;276(6):453–9.
3. Saigal S, Ferro MA, Van Lieshout RJ, et al. Health-related quality of life trajectories of extremely low birth weight survivors into adulthood. J Pediatr 2016;179: 68–73.e1.
4. Zupancic JAF, Kirpalani H, Barrett J, et al. Characterising doctor-parent communication in counselling for impending preterm delivery. Arch Dis Child Fetal Neonatal Ed 2002;87(2):F113–7.
5. Zupancic JA, Gillie P, Streiner DL, et al. Determinants of parental authorization for involvement of newborn infants in clinical trials. Pediatrics 1997;99(1):E6.
6. Lakshmanan A, Agni M, Lieu T, et al. The impact of preterm birth <37 weeks on parents and families: a cross-sectional study in the 2 years after discharge from the neonatal intensive care unit. Health Qual Life Outcomes 2017;15(1):1–13.
7. Treyvaud K, Lee KJ, Doyle LW, et al. Very preterm birth influences parental mental health and family outcomes seven years after birth. J Pediatr 2014;164(3): 515–21.
8. Saigal S, Burrows E, Stoskopf BL, et al. Impact of extreme prematurity on families of adolescent children. J Pediatr 2000;137(5):701–6.
9. Stinson R, Stinson P. On the death of a baby. J Med Ethics 1981;7(1):5–18.
10. Beam A, Fried I, Palmer N, et al. Understanding the cost of prematurity and low birth weight: a nation-wide study from an insurance database of 45 million lives. PAS 2017.
11. Schiffman J, Dukhovny D, Mowitz M, et al. Quantifying the economic burden of neonatal illness on families of preterm infants in the U.S. and Canada. PAS 2015.
12. Trang S, Zupancic JAF, Unger S, et al. Cost-effectiveness of supplemental donor milk versus formula for very low birth weight infants. Pediatrics 2018. https://doi.org/10.1542/peds.2017-0737.
13. Himmelstein DU, Thorne D, Warren E, et al. Medical bankruptcy in the United States, 2007: results of a national study. Am J Med 2009;122(8):741–6.

14. Dolara A. Invitation to "slow medicine". Ital Heart J Suppl 2002;3(1):100–1 [in Italian].
15. Ho T, Zupancic JAF, Pursley DM, et al. Improving value in neonatal intensive care. Clin Perinatol 2017;44(3):617–25.
16. Ho T, Dukhovny D, Zupancic JAF, et al. Choosing wisely in newborn medicine: five opportunities to increase value. Pediatrics 2015;136(2):e482–9.

Public Health Implications of Very Preterm Birth

Wanda D. Barfield, MD, MPH, RADM

KEYWORDS

- Very preterm birth • Public health implications • Disparities • Extreme preterm birth
- Neurodevelopmental outcomes

KEY POINTS

- Although very preterm births (<32 weeks gestation) represent approximately 1.6% of all US live births, they account for 52% of infant deaths, substantial medical complications, neurodevelopmental disability, and associated health care costs.
- Clinicians and health systems should be aware of population-based risks, including disparities, associated with very preterm birth and data available to inform decision-making.
- Public health engagement and collaboration offers opportunities to address social determinants to improve the quality of care and health of reproductive-age women and their newborns.

INTRODUCTION/BACKGROUND
Epidemiology of Very Preterm Birth

Infants born very preterm (<32 weeks gestation) are at increased risk for death, medical complications, and neurodevelopmental sequelae. The World Health Organization defines preterm birth before 37 weeks gestation with subcategories including very preterm birth, and extreme preterm birth (<28 weeks gestation).[1] Worldwide, it is estimated more than 1 in 10 infants were born preterm in 2013, accounting for approximately 15 million premature babies.[2] Among these, 1 million children younger than age 5 die annually because of complications related to preterm birth.[2] In developing countries, the measurement of very preterm birth and extreme preterm birth is more challenging and mortality is extremely high.[3]

In the United States, rates of overall preterm birth (<37 weeks gestation), calculated by last menses, increased from 10.6% in 1990 to a high of 12.8% of all live births in

---

Disclaimer: The findings and conclusions in this article are those of the author and do not necessarily represent the official position of the Centers for Disease Control and Prevention (CDC).

Division of Reproductive Health, National Center for Chronic Disease Prevention and Health Promotion, Centers for Disease Control and Prevention, 4770 Buford Highway, MS F-74, Atlanta, GA 30341, USA
E-mail address: wjb5@cdc.gov

2006, and 12.7% in 2007. These increases were primarily caused by a rise in late pre-term births.[4,5] Based on revised measures to improve the accuracy of gestational age, the National Center for Health Statistics revised this measure of pregnancy length from last menses to obstetric estimate.[6] Subsequently preterm birth rates were adjusted based on obstetric estimate. Based on obstetric estimate, preterm birth was esti-mated at 10.4% in 2007, declining to a rate of 9.6% of all births in 2014.[6,7] This decline in overall preterm birth reflected successful clinical and public health efforts to decrease late preterm birth.[8] However, recent data show new increases in overall pre-term births in 2015, 2016, and early 2017 to be 9.6%, 9.8%, and 9.9%, respectively, caused primarily by increases in late preterm births.[9–11] Nearly 400,000 preterm births occur annually among the nearly 4 million births in the United States.[9]

Preterm births less than 32 weeks gestation represent more than 60,000 births annually, yet the United States has seen little change in these rates over time.[12] In 2015, very preterm birth represented approximately 1.6% of live births but was asso-ciated with 52% of infant deaths in the United States; extreme preterm births repre-sented 0.67% of live births and 45% of infant deaths (**Table 1**).[13] The lack of change in the distribution of very preterm birth may be one reason why infant mortality declines are slow and disparate. In fact, a study by Callaghan and colleagues[12] explained that although infant mortality rates declined from 2007 to 2014, the very pre-term birth weight distribution did not; yet birth weight–specific mortality rates for these tiny infants continued to decline. Causes of very preterm birth are not clear, but most are associated with premature rupture of membranes, preterm labor, and maternal medical conditions (**Box 1**).[14]

Mortality, Morbidity, and Neurodevelopmental Sequelae

Worldwide, survival among infants born very preterm varies by available resources for obstetric and neonatal care, and perceptions of viability.[15–17] Preterm survival at the earliest gestational ages has improved dramatically in developed countries, where the limit of viability has extended to 22 to 23 weeks gestation; yet survival at these gestational ages in developing countries is rare.[15] Improvements in the survival of very preterm infants in developed countries are the result of a variety of factors including improved insurance coverage during pregnancy; advanced obstetric and antenatal care; and improved systems of risk-appropriate care, including resuscitation and stabilization of high-risk newborns.[18–20] In a comparison of developed countries in 2010, the United States ranked second compared with 11 European countries in gestational age–specific survival at the earliest gestations (for infants born between 24 and 27 weeks gestation). However, the United States ranked 26th among 29 coun-tries in the Organisation for Economic Co-operation and Development for overall infant survival.[21]

Table 1					
Percent preterm birth by gestational age categories, United States, 2007, 2010, and 2015					
Year	Total Preterm[a]	34–36 wk	32–33 wk	28–31 wk	≤27 wk
2015	9.62	6.87	1.17	0.91	0.68
2010	9.98	7.15	1.18	0.94	0.71
2007	10.44	7.51	1.22	0.97	0.74

[a] Preterm defined as <37-wk gestation.

Data from Centers for Disease Control and Prevention. User guide to the 2015 period linked birth/infant death public use file. Available at: ftp://ftp.cdc.gov/pub/Health_Statistics/NCHS/Dataset_Documentation/DVS/periodlinked/LinkPE15Guide.pdf. Accessed January 31, 2018.

Box 1
Risks associated with preterm delivery

Maternal demographic characteristics

- Young or advanced maternal age
- Black race
- Low socioeconomic status

Unhealthy lifestyle

- Tobacco use
- Substance abuse
- Low or high prepregnancy body mass index

Pregnancy history

- Short interpregnancy interval
- Previous preterm delivery
- Multiple gestations

Pregnancy complications

- Placental abruption or previa
- Polyhydramnios
- Oligohydramnios

Maternal medical disorders

- Thyroid disease
- Obesity
- Asthma
- Diabetes
- Hypertension

Mental health

- Psychological or social stress
- Depression

Fertility treatments

- Assisted-reproductive technology
- Nonassisted-reproductive technology fertility treatments

Intrauterine infection

- Premature rupture of membranes

Fetal factors

- Fetal anomalies

Adapted from Shapiro-Mendoza CK, Barfield WD, Henderson Z, et al. CDC grand rounds: public health strategies to prevent preterm birth. MMWR Morb Mortal Wkly Rep 2016;65:828; with permission.

Because immature gestational age affects a variety of organ systems, very preterm infants are at risk for longer term medical morbidity and adverse neurodevelopmental outcomes to include motor, neurosensory, cognitive, and behavioral deficits (**Box 2**).[22,23] Adverse medical and neurodevelopmental outcomes are inversely

---

Box 2
Medical complications of preterm birth

Respiratory

Respiratory distress syndrome

Transient tachypnea

Bronchopulmonary dysplasia

Pneumonia

Apnea and bradycardia

Pulmonary interstitial emphysema

Cardiovascular

Patent ductus arteriosus

Gastrointestinal/hepatic

Jaundice

Feeding intolerance

Necrotizing enterocolitis

Immune/infectious

Infection/sepsis

Meningitis

Central nervous system

Retinopathy of prematurity

Intraventricular hemorrhage

Posthemorrhagic hydrocephalus

Periventricular leukomalacia

Cerebral palsy

General

Inability to regulate body heat

Anemia

---

correlated with gestational age. Black infants are more likely to experience preterm birth; for example, infants born to black mothers' experience 2.5 times the rate of very preterm birth compared with white infants.[10] Therefore, black infants, from a population perspective, may be more likely to experience adverse sequelae. Additional sociodemographic, genetic, and environmental risks may further affect the distribution of very and extreme preterm birth and subsequent morbidity and mortality.[22] Risks for preterm delivery may occur within families (eg, female siblings), between pregnancies, and over generations. This may be caused by shared environmental, biologic, and/or genetic factors.[22] Ultimately, prevention of very preterm birth is essential to reducing racial disparities in medical and neurodevelopmental sequelae from birth through adulthood and in subsequent generations.

Very preterm births incur high medical costs. The Institute of Medicine, in its 2007 report on preterm birth, estimated that infant born less than 32 weeks gestation accounted for $11 billion of excess medical costs out of the total $16 billion for all preterm infants.[24] Very preterm infants insured through Medicaid seem to incur higher costs than those covered by commercial insurance and have higher rates of readmission after birth hospitalization, because of higher rates of morbidity.[25] In the United States, nearly 50% of pregnancies are paid for by Medicaid and these proportions vary by state (ranging from 69% in Louisiana to 24% in Hawaii).[26]

PUBLIC HEALTH'S ROLE IN THE PREVENTION OF VERY PRETERM BIRTH

Public health efforts to reduce preterm birth have focused primarily on the prevention of late preterm (between 34 and 36 6/7 weeks gestation) and early term birth (between 37 and 38 6/7 weeks gestation) using public health campaigns and policies aimed at the elimination of early elective deliveries, or nonmedically indicated deliveries before 39 weeks gestation. State, regional, and national collaborations successfully reduced late preterm births through rapid data reporting, changes in clinical practice and recommendations, and policies for reimbursement.[27–32]

Public health efforts to prevent preterm birth at earlier gestations (<34 weeks), however, have not been as robust, likely because of limited understanding of the complex causes of very preterm birth. However, innovative public health efforts can help reduce very preterm birth and associated morbidity and mortality in several ways.[33,34]

Improved Data Systems

Timely population-based surveillance systems are important to monitor trends in preterm births, associated risk factors, and outcomes. The National Center for Health Statistics now reports selective preliminary national vital statistics data, including information on gestational age, on a quarterly timeline.[11] This has been important in monitoring national trends in preterm birth more rapidly. The Pregnancy Risk Assessment Monitoring System collects state-level data on maternal experiences before, during, and shortly after pregnancy. The Pregnancy Risk Assessment Monitoring System, which is linked with vital records, can also be linked with other administrative and program data (eg, Medicaid, hospital discharge, Healthy Start, and Early Intervention registries) to monitor interventions and outcomes.[35,36] Using multiple linked data systems can inform and evaluate prevention efforts at the local, state, and national level. Statistical techniques, such as multilevel modeling, are used to assess birth outcomes caused by policies or practices.

Longitudinally Linked Data

Data systems linked over the lifespan of the mother and child can help to identify risks associated with very preterm birth and short- and long-term outcomes, assess the effectiveness of interventions, and inform strategies for improvement. Much of the research that identified the short- and long-term complications and costs associated with late preterm birth came from longitudinally linked data systems in California, Michigan, and Massachusetts, which linked vital records, maternal and infant hospital data, and program data longitudinally.[37–41] These innovative data systems help to identify the risk for infant and maternal mortality and morbidity, readmission, and developmental disabilities, and access to care.

Improving Preconception Health

Behavioral factors that are usually initiated before pregnancy, such as tobacco, alcohol, and illicit drug use, are associated with preterm birth.[22] Much chronic disease also plays a role in the risk of preterm birth, with such conditions as hypertension, diabetes, and obesity affecting maternal and fetal well-being. Shifts in the average maternal age at delivery in the United States has also increased the risk of preterm birth because mothers are more likely to be older and more likely to have a chronic medical condition.[42,43] Regardless of age, improving the health of women before pregnancy and reducing disparities in preterm birth requires a robust system of surveillance to assess preconception behaviors and access to insurance, primary care, and preventive services.[44]

Preventing Teenage and Unintended Pregnancies and Improving Pregnancy Spacing

Forty-five percent of pregnancies in the United States are unintended and nearly three-quarters of teenage births are unintended.[45] Unintended pregnancies and short interpregnancy interval (a second birth within 18 months) are associated with increased preterm birth.[46] Teenage pregnancies are at 17% higher risk for preterm birth, and teenage mothers are more likely to have a short interpregnancy interval resulting in further preterm birth risks.[47,48] Although the US birth rate for teenagers aged 15 to 19 has declined 51% since 2007 (down to 20.3 live births per 1000 women in 2016[10]), efforts to reduce teenage pregnancy need to continue, especially in African American and Hispanic communities where teenage and preterm birth rates are highest.[49] Access to a full range of effective contraceptive methods, including long-acting reversible contraception, is important to prevent unintended pregnancies, improve birth spacing, and reduce preterm birth.[50,51] Perinatal providers can help to reduce barriers to postpartum contraception access, even among mothers whose infants are in the neonatal intensive care unit, by understanding issues of availability, safety, and cost.[52,53]

Reducing the Risk of Higher-Order Multiples in Assisted-Reproductive Therapies

Use of fertility therapy may result in births to twins, triplets, or higher-order multiple births, which generally deliver at an earlier gestational age than singleton birth births.[22] In 2015, more than one out of every two twins and more than 9 out of every 10 triplets were born preterm or low birth weight.[9] From 2014 to 2015, the twin birth rate declined from an all-time high of 33.9 to 33.5 per 1000 live births. In addition, the triplet and higher-order multiple birth rate declined 9% from 2014 to 2015 to 103.6 per 100,000 live births. The triplet and higher-order birth rate has declined more than 40% from 1998 to 2015.[9,54] In 2014, assisted-reproductive technology in the United States contributed to 18.3% of all multiple births, 4.7% of all preterm births, and 5.0% of all very preterm births.[55] However, states with high use of assisted-reproductive therapy use had higher preterm birth rates. For example, in Massachusetts, 13.4% of all preterm and 14.7% of all very preterm births were associated with assisted-reproductive therapy use.[55] Approaches, such as elective single embryo transfer during assisted-reproductive therapy, can reduce multiple births and the risk for prematurity.[56] Understanding the contributions of other fertility therapies to multiple births is more elusive. In a study by Kulkarni and colleagues[57] in 2011, a total of 36% of twin births and 77% of triplet and higher-order births in the United States resulted from conception assisted by nonassisted-reproductive therapy fertility treatments. Payment strategies, such as broader insurance coverage for fertility therapies, may also reduce the risk of higher-order multiples and preterm birth by reducing costs related to infertility treatment, which may in turn encourage use of treatments that result in singleton births.[58]

Improved Quality and Systems of Care

In 2016, slightly more than three out of four US women (77.2%) began prenatal care in the first trimester.[10] However, only 66.6% of black women and 63.0% of American Indian or Alaska Native women began first trimester prenatal care compared with 82.3% of white women and 80.6% of Asian women. Less than 1 in 10 (6.2%) US women had late (beginning in the third trimester) or no prenatal care.[10] Innovative group prenatal care models have held promise to reduce the risk of preterm birth. However, a recent meta-analysis showed that pregnant women who participated in group prenatal care had similar rates of preterm birth compared with traditional prenatal care models.[59] More research is needed on the content and quality of prenatal care to better understand how it might reduce the risk for early deliveries.

Access to risk-appropriate care is a proven approach to reducing death and neurodevelopmental morbidity associated with very preterm births.[60] In a meta-analysis of more than 30 years of data, Lasswell and colleagues[19] found that very preterm newborns delivered outside of level III or higher facilities were at a 60% increased odds of death. One major step toward lowering death and disability to very preterm infants is to ensure an organized system of care that ensures facilities have appropriate staffing, equipment, and experience that match patient needs. Pregnant women and newborns need to receive the right care at the right place, and the right time.[61,62] Unfortunately, many very preterm infants are not delivered at appropriate facilities to meet their complex medical needs. Additionally, recent studies have demonstrated considerable variation in the quality of care among different racial/ethnic groups based on where they reside.[63,64]

Women at risk for preterm delivery need to be identified early and offered access to effective treatments to prevent preterm birth.[43,65] For example, women who have had a spontaneous preterm delivery, are at a two-fold risk for subsequent preterm deliveries. Among women with a history of spontaneous preterm birth and a singleton pregnancy, the use of 17α-hydroxyprogesterone caproate can reduce the risk of preterm birth by approximately 30%.[66] Public health collaboration with clinical providers and insurers can help identify pregnant women at risk and reduce barriers to access and use. For example, in Ohio, the state quality improvement collaborative focused on low-income women at high risk for preterm birth, with either a prior preterm birth or shortened cervix during pregnancy and provided them access to progesterone through Medicaid. This "progesterone project" aims to reduce rates of preterm birth less than 32 weeks gestation by June 2018.[67] To date, rates of progesterone administration increased from 2013 to 2016 across all races and ethnicities in Medicaid, with the highest rate being achieved in high-risk black women in 2016 (http://www.medicaid.ohio.gov/Portals/0/Resources/Reports/PWIC/PWIC-Report-2017.pdf?ver=2017-12-29-112608-887).

Although the American College of Obstetricians and Gynecologists recommends that mothers at risk for preterm delivery should be offered antenatal corticosteroids, its use is variable. Profit and colleagues[64] found that white infants generally received higher scores on the receipt of antenatal steroids within and between facilities, although these process measures should not have varied by race/ethnicity. Antenatal corticosteroids are highly effective in increasing lung maturity and has been proven to reduce respiratory distress syndrome by 66%, necrotizing enterocolitis by 46%, intraventricular hemorrhage by 54%, and death by 69% with a single course of therapy compared with control subjects.[66] Further research on more effective provider acceptance and use is needed to improve implementation of this effective intervention more equitably to diverse populations.

Perinatal quality collaboratives, through states and networks, can help to identify mothers at risk for preterm birth because of medical conditions, and/or risk for repeat preterm deliveries.[67] Approaches include[68]

- Identifying evidence-based clinical practices and processes to improve pregnancy outcomes.
- Improving maternal and fetal well-being and outcomes in the presence of maternal diseases (eg, hypertension and diabetes).
- Identifying effective interventions that may reduce the risk of very preterm birth and bring these interventions to scale (eg, use of 17-hydroxyprogesterone acetate and antenatal corticosteroids in preterm pregnancies (including late stage of labor and imminent delivery) and the use of low-dose aspirin in the prevention of preeclampsia and subsequent preterm birth).
- Improving early pregnancy assessment to improve the precision of determining gestational age to improve measurement of population-based outcomes.

Improving Social Determinants of Health

A study of preterm infants in the United Kingdom found that preterm infants living in a family with low socioeconomic status tended to score lower on cognitive assessments at 3, 5, and 7 years of age compared with term infants. But the researchers also found that the effects of low socioeconomic status and preterm birth were additive, with little or no evidence of effect modification. Additionally, they found that the magnitude of the estimate effect of poverty was so strong that term children who were living in families with poverty had lower cognitive scores than preterm children who were not living in poor families.[68]

Social determinants of health, the factors that affect health based on where an individual lives, learns, works, and ages, can influence preterm birth rates and preterm birth outcomes, by influencing health well before pregnancy.[69] This life-course perspective on birth outcomes implies that prevention of adverse pregnancy outcomes, including very and extreme preterm birth, must happen before conception and prenatal care. Although the mechanism is not completely clear, it is thought that adverse social determinants may contribute to acute and chronic stress for pregnant women possibly affecting neuroendocrine and immune pathways, leading to indolent inflammation or susceptibility to infection and an increased risk for preterm birth.[22,70]

Adverse social conditions can influence health through such factors as neighborhood poverty and hypersegregation; high crime rates; lack of goods, services, and recreational activities; limited access to quality health care; and limited opportunities for education, employment, living wages, and affordable housing.[71] Poverty is associated with chronic conditions, such as diabetes, hypertension, and obesity, and such behaviors as tobacco and illicit drug use, all of which contribute to poor pregnancy outcomes.[22] Addressing broader social issues, such as racism, discrimination, housing, employment, and education, to improve the health of mothers, particularly in African American and other communities at high risk, could possibly reduce preterm birth and associated disparities.[72] Lastly, clinical and public health interventions may operate in a social context such that implementation may be ineffective or insufficient (eg, poor access to care or lower quality of care), resulting in missed opportunities to prevent early delivery.[63,64,70]

In a commentary, Lorch[73] noted the challenges of combining health equity goals with the measurement of health care quality in perinatal care. By monitoring indicators stratified by indicators of social determinants (race/ethnicity, insurance, urban/rural), quality improvement collaboratives have the potential to improve health care quality, address health equity, and reduce disparities with thoughtful intent in the appropriate cultural context.

Enriching Postnatal Infant Development

Health care providers should be aware of the variety of public health resources available to families of preterm infants to support postnatal infant development, particularly for low-income families. Programs include the following:

- Breastfeeding support
- Special Supplemental Nutrition Program for Women, Infants, and Children (WIC)
- Early intervention services
- Healthy Start
- Home visitation programs
- Head Start
- Literacy initiatives (eg, Reach out and read)

SUMMARY

Preterm birth is a global public health priority. Developed countries have seen dramatic improvements in the survival of very preterm infants with declines in infant mortality. Yet, in the United States, total preterm birth rates are rising while the proportion of very preterm infants born in the United States has not changed substantially over the last several decades. To continue to reduce infant mortality and associated medical and neurodevelopmental disability, the complex issue of early preterm birth and associated racial/ethnic disparities need to be addressed. Public health approaches in collaboration with diverse stakeholders can improve population-based data and identify effective interventions with impact to improve the health of women before, during, and after pregnancy and reduce death and disability among newborns.

Several national organizations are leading initiatives to reduce preterm birth:

- March of Dimes (MOD) (www.marchofdimes.org). MOD has established five multidisciplinary centers to research the complex causes of preterm birth. In 2017, MOD launched the Prematurity Collaborative, a national effort to reduce preterm birth through improving health equity. The Collaborative has more than 200 members with focused strategies on equity, research, clinical and public health interventions, policy, and communications. Lastly, the MOD's "Roadmap to 2020 and 2030 Goals" identified 16 states with preterm birth rates greater than 11.5% with substantial racial/ethnic disparities and approximately 100,000 births per year to reduce modifiable risk factors by bundling various interventions through the Healthy Babies are Worth the Wait Community Program.
- Association of State and Territorial Health Officials Healthy Babies Initiative (www.astho.org):
- Collaboration on Innovation and Improvement Network (www.mchb.org):
- National Network of Perinatal Quality Collaboratives (https://www.cdc.gov/reproductivehealth/maternalinfanthealth/pqc.htm)

REFERENCES

1. WHO: preterm birth fact sheet. Available at: www.who.int/mediacentre/factsheet/fs363/en/. Accessed January 15, 2018.

2. Liu L, Oza S, Hogan D, et al. Global, regional, and national causes of under-5 mortality in 2000-15: an updated systematic analysis with implications for the sustainable development goals. Lancet 2016;388(10063):3027–35.

3. Blencowe H, Cousens S, Chou D, et al. Born too soon: the global epidemiology of 15 million preterm births. Reprod Health 2013;10(suppl1):S2.

4. Hamilton BE, Martin JA, Ventura SJ, et al. Births: final data for 2007. Natl Vital Stat Rep 2010;58:24. Available at: http://www.cdc.gov/nchs/data/nvsr/nvsr58/nvsr58_24.pdf.

5. Davidoff MJ, Dias T, Damus K, et al. Changes in the gestational age distribution among U.S. singleton births: impact on rates of late preterm birth, 1992 to 2002. Semin Perinatol 2006;30:8.

6. Martin JA, Osterman MJ, Kirmeyer SE, et al. Measuring gestational age in vital statistics data: transitioning to the obstetric estimate. Natl Vital Stat Rep 2015; 64:1.

7. Hamilton BE, Martin JA, Osterman MJK, et al. Births: final data for 2014. Natl Vital Stat Rep 2015;64(12):1–64.

8. Harai AH, Sappenfield WM, Ghandour RM, et al. The Collaborative Improvement and Innovation Network (CoIIN) to reduce infant mortality: an outcome evaluation from the US South, 2011 to 2014. Am J Public Health 2018;108(6): 815–21.

9. Martin JA, Hamilton BE, Osterman MJK, et al. Births: final data for 2015. Natl Vital Stat Rep 2017;66(1):1–70.

10. Martin JA, Hamilton BE, Osterman MJK, et al. Births: final data for 2016. Natl Vital Stat Rep 2018;67(1):1–55.

11. National Center for Health Statistics. National Vital Statistics System, Vital Statistics Rapid Release, Quarterly Provisional Estimates. Available at: www.cdc.gov/nchs/nvss/vsrr/natality-dashboard.htm#. Accessed January 15, 2018.

12. Callaghan WM, MacDorman MF, Shapiro-Mendoza CK, et al. Explaining the recent decrease in US infant mortality rate, 2007-2013. Am J Obstet Gynecol 2017;216:73.e1–8.

13. Centers for Disease Control and Prevention. User guide to the 2015 period linked birth/infant death public use file. Available at: ftp://ftp.cdc.gov/pub/Health_Statistics/NCHS/Dataset_Documentation/DVS/periodlinked/LinkPE15Guide.pdf. Accessed January 31, 2018.

14. Goldenberg RL, Culhane JF, Iams JD, et al. Epidemiology and causes of preterm birth. Lancet 2008;371:75.

15. Schoen CN, Tabbah S, Iams JD, et al. Why the United States preterm birth rate is declining. Am J Obstet Gynecol 2015;213:175–80.

16. Raju TN, Mercer BM, Burchfield DJ, et al. Periviable birth: executive summary of a joint workshop by the Eunice Kennedy Shriver National Institute of Child Health and Human Development, Society for Maternal-Fetal Medicine, American Academy of Pediatrics, and American College of Obstetricians and Gynecologists. Obstet Gynecol 2014;123(5):1083–96.

17. Backes CH, Rivera BK, Haque U, et al. A proactive approach to neonates born at 23 weeks of gestation. Obstet Gynecol 2015;126:930–46.

18. Stoll BJ, Hansen NI, Bell EF, et al. Trends in care practices, morbidity, and mortality of extremely preterm neonates. 1993-2012. JAMA 2013;314:1039–51.

19. Lasswell SM, Barfield WD, Rochat RW, et al. Perinatal regionalization for very low-birth-weight and very preterm infants: a meta-analysis. JAMA 2010;304: 992–1000.

20. Engle WA, American Academy of Pediatrics Committee on Fetus and Newborn. Surfactant replacement therapy for respiratory distress in the preterm and term neonate. Pediatrics 2008;121:419.
21. MacDorman MF, Mathews TJ, Mohangoo AD, et al. International comparisons of infant mortality and related factors: United States and Europe, 2010. Natl Vital Stat Rep 2014;63(5):1–6.
22. Behrman RE, Butler AS, Institute of Medicine (US) Committee on Understanding Premature Birth and Assuring Healthy Outcomes. Preterm birth: causes, consequences, and prevention. Washington, DC: National Academies Press (US); 2007.
23. Rogers EE, Hintz SR. Early neurodevelopmental outcomes of extremely preterm infants. Semin Perinatol 2016;40:497–509.
24. Institute of Medicine (US) Committee on Understanding Premature Birth and Assuring Healthy Outcomes, Behrman RE, Butler AS, editors. Preterm birth: causes, consequences, and prevention. Washington, DC: National Academies Press (US); 2007. p. 12. Societal Costs of Preterm Birth. Available at: https://www.ncbi.nlm.nih.gov/books/NBK11358/.
25. Barradas DT, Wasserman MP, Daniel-Robinson L, et al. Hospital utilization and costs among preterm infants by payer: nationwide inpatient sample, 2009. Matern Child Health J 2016;20(4):808–18.
26. Markus AR, Andres E, West KD, et al. Medicaid covered births, 2008 through 2010, in the context of the implementation of health reform. Womens Health Issues 2013;23(5):e273–80.
27. March of Dimes. Healthy babies are worth the wait. Available at: https://www.marchofdimes.org/professionals/healthy-babies-are-worth-the-wait.aspx. Accessed January 15, 2018.
28. American College of Obstetricians and Gynecologists. ACOG committee opinion no. 560: medically indicated late-preterm and early-term deliveries. Obstet Gynecol 2013;121(4):908. Reaffirmed July 2017.
29. American College of Obstetricians and Gynecologists. ACOG committee opinion no. 561: nonmedically indicated early-term deliveries. Obstet Gynecol 2013;121:911. Reaffirmed July 2017.
30. Association of State and Territorial Health Officials. States Accepting the Healthy Babies President's Challenge. Available at: http://www.astho.org/Programs/Access/Maternal-and-Child-Health/ASTHO-March-of-Dimes-Partnership/. Accessed January 31, 2018.
31. Health Services Resources Administration, Maternal Child Health Bureau. Collaborative Improvement and Innovation Networks. Available at: https://mchb.hrsa.gov/maternal-child-health-initiatives/collaborative-improvement-innovation-networks-coiins. Accessed January 15, 2018.
32. National Conference of State Legislators. Early elective deliveries. Available at: http://www.ncsl.org/research/health/early-elective-deliveries-postcard.aspx. Accessed January 15, 2018.
33. Howse JL, Katz M. Conquering prematurity. Pediatrics 2013;131(1):1–2.
34. Shapiro-Mendoza CK, Barfield WD, Henderson Z, et al. CDC grand rounds: public health strategies to prevent preterm birth. MMWR Morb Mortal Wkly Rep 2016;65(32):826–30.
35. Centers for Disease Control and Prevention. Pregnancy Risk Assessment Monitoring System (PRAMS). Available at: www.cdc.gov/prams. Accessed January 31, 2018.
36. Kotelchuck M. Pregnancy Risk Assessment Monitoring System (PRAMS): possible new roles for a national MCH data system. Public Health Rep 2006;121(1):6–10.

37. Gould JB. The role of regional collaboratives: the California Perinatal Quality Care Collaborative model. Clin Perinatol 2010;37:71–86.
38. Kotelchuck M, Hoang L, Stern JE, et al. The MOSART database: linking the SART CORS clinical database to the population-based Massachusetts PELL reproductive public health data system. Matern Child Health J 2014;18(9):2167–78.
39. Shapiro-Mendoza C, Kotelchuck M, Barfield W, et al. Enrollment in early intervention programs among infants born late preterm, early term, and term. Pediatrics 2013;131(1):e61–9.
40. Underwood MA, Danielsen B, Gilbert WM. Cost, causes and rates of rehospitalization of preterm infants. J Perinatol 2007;27:614.
41. Hafstrom M, Kallen K, Serenius F, et al. Cerebral palsy in extremely preterm infants. Pediatrics 2018;141(1):e20171433.
42. Ferre C, Callaghan W, Olson C, et al. Effects of maternal age and age-specific preterm birth on overall preterm birth rates—United States, 2007 and 2014. MMWR Morb Mortal Wkly Rep 2016;65(43):1181–4.
43. Committee on Practice Bulletins—Obstetrics, The American College of Obstetricians and Gynecologists. Practice bulletin no. 130: prediction and prevention of preterm birth. Obstet Gynecol 2012;120:964–73.
44. Robbins C, Boulet SL, Morgan I, et al. Disparities in preconception health indicators: behavioral risk factor surveillance system, 2013-2015, and pregnancy risk assessment monitoring system, 2013-2014. MMWR Surveill Summ 2018;67(1):1–16.
45. Finer LB, Zolner MR. Declines in unintended pregnancy in the United States, 2008-2011. N Engl J Med 2016;374:843–52.
46. Orr ST, Miller CA, James SA, et al. Unintended pregnancy and preterm birth. Paediatr Perinat Epidemiol 2000;14(4):309–13.
47. Nerlander LM, Callaghan WM, Smith RA, et al. Short interpregnancy interval associated with preterm birth in US adolescents. Matern Child Health J 2015;19(4):850–8.
48. Gavin L, Warner L, O'Neil ME, et al. Vital signs: repeat births among teens—United States, 2007–2010. MMWR Morb Mortal Wkly Rep 2013;62(13):249–55.
49. Romero L, Pazol K, Warner L, et al. Reduced disparities in birth rates among teens aged 15–19 years—United States, 2006–2007 and 2013–2014. MMWR Morb Mortal Wkly Rep 2016;65:409–14.
50. Gavin L, Moskosky S, Carter M, et al. Providing quality family planning services: recommendations of CDC and the U.S. Office of Population Affairs. MMWR Recomm Rep 2014;63(Rr-04):1–54.
51. Zuckerman B, Nathan S, Mate K. Preventing unintended pregnancy: a pediatric opportunity. Pediatrics 2014;133(2):181–3.
52. American Academy of Pediatrics, Committee on Adolescence. Contraception for adolescents. Pediatrics 2014;134(4):e1244–56.
53. American College of Obstetricians and Gynecologists. Practice bulletin no. 186. Long-acting reversible contraception: implants and intrauterine devices. Obstet Gynecol 2017;187(30):e251–69.
54. Martin JA, Osterman MJK, Thoma ME. Declines in triplet and higher-order multiple births in the United States, 1998–2014. Hyattsville (MD): National Center for Health Statistics; 2016. NCHS data brief, no 243.
55. Sunderam S, Kissin DM, Crawford SB, et al. Assisted reproductive technology surveillance—United States, 2014. MMWR Surveill Summ 2017;66(No. SS-6):1–24.
56. Luke B, Brown MB, Wantman E, et al. Application of a validated prediction model for in vitro fertilization: comparison of live birth rates and multiple birth rates with 1

embryo transferred over 2 cycles vs 2 embryos in 1 cycle. Am J Obstet Gynecol 2015;212:676.e1-e7.

57. Kulkarni AD, Jamieson DJ, Jones HW, et al. Fertility treatments and multiple births in the United States. N Engl J Med 2013;369:2218–25.
58. Crawford S, Boulet S, Mneimneh A, et al. Costs of achieving live birth from assisted reproductive technology: a comparison of sequential single and double embryo transfer approaches. Fertil Steril 2016;105:444–50.
59. Carter EB, Temming LA, Akin J, et al. Group prenatal care compared with traditional prenatal care: a systematic review and meta-analysis. Obstet Gynecol 2016;128:551–61.
60. March of Dimes Foundation. Toward improving the outcome of pregnancy III: enhancing perinatal health through quality, safety and performance initiatives. White Plains (NY): March of Dimes; 2010.
61. American Academy of Pediatrics. Policy statement—levels of neonatal care. Pediatrics 2012;130:587–97.
62. American College of Obstetricians and Gynecologists and the Society for Maternal-Fetal Medicine, Menard MK, et al. Obstetric care consensus No. 2: levels of maternal care. Obstet Gynecol 2015;125:502–15.
63. Howell EA, Janevic T, Hebert PL, et al. Differences in morbidity and mortality rates in black, white, and Hispanic very preterm infants among New York City hospitals. JAMA Pediatr 2018;172:269–77.
64. Profit J, Gould JB, Bennett M, et al. Comprehensive assessment of racial/ethnic disparity in NICU quality of care delivery. Pediatrics 2017;140(3):e20170918.
65. American College of Obstetricians and Gynecologists, Committee on Practice Bulletins—Obstetrics. ACOG practice bulletin no. 127: management of preterm labor. Obstet Gynecol 2012;119:1308–17.
66. Brownfoot FC, Gagliardi DI, Bain F, et al. Different corticosteroids and regimens for accelerating fetal lung maturation for women at risk of preterm birth. Cochrane Database Syst Rev 2013;(8):CD006764.
67. Centers for Disease Control and Prevention. Perinatal Quality Improvement Collaboratives. Available at: https://www.cdc.gov/reproductivehealth/maternalinfanthealth/pqc.htm. Accessed April 29, 2018.
68. Beauregard JL, Drews-Botsch C, Sales JM, et al. Preterm birth, poverty, and cognitive development. Pediatrics 2018;141(1):e20170509.
69. Lu MC, Halfon N. Racial and ethnic disparities in birth outcomes: a life-course perspective. Matern Child Health J 2003;7(1):13–30.
70. Lorch SA, Enlow E. The role of social determinants in explaining racial/ethnic disparities in perinatal outcomes. Pediatr Res 2016;79(1–2):141–7.
71. Institute of Medicine (US) Committee on understanding and eliminating racial and ethnic disparities in health care. In: Smedley BD, Stith AY, Nelson AR, editors. Unequal treatment: confronting racial and ethnic disparities in healthcare. Washington, DC: National Academies Press(US); 2003.
72. Rankin KM, David RJ, Collins JW. African American women's exposure to interpersonal racial discrimination in public settings and preterm birth: the effect of coping behaviors. Ethn Dis 2011;21(3):370–6.
73. Lorch SA. Health equity and quality of care assessment: a continuing challenge. Pediatrics 2017;140(3):e20172213.

Prevention of Prematurity
Advances and Opportunities

Balaji Govindaswami, MBBS, MPH*, Priya Jegatheesan, MD,
Matthew Nudelman, MD, Sudha Rani Narasimhan, MD, IBCLC

KEYWORDS

- Preterm birth prevention • Preterm prevention clinic • Progesterone • Cerclage
- Aspirin • Clindamycin • Clotrimazole • Nifedipine

KEY POINTS

- Preterm birth (PTB) rate varies widely with significant racial and ethnic disparities. Causal mechanisms are ill understood, but phenotype and genotype provide insight into pathways for preventing PTB.
- Varied response to medical interventions is explicable by underlying pharmacogenomics. Prevention should focus on minimizing iatrogenic PTB and risk reduction, especially those with prior PTB.
- Current PTB prevention includes reduction of non-medically indicated delivery less than 39 weeks, smoking cessation, implementation of preterm prevention clinic and appropriate use of cerclage and medications (progesterone, antimicrobials, and nifedipine). Aspirin and oral magnesium are currently under study.
- Placental health requires optimal management of diseases in pregnancy, smoking cessation, omega 3 supplements if smoking continues during pregnancy, anti-platelet agents, and eliminating non-medically indicated uterine manipulation.
- Future preventive approaches should focus on better understanding of sociodemography, nutrition, dysbiosis, lifestyles, phenotype, risk factors, and underlying individual genetic, pharmacogenomics, and epigenetic variation.

INTRODUCTION

Preterm birth (PTB) occurs with a prevalence ranging from less than 5% to greater than 15% worldwide. The widespread variability is well emphasized in the United Nations/World Health Organization (WHO) report entitled "Born Too Soon."[1] All countries with PTB rates greater than 15% are in sub-Saharan Africa,[2] and PTB rates in African Americans have traditionally been significantly greater than for other ethnic and racial groups. In the United States, the rate increased for 14 consecutive years followed by a

Division of Neonatology, Pediatrics, Santa Clara Valley Medical Center: Hospital and Clinics, 751 South Bascom Avenue, San Jose, CA 95128, USA
* Corresponding author.
E-mail address: Balaji.Govindaswami@hhs.sccgov.org

Clin Perinatol 45 (2018) 579–595
https://doi.org/10.1016/j.clp.2018.05.013
0095-5108/18/© 2018 Elsevier Inc. All rights reserved.
perinatology.theclinics.com

decline for 7 consecutive years. Unfortunately, now US PTB rates have been increasing for 2 consecutive years to 9.84% in 2016.[3]

PREMATURITY PREVENTION AND INSIGHTS INTO CAUSE

Prevention of PTB has been attempted for several decades and in several settings with mixed success,[4–8] most likely related to the poorly understood heterogeneity of disease. Studies in the late 1990s showed some promise of interventions to prevent PTB with the publication of the injectable[9] and vaginal[10] progesterone trials. A population-based, multiethnic, cross-sectional study in 8 countries[11] over a 12-month period examined 60,058 births. Prevalence of PTB ranged from 8.2% in Muscat, Oman and Oxford, England to 16.6% in Seattle, Washington. Twelve PTB clusters were identified using phenotypes that included signs of presentation at hospital admission and a predefined conceptual framework. The distribution of clinical phenotypes in PTB across these multiethnic populations suggests that in 22% of these births, parturition started spontaneously and was unassociated with any of the phenotypes considered. A current genome-wide association study of 43,568 women with greater than 97% European ancestry demonstrates putative genetic and mechanistic insights into prematurity.[12] Six maternal genomic loci identified and replicated were robustly associated with gestational duration and contain genes whose established functions are consistent with a role in the timing of birth. Three of these loci are also associated with PTB with genome-wide significance. Furthermore, it is known that some of the variation in response to medications used in PTB prevention and treatment may be attributable to pharmacogenomic effects. Currently, greater than 50 genes are implicated in genomic biomarkers most commonly pertaining to polymorphisms in cytochrome p450 (CYP) enzyme metabolism. Polymorphisms in CYP enzymes are relatively common. For example, CYP2D6 is estimated to metabolize ~25% of drugs (including fluoxetine, metoprolol, codeine), and greater than 70 alleles have been identified in this highly polymorphic gene. As a result, CYP2D6 activity ranges widely even within populations, and up to 8% of European Americans may be identified as poor metabolizers.[13] Specific to 17-hydroxy progesterone caproate (17-OHPC) metabolism, Caritis and colleagues[14] examined plasma concentrations in 315 women at 25 to 28 weeks' gestation and grouped their 17-OHPC levels into quartiles. Women in the lowest quartile were significantly more likely to have recurrent PTB than those in the upper 3 quartiles (46% vs 29%; $P = .03$). Lowest PTB rates were seen when median 17-OHPC concentrations exceeded 6.4 ng/mL. Women in the second, third, or fourth quartiles had a 50% reduction in delivering preterm (hazard ratio: 0.48; 95% confidence interval [CI] 0.31–0.75; $P = .001$). Two specific pharmacogenomics studies have been performed to study the relationship between genotype and the response to 17-OHPC. Similarly, Nifedipine concentrations linked to CYP3A5 genotype are correlated with high clearance of Nifedipine and thus lower levels.[15] Women with high expression of CYP3A5 had less improvement in contraction frequency at several time points, including after the loading dose, at the steady state, and in the first hour after study dose.[16] No pharmacogenomics data are currently available for indomethacin or magnesium sulfate, although it is known that indomethacin is metabolized in the liver by polymorphic CYP2C9 and CYP2C19. Maternal and fetal genetic variance in several single nucleotide polymorphisms including CYP3A5 and CYP3A7*1E are associated with variation in neonatal respiratory outcomes, including need for surfactant and ventilator support. Thus, it has been surmised that genetic variation in betamethasone genes can be associated with severity of respiratory morbidity.[17] In conclusion, these data suggest that genotype may influence response to commonly used therapies in PTB prevention and treatment.

CURRENT OPPORTUNITIES FOR PRETERM BIRTH PREVENTION

Several strategies exist to target PTB risk reduction and prevention. Included among these are nonmedically indicated PTB that might be an early target for studying practice-based variation. **Box 1** provides strategies for PTB prevention, which serves as an outline for this article.

PRECONCEPTION STRATEGIES
Optimal Maternal Body Composition

It is known that extremes of body mass index (BMI, kg/m^2) increase the risk of PTB. Data from Poland[18] and 21 states in the United States[19] show PTB rates are increased with prepregnancy BMI less than 19.8 and in women with poor weight gain during pregnancy. These findings have been reiterated in more recent data from California, including almost a million live births.[20] Furthermore, this study also shows BMI greater

---

Box 1
Preterm birth prevention opportunity

Preconceptional and public health strategies

1. Optimal maternal body composition

2. Optimal IPI and exclusive breastfeeding

3. Tobacco avoidance and cessation, omega-3 supplements

4. Periodontal disease prevention

5. Dedicated PPC

6. Public health strategies

Minimize iatrogenic contributions to PTB

1. Judicious use of fertility treatment

2. Eliminate elective induction less than 39 weeks

3. Lower CS rates

Medical

1. Antiplatelet agents

2. Vaginal and injectable progesterone

3. Magnesium

4. Antimicrobials

5. Tocolytics

6. Ethanol, oxytocin receptor antagonists, Cox inhibitors

7. Nutritional supplements

8. Ongoing trials

Surgical

1. Cerclage

2. Pessary

than 30 is associated with increased risk of PTB with the highest risk of PTB less than 24 weeks in non-Hispanic white women followed by non-Hispanic black and then Hispanic women. Thus it is important to optimize maternal BMI before conception with lifestyle interventions, including diet and exercise, as a critical prevention strategy.

Optimal Interpregnancy Interval and Exclusive Breastfeeding

Interpregnancy interval (IPI), defined as the time between the birth of one child and conception of the next child, may affect pregnancy risk of adverse perinatal/neonatal outcomes. Based on information up to 2005, WHO recommended an optimal IPI to be at least 24 months to reduce risk of adverse maternal, perinatal, and infant outcomes.[21,22] Studies have shown that infants born after IPI less than 6 months had increased risk of adverse neonatal outcomes including PTB (odds ratio [OR] = 1.40, 95% CI 1.24–1.58), small for gestational age (OR = 1.26, 95% CI 1.18–1.33), and low birth weight (LBW) (OR = 1.61, 95% CI 1.39–1.86) when compared with IPI of 18 to 24 months.[22,23] However, controversies still exist. Recent studies from Perth, Australia and British Columbia, Canada, using matched controls, question the possible causal relationship between IPI and pregnancy risk.[24,25] The applicability of these studies in the US population require further validation. Data from several studies including in sub-Saharan Africa suggest long IPIs (60 months or more) are also associated with higher risk of adverse outcomes in maternal and infant health, including PTB.[26] Despite recommendations of optimal IPI, data from the 2015 National Vital Statistics Report and National Survey of Family Growth show 30% of women in the United States have IPIs less than 18 months.[27] The recommended optimal IPI is in alignment with the WHO's recommendation for breastfeeding duration of 2 years or more. Not only does breastfeeding provide infant benefit (including reductions in infections and improved long-term neurodevelopmental outcomes),[28–30] nursing mothers may also benefit from lactational amenorrhea for 6 months postdelivery if they continuously and exclusively breastfeed (feeding at least every 4 hours during the day and at least every 6 hours at night).[28,31] This method of contraception, although effective, is temporary. Thus, health care providers need to be proactive in following and counseling new mothers on the recommended IPI to reduce potential perinatal risks, including PTB.

Tobacco Avoidance and Cessation, Omega-3 Supplements

It has been recognized for decades that maternal cigarette smoking increases risk of PTB as well as LBW. Compared with women who continue to smoke, PTB risk is reduced in women who stop smoking in the first trimester of pregnancy. Data from 4876 women who delivered within 6 years of a 1988 US National Health Interview Survey showed that nonsmokers had a PTB rate of 5.9% versus 8.9% for smokers ($P = .003$).[32] More recently, data from Sweden (1999–2012) show tobacco use increases risk of extremely PTB. Although snuff use doubled the risk of medically indicated extremely PTB, smoking was associated with an increased risk of both medically indicated and spontaneous extremely PTB.[33] Other novel treatments like omega-3 supplementation have been shown to reduce PTB in smokers but not in nonsmokers.[34]

Periodontal Disease Prevention

A large prospective study from Birmingham, Alabama showed significant association between PTB and periodontitis between 21 and 24 weeks' gestation. In a group of high-risk women stratified by risk factors of either prior history of spontaneous PTB less than 35 weeks or BMI less than 19.8/bacterial vaginosis, a pilot intervention of scaling and dental root planing as a treatment intervention in women (85% African American) with periodontitis between 21 and 25 weeks' gestation reduced the risk of PTB less than 35 weeks. The addition of Metronidazole to this intervention when compared with placebo, however, did not reduce risk of PTB less than 35 weeks.[35] More recently, it has been reiterated that periodontal treatment during pregnancy decreases risk of PTB.[36] Current evidence provides an interesting clinicopathologic correlate that the biome of the placenta is most similar to the maternal oral cavity.[37] More current and comprehensive reviews from India[38] and Africa[39] also suggest "the promotion of early detection and treatments of periodontal disease in young women before and during pregnancy will be beneficial, especially for women at risk."[38] However, more recent meta-analysis question the risk reduction in PTB less than 35 weeks in women treated for periodontal disease in pregnancy.[40]

Dedicated Preterm Prevention Clinic

In reviewing 6 randomized control trials (RCT), the effectiveness of PTB prevention educational programs in high-risk mothers showed no significant benefit in preventing death, LBW, or PTB rates. The only difference shown was an increase in the frequency of preterm labor diagnosis.[41]

Because the cause of spontaneous preterm labor is heterogeneous, inclusion criteria for women who should attend preterm prevention clinic (PPC) are important. Some have recommended excluding women with a multiple pregnancy, those with previous elective indicated PTB (due to preeclampsia, maternal reasons, intrauterine growth restriction), and those with previous intrauterine fetal demise without labor.[42] Utah Intermountain Health instituted a PPC with 3 visits wherein PTB risk assessment was done. Women were offered 17-OHPC as well as screened for bacterial vaginosis and urinary tract infection, and treated if positive. With this intervention, they showed fewer women enrolled in the PPC delivered before 37 weeks (49% vs 63% $P = .04$). The neonatal intensive care unit admission rate was the same, but neonatal morbidity, including intraventricular hemorrhage, sepsis, or death, was significantly lower in the PPC group (6% vs 16%, $P = .03$). More women in PPC received 17-OHPC (68.6% vs 39.1%, $P<.01$), but the use of progesterone was not associated with reduction of PTB.[43] In studying pregnant women's preferences and concerns[44] regarding PTB, 311 women completed a survey at median gestation of 32 weeks. If they were told that they were at increased risk for PTB, they preferred not to use PTB prevention methods, but chose close monitoring or nothing. They were most likely to follow use of 17-OHPC and least likely to follow recommendations for cerclage. They also report the women preferred to use sources other than their provider to seek information and learn about PTB, such as the Internet.

The following are suggested minimum criteria of those in pregnancy who should be referred to a dedicated PTB prevention clinic:

- Systemic maternal disease associated with PTB
- Poorly controlled diabetes
- Chronic hypertension with associated renal or cardiac disease
- Fetal anomaly
- Fetal arrhythmia
- Certain types of isoimmunization (C, D, E, Kell)
- Monochorionic twins
- Triplets or greater
- Placenta accreta
- Mothers exposed to substance associated with PTB
- Severe or early intrauterine growth restriction
- History of cervical insufficiency

- History of spontaneous PTB
- Polyhydramnios greater than 30 cm
- Multiple CSs (3 or more)
- Recurrent loss (3 or more)
- History of preeclampsia

Preconceptional and Public Health Strategies

The overwhelming majority of Utah women in a prospective convenience sample studied in a state infant follow-up clinic (2010–2012) who had prior PTB were not educated on medical strategies to prevent future PTB,[45] thus providing opportunity for health promotion and PTB prevention through education in this very high-risk population. A variety of other effective public health approaches to PTB risk reduction have been explored in different populations. For example, an Ohio statewide collaborative consisting of 20 maternity hospitals achieved a 6.6% reduction in singleton births less than 32 weeks through greater progesterone access for at-risk pregnancies. Improved progesterone access was accomplished through expanding Medicaid eligibility, maintaining Medicaid coverage during pregnancy, improving communication, and adopting uniform data collection and efficient treatment protocols.[46] Similar examples are found in an Australian prospective population-based cohort study that found a 7.6% reduction in PTB within 1 year following implementation of a multifaceted PTB prevention program aimed at both health care practitioners and the general public, operating within the environment of a government-funded universal health care system.[47]

MINIMIZE IATROGENIC CONTRIBUTIONS TO PRETERM BIRTH
Judicious Use of Fertility Treatment

Between 1996 and 2014, the number of assisted reproductive technology (ART) procedures in the United States and the resultant births has nearly tripled. Although 17 reporting European nations had 81% of in vitro fertilization deliveries being singleton, the United States had a 72% comparable singleton rate. The 1.6% of US live births in 2014 who were ART-conceived had a singleton PTB rate of 13.2% and LBW rate of 8.9% compared with 9.7% PTB rate and 6.3% LBW rate of all singleton US births. Careful monitoring of rates of multiple embryo transfers and early single embryo transfer rates in addition to knowledge of infant outcomes can guide judicious use and evaluation of fertility treatment. The Centers for Disease Control and Prevention's National Center for Health Statistics plans to include information on the use of ART and non-ART treatments and birth outcomes from US birth certificate data year 2016.[48]

Eliminate Nonmedically Indicated Induction less than 39 weeks

Elimination of nonmedically indicated deliveries could potentially decrease PTB. Using a toolkit from California's Maternal Quality Care Collaborative, 26 hospitals in the "big 5" states (California, Florida, Illinois, New York, Texas) effectively reduced elective early-term deliveries (37–38 weeks) from 27.8% to 4.8%, an 83% decline within 1 year.[49]

Eliminate Nonmedically Indicated Cesarean Section Rates

Minimizing the primary cesarean section (CS) rate is the single best way to lower risk of repeated CS. Multiple CSs are associated with abnormal placentation, which can lead to increased risk of medically indicated CS and PTB. Cesarean scar pregnancies are associated with morbidly adherent placentas, which increase risk of PTB and have serious implications for maternal fertility.[50]

MEDICAL
Antiplatelet Agents

Multiple studies have evaluated the use of antiplatelet agents (low-dose aspirin–dipyridamole) to treat preeclampsia. A recent individual patient data (IPD) meta-analysis included 17 trials with 28,797 pregnant women at risk for pregnancy-induced hypertension showed a lower risk of PTB in those who received antiplatelet agents.[51] Currently, a multicenter RCT evaluating the efficacy of low-dose aspirin in preventing PTB in pregnant women with history of PTB is underway in The Netherlands and Australia.[52]

Vaginal and Injectable Progesterone

A matched sample comparison of intramuscular (IM) versus vaginal micronized progesterone for PTB prevention[53] studied 168 pregnant women at high risk of PTB randomized at 20 to 24 weeks' gestation to receive micronized progesterone tablets (200 mg) vaginally daily or 100 mg IM every 3 days: PTB rates were 20% and 27.5% in the vaginal and IM groups, respectively. The study concluded that although both therapies were nearly equally effective, vaginal progesterone had less undesirable side effects.

Progesterone in singletons

Vaginal progesterone 100 to 200 mg daily[54,55] and 250 mg weekly of IM 17-OHPC[9] have been used in women with singleton pregnancy at risk for PTB. Meta-analysis of RCTs has shown that progesterone decreases PTB risk at less than 37 weeks' gestation.[56–58] A recent network meta-analysis[58] of studies that evaluated progesterone, cerclage, and pessary as PTB risk-lowering treatment modalities showed progesterone is effective in lowering PTB risk less than 34 weeks' gestation (OR 0.44; 95% CI 0.22–0.79; low quality), less than 37 weeks' gestation (OR 0.58; 95% CI 0.41–0.79; moderate quality), and reducing neonatal death (OR 0.50; 95% CI 0.28–0.85; high quality). In subgroup analysis, vaginal progesterone was more effective than 17-OHPC in preventing PTB, and cerclage was effective in reducing PTB risk in those with short cervical length.

Progesterone in twin pregnancies

Even though multiple pregnancies account only for 1% to 2% of live births, they are overrepresented in PTB. Hence, numerous studies have evaluated the use of both 17-OHPC and vaginal progesterone use to reduce PTB risk in multiple pregnancies. IPD meta-analysis of 13 RCTs with 3768 women with twin pregnancies did not show a benefit in reduction of adverse perinatal outcome with the use of 17-OHPC.[59] However, in a subset of women with short cervical length less than 25 mm, the use of vaginal progesterone was associated with reduction in PTB. Another IPD meta-analysis of 6 trials with 447 asymptomatic women with twin pregnancies and short cervical length less than 25 mm showed that vaginal progesterone reduced the rate of PTB less than 33 weeks' gestation (OR 0.69, 95% CI 0.51–0.93, $P = .01$) and neonatal mortality and morbidity (respiratory distress syndrome, use of mechanical ventilation, birth weight <1500 g).[60] A recent network meta-analysis[61] comparing 17-OHPC, cerclage, and pessary did not show a significant benefit in reducing PTB with any of these interventions. However, a subgroup analysis showed that in women with short cervix vaginal progesterone was effective in reducing neonatal outcomes of very LBW and mechanical ventilation.

Progesterone pharmacogenomics

Whole-exome sequencing in pregnant women with a history of recurrent PTB shows key genetics differences in efficacy of 17-OHPC treatment between those who had success or lack thereof.[13] Success/nonsuccess was defined as either difference in gestational age at delivery between 17-OHPC-treated and untreated pregnancies (success: delivered ≥3 weeks later with 17-OHPC) or success/nonsuccess based on reaching term (success: delivered at term with 17-OHPC).

Magnesium

RCTs in the 1990s investigating magnesium sulfate for PTB prevention have concluded it was ineffective.[62] Currently, maternal magnesium sulfate is used for its infant neuroprotective benefit in those at risk for preterm delivery. Oral magnesium sulfate is being studied for its potential in PTB prevention in an RCT in Brazil in women at risk for placental dysfunction.[63]

Antimicrobials

Multiple pathologic processes are involved in infection contributing to PTB. Although the molecular mechanisms are identified, there is a lack of consensus on effective antibiotics for bacterial vaginosis or related organisms, used early in pregnancy to reduce PTB.[64,65] Antibiotic treatment in women with preterm premature rupture of membranes (PPROM) <34 weeks has been associated with prolongation of pregnancy[66] but not in those with preterm labor. Early treatment of abnormal vaginal colonization with Clindamycin was associated with lower risk of PTB less than 37 weeks.[67] However, a meta-analysis of 17 trials using prophylactic antibiotics to prevent PTB did not show any benefit.[68,69] A meta-analysis of 2 trials (one was from a post hoc subgroup analysis) with 685 women showed treatment of asymptomatic vulvovaginal candidiasis significantly reduced PTB risk.[70] Although further discussion of antimicrobials is beyond the scope of this article, a recent comprehensive review of antibiotics and PTB is recommended reading.[69]

Tocolytics

Calcium channel blockers, mainly Nifedipine, are beneficial in postponement of birth by a mean of 4.38 days (95% CI 0.25–8.52) and a Cochrane review[71] showed reduction in PTB (relative risk [RR] 0.64, 95% CI 0.47–0.89). This short postponement demonstrated benefits in allowing opportunity for antenatal steroids and transfer to higher level of care. The review also recommends future trials to use blinding of the intervention and assessment of long-term childhood outcomes and costs.

Terbutaline for PTB prevention is not recommended, and its use should be limited to research settings because of several cases of maternal deaths and cardiovascular events in patients receiving terbutaline tocolysis.[72]

Cochrane Reviews of Nonbeneficial Interventions: Probiotics, Relaxation Therapy, Hydration Therapy, Magnesium Therapy, Oxytocin Receptor Antagonists, Cox Inhibitors, Ethanol

Several therapies are known to be ineffective in reducing the risk of PTB according to Cochrane reviews in the last decade,[73–79] although some ambitious new trials[52,63] are underway.

Nutritional Supplements

Vitamin C deficiency may lead to premature rupture of membrane (PROM). North Carolina women with total vitamin C intakes less than the 10th percentile preconceptionally had twice the risk of PTB associated with PROM (RR 2.2; 95% CI 1.1, 4.5). The elevated risk of PPROM was greatest for women with a low vitamin C intake during both preconception and in the second trimester.[80] In a secondary analysis of a double-masked, placebo RCT in low-risk nulliparous women (10,154 women randomized, outcome data available on 9968; 4992 vitamin group and 4976 placebo group) administered 1000 mg vitamin C and 400 IU vitamin E or placebo daily from 9 to 16 weeks' gestation until delivery, no differences were noted in PTB attributable to PROM less than 37 and less than 35 weeks' gestation but were less frequent at less than 32 weeks' gestation (0.3% vs 0.6% adjusted OR 0.3–0.9).[81] The role of supplemental vitamin C in PPROM has shown some promise in an Iranian RCT that randomized 170 pregnant women with singleton pregnancy with history of PPROM to daily 100 mg vitamin C or placebo starting at 14 weeks' gestation.[82] It is unclear if this high-risk population in Iran was deficient in vitamin C. A current review[83] highlights other deficiencies of micronutrients such as zinc[84] and vitamin D in nutritionally deprived populations that may affect PTB rates. A Cochrane review inclusive of 3 trials involving 477 women suggest that vitamin D supplementation during pregnancy reduces the risk PTB (RR 0.36; 95% CI 0.14–0.93, moderate quality). The benefits of omega 3 supplementation in PTB reduction in smokers have been previously stated.[34]

In summary, these observations suggest the need to further understand nutritional deficiencies and their role in the variation of PTB prevalence, both endemic deficiencies and those peculiar to high-risk populations.

Ongoing Trials

Currently, multiple studies are underway comparing different treatments for PTB: vaginal progesterone versus cerclage versus pessary in pregnant women with short cervix[85]; progesterone versus pessary[86,87]; and pessary versus cerclage.[88] Studies evaluating novel treatments like low-dose aspirin and oral magnesium to decrease PTB are also underway.[52,63]

SURGICAL
Cerclage

A retrospective cohort study of 444 women who received 1 or 2 stitches during transvaginal cervical cerclage in PTB prevention did not show differences in PTB or pregnancy outcome, regardless of whether cerclage was indicated for prior history of PTB or cervical ultrasound changes.[89]

A systematic review of adjunctive therapies to cerclage in the prevention of PTB[90] identified 305 studies for review, of which only 12 studies compared use of adjunctive therapy with cerclage to cerclage alone. None of the 12 studies were prospective RCTs, and none of them demonstrated clear benefit of any adjunctive therapy used with cerclage or cerclage alone. In singletons, cerclage has been shown to reduce the risk of PTB in meta-analysis of 15 trials with 3490 pregnant women.[91] Subgroup analysis in a network meta-analysis showed cerclage was effective in reducing PTB risk in those with short cervical length[61] but not in all. In 2 separate meta-analyses, cerclage has not been shown to be effective in twin pregnancies.[61,92]

Pessary

A meta-analysis of 3 RCTs of cervical pessary in 1412 asymptomatic women with short cervix did not show a reduction in PTB or neonatal mortality or morbidity.[93]

Table 1 summarizes the most promising interventions to prevent PTB.

FUTURE CONSIDERATIONS

Answering clinically important questions related to relatively rare outcomes or very small subgroup populations is difficult in a single RCT. Critical evaluation of evidence examining progesterone for the prevention of PTB shows studies of variable quality.[94] A cumulative meta-analysis showed that progesterone treatment benefit for the

Table 1
Summary of promising interventions to prevent preterm birth

Intervention	Detail	Effect RR (95% CI)	Reference
Progesterone: Singletons			
17-OHP 250 mg weekly	History of preterm delivery n = 463	PTB <37 wk 0.66 (0.54–0.81) PTB <35 wk 0.67 (0.48–0.93)	Meis et al,[9] 2003
Vaginal progesterone 100 mg daily	At risk for PTB n = 142	PTB <37 wk 0.48 (13.8% vs 28.5%) P = .03	da Fonseca,[10] 2003
Vaginal progesterone 200 mg daily	At risk for PTB n = 1228	PTB <35 wk 0.86 (0.61–1.22)	Norman,[55] 2012
Vaginal progesterone	Asymptomatic women with short cervix, IPDMA, 5 trials, n = 775	PTB <35 wk RR 0.66 (0.52–0.83) NNT 11	Romero,[56,57] 2012, 2016
Progesterone	Network meta-analysis in singletons, 10 trials, n = 2850	PTB <34 wk 0.44 (0.22–0.79) NNT 9	Jarde,[58] 2017 singletons
Progesterone: Multiples			
Vaginal progesterone	Network analysis in twins, 16 trials	BW <1500 g 0.71 (0.52–0.98) Mechanical ventilation 0.61 (0.45–0.82)	Jarde,[61] 2017 twins
Vaginal progesterone	Twins with short cervix, IPDMA, 13 trials, n = 3768	PTB <33 wk 0.69 (0.51–0.93)	Schui,[59] 2015; Romero,[60] 2017
Antiplatelet agents	At risk for preeclampsia, gestational hypertension, intrauterine growth restriction IPDMA 17 trials, n = 28,797	PTB <37 wk 0.93 (0.86–0.996) PTB <34 wk 0.86 (0.76–0.99)	van Vliet,[51] 2017
Antimicrobials			
Latency antibiotics	PPROM, 5 trials, n = 3226	Latency days 0.33 (0.17–0.5)	Hutzal,[66] 2008
Clindamycin	Asymptomatic bacterial vaginosis or abnormal vaginal fora <22 wk, 5 trials, n = 2346	PTB <37 wk 0.6 (0.42–0.86)	Lamont,[67] 2011
Clotrimazole	Asymptomatic vulvovaginal candidiasis, 2 trials, n = 685	PTB <37 wk 0.36 (0.17–0.75)	Roberts,[70] 2015
Cerclage	At high risk of PTB or ultrasound evidence of need for cerclage, 9 trials, n = 2415	PTB <34 wk 0.77 (0.66–0.89)	Alfrevic,[91] 2017

Abbreviation: IPDMA, individual participant data meta-analysis.

outcome PTB less than 37 weeks had a $P<.01$ in 1975. By 1985, the P value was less than .001 and by 2003 it was less than .0001. Another cumulative meta-analysis limited to just the highest quality trials showed significant benefit with OR 0.47; 95% CI 0.33, 0.66; $P<.0001$. Recently, a group of statisticians and scientists have suggested using a $P<.005$ as the threshold for statistical significance instead of $P<.05$ in an effort to increase the reproducibility of study results. Increasing the sample size and other methods of summarizing data such as using Bayesian factor instead of *P* value have also been recommended. Future studies should consider such statistical methods to optimize the reproducibility of study results.[95] IPD meta-analyses have been helpful in answering clinical questions in smaller subgroup populations.[96,97] Such meta-analyses are possible when the studies have recorded all relevant outcomes with standardized definitions and the inclusion criteria have included subgroups of populations of interest. It is important for future trials to proactively consider including heterogeneous clinical subgroups, instead of having comprehensive exclusion criteria, to provide the opportunity for IPD meta-analysis to answer clinically important questions. Network meta-analysis evaluating comparative effectiveness of the different interventions provides an opportunity to identify the most effective interventions. It has been pointed out that several limitations in meta-analysis peculiar to nutrition research[98] merit consideration. It will be interesting to see how the future incorporates current nutritional trials such as Docosahexaenoic acid supplements to decrease the frequency of PTB less than 34 weeks using Bayesian adaptive randomization design[99] into novel meta-analytic frameworks in nutrition research. Integrating genomic factors with the phenotypic risk factors to identify the most effective treatment of each patient is essential to ensure successful clinical outcomes as highlighted by the Precision Medicine Initiative.[100]

Best Practices

What is the current practice?

Recognize higher risk of preterm birth as early as possible before or during pregnancy

Objective: To minimize risk of preterm birth, optimize management during preterm labor, and mitigate perinatal morbidity and mortality for both mother and infant

What changes in current practice are likely to improve outcomes?

Early recognition of risk factors for preterm birth and mitigation at the appropriate phase, be it before conception, during pregnancy, in preterm labor, or after preterm rupture of membrane

Major recommendations

Preconception strategies
  I. Avoid BMI less than 19.8 or greater than 30
 II. Optimal interpregnancy interval of 18 to 24 months and exclusive breastfeeding for ≥ 6 months
III. Tobacco avoidance and cessation, omega-3 supplements
 IV. Periodontal disease prevention
  V. Dedicated preterm prevention clinic for women with prior preterm birth

Minimize iatrogenic contributions to preterm birth
  I. Judicious use of ART fertility treatment and limiting number of embryos transferred
 II. Eliminate nonmedically indicated induction less than 39 weeks
III. Eliminate nonmedically indicated cesarean section rates

Medical
  I. Vaginal progesterone/17-OHPC in singletons
     a. Decreases risk of PTB at less than 34, less than 37 weeks' gestation and neonatal death
     b. Vaginal progesterone was more effective than 17-OHPC in preventing PTB
 II. Vaginal progesterone in twins
     a. Decreases risk of PTB at less than 33 weeks' gestation and neonatal mortality and morbidity in those with short cervical length less than 25 mm

Summary statement

Reexamine data for effectiveness of progesterone in preterm birth prevention and in high-risk subgroup populations. Long-term safety data on progesterone use for preterm birth prevention.

ACKNOWLEDGMENTS

This article is dedicated to all the great obstetricians who teach us so much and do so much for our women, children, and families. Special thanks to Drs James Byrne, Jin Chang-Yu, Iris Colon, Bonnie Dwyer, Matthew Garabedian, Kim Gregory, Andrea Jelks, Liza Kunz, Deborah Krakow, Anthony Ogundipe, and Neil Silverman.

REFERENCES

1. Howson CP, Kinney MV, Lawn JE, editors. Born too soon: the global action report on preterm birth. Geneva (Switzerland): March of Dimes, PMNCH, Save the Children, WHO; 2012.
2. Blencowe H, Cousens S, Oestergaard MZ, et al. National, regional, and worldwide estimates of preterm birth rates in the year 2010 with time trends since 1990 for selected countries: a systematic analysis and implications. Lancet 2012;379(9832):2162–72.
3. Rossen LM, Osterman MJK, Hamilton BE, et al. Quarterly provisional estimates for selected birth indicators, 2015-Quarter 1, 2017. Available at: https://www.cdc.gov/nchs/data/vsrr/report004.pdf. Accessed September 18, 2017.
4. Goldenberg RL, Andrews WW. Intrauterine infection and why preterm prevention programs have failed. Am J Public Health 1996;86(6):781–3.
5. Goldenberg RL, Davis RO, Copper RL, et al. The Alabama preterm birth prevention project. Obstet Gynecol 1990;75(6):933–9.
6. Hobel CJ, Ross MG, Bemis RL, et al. The West Los Angeles preterm birth prevention project. I. Program impact on high-risk women. Am J Obstet Gynecol 1994;170(1 Pt 1):54–62.
7. Gomez-Olmedo M, Delgado-Rodriguez M, Bueno-Cavanillas A, et al. Prenatal care and prevention of preterm birth. A case-control study in southern Spain. Eur J Epidemiol 1996;12(1):37–44.
8. Holzman C, Paneth N. Preterm birth: from prediction to prevention. Am J Public Health 1998;88(2):183–4.
9. Meis PJ, Klebanoff M, Thom E, et al. Prevention of recurrent preterm delivery by 17 alpha-hydroxyprogesterone caproate. N Engl J Med 2003;348(24):2379–85.
10. da Fonseca EB, Damiao R, Nicholaides K. Prevention of preterm birth based on short cervix: progesterone. Semin Perinatol 2009;33(5):334–7.
11. Barros FC, Papageorghiou AT, Victora CG, et al. The distribution of clinical phenotypes of preterm birth syndrome: implications for prevention. JAMA Pediatr 2015;169(3):220–9.
12. Zhang G, Feenstra B, Bacelis J, et al. Genetic associations with gestational duration and spontaneous preterm birth. N Engl J Med 2017;377(12):1156–67.
13. Manuck TA, Watkins WS, Esplin MS, et al. Pharmacogenomics of 17-alpha hydroxyprogesterone caproate for recurrent preterm birth: a case-control study. BJOG 2018;125(3):343–50.
14. Caritis SN, Venkataramanan R, Thom E, et al. Relationship between 17-alpha hydroxyprogesterone caproate concentration and spontaneous preterm birth. Am J Obstet Gynecol 2014;210(2):128.e1-6.
15. Haas DM, Quinney SK, Clay JM, et al. Nifedipine pharmacokinetics are influenced by CYP3A5 genotype when used as a preterm labor tocolytic. Am J Perinatol 2013;30(4):275–81.
16. Haas DM, Quinney SK, McCormick CL, et al. A pilot study of the impact of genotype on nifedipine pharmacokinetics when used as a tocolytic. J Matern Fetal Neonatal Med 2012;25(4):419–23.

17. Haas DM, Dantzer J, Lehmann AS, et al. The impact of glucocorticoid polymorphisms on markers of neonatal respiratory disease after antenatal betamethasone administration. Am J Obstet Gynecol 2013;208(3):215.e1-6.
18. Omanwa K, Zimmer M, Tlolka J, et al. Is low pre-pregnancy body mass index a risk factor for preterm birth and low neonatal birth weight? Ginekol Pol 2006; 77(8):618–23 [in Polish].
19. Dietz PM, Callaghan WM, Cogswell ME, et al. Combined effects of prepregnancy body mass index and weight gain during pregnancy on the risk of preterm delivery. Epidemiology 2006;17(2):170–7.
20. Shaw GM, Wise PH, Mayo J, et al. Maternal prepregnancy body mass index and risk of spontaneous preterm birth. Paediatr Perinat Epidemiol 2014;28(4): 302–11.
21. Marston C. Research Technical Consultation and Scientific Review of Birth Spacing. Report of a WHO technical consultation on birth spacing: World Health Organization. 2005. Available at: http://apps.who.int/iris/bitstream/handle/10665/69855/WHO_RHR_07.1_eng.pdf?sequence=1&isAllowed=y. Accessed July 2, 2018.
22. Conde-Agudelo A, Rosas-Bermudez A, Kafury-Goeta AC. Birth spacing and risk of adverse perinatal outcomes: a meta-analysis. JAMA 2006;295(15): 1809–23.
23. Conde-Agudelo A, Belizan JM, Norton MH, et al. Effect of the interpregnancy interval on perinatal outcomes in Latin America. Obstet Gynecol 2005;106(2): 359–66.
24. Ball SJ, Pereira G, Jacoby P, et al. Re-evaluation of link between interpregnancy interval and adverse birth outcomes: retrospective cohort study matching two intervals per mother. BMJ 2014;349:g4333.
25. Hanley GE, Hutcheon JA, Kinniburgh BA, et al. Interpregnancy interval and adverse pregnancy outcomes: an analysis of successive pregnancies. Obstet Gynecol 2017;129(3):408–15.
26. Mahande MJ, Obure J. Effect of interpregnancy interval on adverse pregnancy outcomes in northern Tanzania: a registry-based retrospective cohort study. BMC Pregnancy Childbirth 2016;16(1):140.
27. Copen CE, Thoma ME, Kirmeyer S. Interpregnancy intervals in the United States: data from the birth certificate and the national survey of family growth. Natl Vital Stat Rep 2015;64(3):1–10.
28. Bar S, Milanaik R, Adesman A. Long-term neurodevelopmental benefits of breastfeeding. Curr Opin Pediatr 2016;28(4):559–66.
29. Kramer MS, Aboud F, Mironova E, et al. Breastfeeding and child cognitive development: new evidence from a large randomized trial. Arch Gen Psychiatry 2008; 65(5):578–84.
30. Belfort MB, Anderson PJ, Nowak VA, et al. Breast milk feeding, brain development, and neurocognitive outcomes: a 7-year longitudinal study in infants born at less than 30 weeks' gestation. J Pediatr 2016;177:133–9.e1.
31. Sridhar A, Salcedo J. Optimizing maternal and neonatal outcomes with postpartum contraception: impact on breastfeeding and birth spacing. Matern Health Neonatol Perinatol 2017;3:1.
32. Mainous AG 3rd, Hueston WJ. The effect of smoking cessation during pregnancy on preterm delivery and low birthweight. J Fam Pract 1994;38(3):262–6.
33. Dahlin S, Gunnerbeck A, Wikstrom AK, et al. Maternal tobacco use and extremely premature birth - a population-based cohort study. BJOG 2016; 123(12):1938–46.

34. Kuper SG, Abramovici AR, Jauk VC, et al. The effect of omega-3 supplementation on pregnancy outcomes by smoking status. Am J Obstet Gynecol 2017; 217(4):476.e1–6.

35. Jeffcoat MK, Hauth JC, Geurs NC, et al. Periodontal disease and preterm birth: results of a pilot intervention study. J Periodontol 2003;74(8):1214–8.

36. Novak T, Radnai M, Gorzo I, et al. Prevention of preterm delivery with periodontal treatment. Fetal Diagn Ther 2009;25(2):230–3.

37. Aagaard K, Ma J, Antony KM, et al. The placenta harbors a unique microbiome. Sci Transl Med 2014;6(237):237ra265.

38. Walia M, Saini N. Relationship between periodontal diseases and preterm birth: recent epidemiological and biological data. Int J Appl Basic Med Res 2015;5(1): 2–6.

39. Teshome A, Yitayeh A. Relationship between periodontal disease and preterm low birth weight: systematic review. Pan Afr Med J 2016;24:215.

40. Iheozor-Ejiofor Z, Middleton P, Esposito M, et al. Treating periodontal disease for preventing adverse birth outcomes in pregnant women. Cochrane Database Syst Rev 2017;(6):CD005297.

41. Hueston WJ, Knox MA, Eilers G, et al. The effectiveness of preterm-birth prevention educational programs for high-risk women: a meta-analysis. Obstet Gynecol 1995;86(4 Pt 2):705–12.

42. Lamont RF. Setting up a preterm prevention clinic: a practical guide. BJOG 2006;113(Suppl 3):86–92.

43. Manuck TA, Henry E, Gibson J, et al. Pregnancy outcomes in a recurrent preterm birth prevention clinic. Am J Obstet Gynecol 2011;204(4):320.e1-6.

44. Ha V, McDonald SD. Pregnant women's preferences for and concerns about preterm birth prevention: a cross-sectional survey. BMC Pregnancy Childbirth 2017;17(1):49.

45. Clark EA, Esplin S, Torres L, et al. Prevention of recurrent preterm birth: role of the neonatal follow-up program. Matern Child Health J 2014;18(4):858–63.

46. Iams JD, Applegate MS, Marcotte MP, et al. A statewide progestogen promotion program in Ohio. Obstet Gynecol 2017;129(2):337–46.

47. Newnham JP, White SW, Meharry S, et al. Reducing preterm birth by a statewide multifaceted program: an implementation study. Am J Obstet Gynecol 2017; 216(5):434–42.

48. Sunderam S, Kissin DM, Crawford SB, et al. Assisted reproductive technology surveillance - United States, 2014. MMWR Surveill Summ 2017;66(6):1–24.

49. Oshiro BT, Kowalewski L, Sappenfield W, et al. A multistate quality improvement program to decrease elective deliveries before 39 weeks of gestation. Obstet Gynecol 2013;121(5):1025–31.

50. Timor-Tritsch IE, Monteagudo A, Cali G, et al. Cesarean scar pregnancy is a precursor of morbidly adherent placenta. Ultrasound Obstet Gynecol 2014;44(3): 346–53.

51. van Vliet EO, Askie LA, Mol BW, et al. Antiplatelet agents and the prevention of spontaneous preterm birth: a systematic review and meta-analysis. Obstet Gynecol 2017;129(2):327–36.

52. Visser L, de Boer MA, de Groot CJM, et al. Low dose aspirin in the prevention of recurrent spontaneous preterm labour - the APRIL study: a multicenter randomized placebo controlled trial. BMC Pregnancy Childbirth 2017;17(1):223.

53. El-Gharib MN, El-Hawary TM. Matched sample comparison of intramuscular versus vaginal micronized progesterone for prevention of preterm birth. J Matern Fetal Neonatal Med 2013;26(7):716–9.

54. da Fonseca EB, Bittar RE, Carvalho MH, et al. Prophylactic administration of progesterone by vaginal suppository to reduce the incidence of spontaneous preterm birth in women at increased risk: a randomized placebo-controlled double-blind study. Am J Obstet Gynecol 2003;188(2):419–24.

55. Norman JE, Shennan A, Bennett P, et al. Trial protocol OPPTIMUM– does progesterone prophylaxis for the prevention of preterm labour improve outcome? BMC Pregnancy Childbirth 2012;12:79.

56. Romero R, Nicolaides K, Conde-Agudelo A, et al. Vaginal progesterone in women with an asymptomatic sonographic short cervix in the midtrimester decreases preterm delivery and neonatal morbidity: a systematic review and metaanalysis of individual patient data. Am J Obstet Gynecol 2012; 206(2):124.e1-9.

57. Romero R, Nicolaides KH, Conde-Agudelo A, et al. Vaginal progesterone decreases preterm birth </= 34 weeks of gestation in women with a singleton pregnancy and a short cervix: an updated meta-analysis including data from the OPPTIMUM study. Ultrasound Obstet Gynecol 2016;48(3):308–17.

58. Jarde A, Lutsiv O, Park CK, et al. Effectiveness of progesterone, cerclage and pessary for preventing preterm birth in singleton pregnancies: a systematic review and network meta-analysis. BJOG 2017;124(8):1176–89.

59. Schuit E, Stock S, Rode L, et al. Effectiveness of progestogens to improve perinatal outcome in twin pregnancies: an individual participant data meta-analysis. BJOG 2015;122(1):27–37.

60. Romero R, Conde-Agudelo A, El-Refaie W, et al. Vaginal progesterone decreases preterm birth and neonatal morbidity and mortality in women with a twin gestation and a short cervix: an updated meta-analysis of individual patient data. Ultrasound Obstet Gynecol 2017;49(3):303–14.

61. Jarde A, Lutsiv O, Park CK, et al. Preterm birth prevention in twin pregnancies with progesterone, pessary, or cerclage: a systematic review and meta-analysis. BJOG 2017;124(8):1163–73.

62. Cox SM, Sherman ML, Leveno KJ. Randomized investigation of magnesium sulfate for prevention of preterm birth. Am J Obstet Gynecol 1990;163(3): 767–72.

63. Alves JG, de Araujo CA, Pontes IE, et al. The BRAzil MAGnesium (BRAMAG) trial: a randomized clinical trial of oral magnesium supplementation in pregnancy for the prevention of preterm birth and perinatal and maternal morbidity. BMC Pregnancy Childbirth 2014;14:222.

64. Oliver RS, Lamont RF. Infection and antibiotics in the acause, prediction and prevention of preterm birth. J Obstet Gynaecol 2013;33(8):768–75.

65. Ramsey PS, Lieman JM, Brumfield CG, et al. Chorioamnionitis increases neonatal morbidity in pregnancies complicated by preterm premature rupture of membranes. Am J Obstet Gynecol 2005;192(4):1162–6.

66. Hutzal CE, Boyle EM, Kenyon SL, et al. Use of antibiotics for the treatment of preterm parturition and prevention of neonatal morbidity: a metaanalysis. Am J Obstet Gynecol 2008;199(6):620.e1-8.

67. Lamont RF, Nhan-Chang CL, Sobel JD, et al. Treatment of abnormal vaginal flora in early pregnancy with clindamycin for the prevention of spontaneous preterm birth: a systematic review and metaanalysis. Am J Obstet Gynecol 2011;205(3): 177–90.

68. Simcox R, Sin WT, Seed PT, et al. Prophylactic antibiotics for the prevention of preterm birth in women at risk: a meta-analysis. Aust N Z J Obstet Gynaecol 2007;47(5):368–77.

69. Lamont RF. Advances in the prevention of infection-related preterm birth. Front Immunol 2015;6:566.
70. Roberts CL, Algert CS, Rickard KL, et al. Treatment of vaginal candidiasis for the prevention of preterm birth: a systematic review and meta-analysis. Syst Rev 2015;4:31.
71. Flenady V, Wojcieszek AM, Papatsonis DN, et al. Calcium channel blockers for inhibiting preterm labour and birth. Cochrane Database Syst Rev 2014;(6):CD002255.
72. Gaudet LM, Singh K, Weeks L, et al. Effectiveness of terbutaline pump for the prevention of preterm birth. A systematic review and meta-analysis. PLoS One 2012;7(2):e31679.
73. Othman M, Neilson JP, Alfirevic Z. Probiotics for preventing preterm labour. Cochrane Database Syst Rev 2007;(1):CD005941.
74. Khianman B, Pattanittum P, Thinkhamrop J, et al. Relaxation therapy for preventing and treating preterm labour. Cochrane Database Syst Rev 2012;(8):CD007426.
75. Stan CM, Boulvain M, Pfister R, et al. Hydration for treatment of preterm labour. Cochrane Database Syst Rev 2013;(11):CD003096.
76. Han S, Crowther CA, Moore V. Magnesium maintenance therapy for preventing preterm birth after threatened preterm labour. Cochrane Database Syst Rev 2013;(5):CD000940.
77. Reinebrant HE, Pileggi-Castro C, Romero CL, et al. Cyclo-oxygenase (COX) inhibitors for treating preterm labour. Cochrane Database Syst Rev 2015;(6):CD001992.
78. Haas DM, Morgan AM, Deans SJ, et al. Ethanol for preventing preterm birth in threatened preterm labor. Cochrane Database Syst Rev 2015;(11):CD011445.
79. Flenady V, Reinebrant HE, Liley HG, et al. Oxytocin receptor antagonists for inhibiting preterm labour. Cochrane Database Syst Rev 2014;(6):CD004452.
80. Siega-Riz AM, Promislow JH, Savitz DA, et al. Vitamin C intake and the risk of preterm delivery. Am J Obstet Gynecol 2003;189(2):519–25.
81. Hauth JC, Clifton RG, Roberts JM, et al. Vitamin C and E supplementation to prevent spontaneous preterm birth: a randomized controlled trial. Obstet Gynecol 2010;116(3):653–8.
82. Ghomian N, Hafizi L, Takhti Z. The role of vitamin C in prevention of preterm premature rupture of membranes. Iran Red Crescent Med J 2013;15(2):113–6.
83. Gernand AD, Schulze KJ, Stewart CP, et al. Micronutrient deficiencies in pregnancy worldwide: health effects and prevention. Nat Rev Endocrinol 2016;12(5):274–89.
84. Ota E, Mori R, Middleton P, et al. Zinc supplementation for improving pregnancy and infant outcome. Cochrane Database Syst Rev 2015;(2):CD000230.
85. Hezelgrave NL, Watson HA, Ridout A, et al. Rationale and design of SuPPoRT: a multi-centre randomised controlled trial to compare three treatments: cervical cerclage, cervical pessary and vaginal progesterone, for the prevention of preterm birth in women who develop a short cervix. BMC Pregnancy Childbirth 2016;16(1):358.
86. van Zijl MD, Koullali B, Naaktgeboren CA, et al. Pessary or progesterone to prevent preterm delivery in women with short cervical length: the Quadruple P randomised controlled trial. BMC Pregnancy Childbirth 2017;17(1):284.
87. Cabrera-Garcia L, Cruz-Melguizo S, Ruiz-Antoran B, et al. Evaluation of two treatment strategies for the prevention of preterm birth in women identified as at risk by ultrasound (PESAPRO Trial): study protocol for a randomized controlled trial. Trials 2015;16:427.
88. Koullali B, van Kempen LEM, van Zijl MD, et al. A multi-centre, non-inferiority, randomised controlled trial to compare a cervical pessary with a cervical

cerclage in the prevention of preterm delivery in women with short cervical length and a history of preterm birth - PC study. BMC Pregnancy Childbirth 2017;17(1):215.

89. Giraldo-Isaza MA, Fried GP, Hegarty SE, et al. Comparison of 2 stitches vs 1 stitch for transvaginal cervical cerclage for preterm birth prevention. Am J Obstet Gynecol 2013;208(3):209.e1-9.

90. Defranco EA, Valent AM, Newman T, et al. Adjunctive therapies to cerclage for the prevention of preterm birth: a systematic review. Obstet Gynecol Int 2013; 2013:528158.

91. Alfirevic Z, Stampalija T, Medley N. Cervical stitch (cerclage) for preventing preterm birth in singleton pregnancy. Cochrane Database Syst Rev 2017;(6):CD008991.

92. Rafael TJ, Berghella V, Alfirevic Z. Cervical stitch (cerclage) for preventing preterm birth in multiple pregnancy. Cochrane Database Syst Rev 2014;(9):CD009166.

93. Jin XH, Li D, Huang LL. Cervical pessary for prevention of preterm birth: a meta-analysis. Sci Rep 2017;7:42560.

94. Coomarasamy A, Thangaratinam S, Gee H, et al. Progesterone for the prevention of preterm birth: a critical evaluation of evidence. Eur J Obstet Gynecol Reprod Biol 2006;129(2):111–8.

95. Benjamin DJ, Berger J, Johannesson M, et al. Redefine statistical significance. Nature Human Behaviour 2018;2:6–10.

96. Berghella V. The power of meta-analysis to address an important clinical question in obstetrics. Am J Obstet Gynecol 2017;216(4):379.e1–4.

97. Broekhuijsen K, Bernardes T, van Baaren GJ, et al. Relevance of individual participant data meta-analysis for studies in obstetrics: delivery versus expectant monitoring for hypertensive disorders of pregnancy. Eur J Obstet Gynecol Reprod Biol 2015;191:80–3.

98. Barnard ND, Willett WC, Ding EL. The misuse of meta-analysis in nutrition research. JAMA 2017;318(15):1435–6.

99. Carlson SE, Gajewski BJ, Valentine CJ, et al. Assessment of DHA on reducing early preterm birth: the ADORE randomized controlled trial protocol. BMC Pregnancy Childbirth 2017;17(1):62.

100. Dzau VJ, Ginsburg GS. Realizing the full potential of precision medicine in health and health care. JAMA 2016;316(16):1659–60.

Moving?

Make sure your subscription moves with you!

To notify us of your new address, find your **Clinics Account Number** (located on your mailing label above your name), and contact customer service at:

Email: journalscustomerservice-usa@elsevier.com

800-654-2452 (subscribers in the U.S. & Canada)
314-447-8871 (subscribers outside of the U.S. & Canada)

Fax number: 314-447-8029

Elsevier Health Sciences Division
Subscription Customer Service
3251 Riverport Lane
Maryland Heights, MO 63043

*To ensure uninterrupted delivery of your subscription, please notify us at least 4 weeks in advance of move.

Moving?

Make sure your subscription moves with you!

To notify us of your new address, find your Clinics Account Number (located on your mailing label above your name), and contact customer service at:

Email: journalscustomerservice-usa@elsevier.com

800-654-2452 (subscribers in the U.S. & Canada)
314-447-8871 (subscribers outside of the U.S. & Canada)

Fax number: 314-447-8029

**Elsevier Health Sciences Division
Subscription Customer Service
3251 Riverport Lane
Maryland Heights, MO 63043**